Nutrients and Cancer Prevention

T0332922

Experimental Biology and Medicine

Nutrients
and
Cancer Prevention

Edited by

Kedar N. Prasad
and
Frank L. Meyskens, Jr.

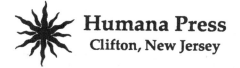 **Humana Press**
Clifton, New Jersey

Library of Congress Cataloging-in-Publication Data

Nutrients and cancer prevention / edited by Kedar N. Prasad and Frank
L. Meyskens, Jr.
  p. cm. — (Experimental biology and medicine)
  Based on the secontd meeting of the International Association for
Vitamins and Nutritional Oncology, held in Charleston, S.C., June
25–29, 1989. sponsored by the Samuel Freeman Charitable Trust and
others.
  Includes index.
  ISBN 0-89603-171-3 : $69.50
  1. Cancer—Surgery —Nutriional aspects—Congresses. 2. Cancer-
-Prevention—Congresses. I. Prasad, Kedar N. II. Meyskens, F. L.
(Frank L.) III. International Association for Vitamins and
Nutritional Oncology, Meeting (2nd : 1989 : Charleston, S.C.)
IV. Samuel Freeman Charitable Trust. V. Series: Experimental
biology and medicine (Clifton, N.J.)
  [DNLM: 1. Clinical trials—congresses. 2. Neoplasms—prevention
and control—congresses. 3. Nutrition—congresses.   QZ 200 N9755
1989]
  RC268.45.N87   1990
  616.99 ' 405—dc20
  DNLM/DLC
  for Library of Congress
                                                                    90-4677
                                                                    CIP

© 1990 The Humana Press Inc.
Crescent Manor
PO Box 2148
Clifton, New Jersey 07015

All rights of any nature reserved.

No part of this book may be reproduced, stored in a retrieval system, or transmitted in any form or by
any means, electronic, mechanical, photocopying, microfilming, recording, computer database entry,
or networking, or in any manner whatsoever without written permission from the Publisher.

Preface

During the last 10 years, the role of specific nutrients in cancer prevention and cancer treatment has been the subject of intense basic, preclinical, and clinical research. At present, the major focus of nutritional oncology is on the mechanisms of carcinogenesis and their modification by nutrients and on cancer prevention studies in animals and humans. Some human epidemiological studies have confirmed the hypothesis, developed on animals, that there is an inverse relationship between the intake and/or level of β-carotene, vitamin A, vitamin E, or vitamin C and the risk of cancer, whereas others have shown no such relationship. This is not unexpected, since the protective effect of individual nutrients may be too small to be detected by epidemiological methodologies in which a single vitamin or mineral is considered as one variable. Conclusive evidence regarding the role of nutrients in human cancer prevention will come from a well-designed human intervention study using one or more nutrients in a population that has a high risk of developing cancer. The involvement of specific nutrients in the regulation of protooncogene expression has just begun. Also, some of the results of human intervention trials are beginning to yield interesting results. A large number of international scientists from various disciplines, including cell biology, molecular biology, nutritional oncology, epidemiology, and public health, reviewed and discussed their most recent findings. The following topics were emphasized:

1. Mechanisms of carcinogenesis;
2. The mechanism of action of carotenoids, retinoids, vitamin E, protease inhibitors, and fatty acids;
3. Prevention of cancer in animals by carotenoids, retinoids, vitamin E, and selenium;
4. Nutritional causes of large-bowel cancer;

5. Preliminary results of intervention trials in China and Italy; and
6. The role of retinoids, vitamin D, and vitamins B6 and B1 in cancer treatment.

This volume provides up-to-date information on basic and clinical research in the area of nutritional oncology and will be useful to nutritionists, oncologists, cell biologists, pharmacologists, and epidemiologists.

The second meeting of the International Association for Vitamin and Nutritional Oncology (IAVNO) was sponsored by the Samuel Freeman Charitable Trust; National Cancer Institute; Henkel Corporation; Cancer Research Institute; BASF Corporation; General Nutrition; Takeda, USA; Rhone-Poulene, Inc.; Hoffman-LaRoche, Inc.; Bristol-Myers Company; and American Cyanamid Company.

Kedar N. Prasad
Frank L. Meyskens, Jr.
November 1989

Contents

Preclinical Studies
in Cancer Prevention and Treatment

Clinical Studies
in Cancer Prevention and Treatment

Nutrition and Cancer

An Overview of Present Reality and Future Goals

Kedar N. Prasad
President of IAVNO

Introduction

I welcome all of you to this second meeting of IAVNO. I am pleased to note that 14 countries have sent their delegations to attend this conference. Since this is my last opportunity to address this distinguished audience as President of IAVNO, I decided to review some well known, some not so well known, and even some controversial issues in order to generate new discussions on these matters. These decisions are deliberate, because I believe that our area of cancer research has an impact on the issue of public health and safety.

Cancer Prevention

In the USA, approx 900,000 new cases of cancer are detected every year, and about 450,000 persons die of this disease each year. In the world, about 8 million new cases of cancer are diagnosed each year, and approx 5 million people die of this disease every year. Therefore, cancer has become one of the major health problems throughout the world. It is estimated that over 90% of the human cancers are caused by environmental, dietary, and life-style-related factors; approx 30% of these are attributed to tobacco smoking and about 40% to dietary factors. From this estimation, it appears that over 70% of human cancers could be prevented if we stopped smoking and modified our diets and life styles based on scientific principles. Such a strategy could also reduce the risk of cancer among humans who are at high risk of developing cancers.

The Cancer Prevention Program at the National Cancer Institute under the leadership of Dr. Peter Greenwald has made remarkable progress during the last five years. We applaud the National Cancer Institute's goal of reducing cancer death by 50% by the year 2000. This is a noble goal, and we must try to achieve it by new fundamental research, clinical studies, and an aggressive public education program. While educating the public, we are faced with the problem of complex human behaviors that exhibit contradiction to the extreme. Humankind can be gentle to a point that we are moved by the suffering of the smallest creatures on our planet, and, at the same time, we can be brutal to a point that we do not hesitate to take self-destructive steps. The latter is reflected by the fact that tobacco smoking has not decreased significantly among the overall US population, in spite of public education programs on this issue. On the other hand, in the developing countries, the incidence of tobacco smoking among young individuals is increasing. We have also failed to convince those industries that are directly or indirectly involved in the manufacture and/or distribution of carcinogenic agents to develop a program that balances economic growth and the public safety. Nevertheless, we must continue to devise novel programs for educating the public and industries on the issue of cancer prevention and treatment.

Some public and private organizations have published guidelines for diets and life styles in order to reduce the risk of human cancer. I believe that they are very useful and should be adopted. However, it must be pointed out that all balanced diets contain cancer-protective substances as well as man-made and naturally occurring carcinogenic substances. In addition, some of the mutagenic and carcinogenic substances are formed during storage, digestion, and metabolism of food. This raises a question of whether the particular diet or the relative amounts of cancer-protective and cancer-causing agents would be more effective in cancer prevention. Numerous animal studies have shown that the dietary supplementation with carotenoids, retinoids, α-tocopherol, or selenium reduces the risk of chemical-induced cancers. Utilizing in vitro transforming cell systems, the role of supplementary β-carotene, α-tocopheryl succinate, and selenium in reducing the frequency of chemical- and radiation-induced transformation has been confirmed. In all animal and in vitro studies, nutrients have been used as a supplemental agent; therefore, the animal hypothesis that certain vitamins and minerals may reduce the risk of cancer can be tested only by intervention trials among the high-risk human populations, utilizing one or more specific nutrients. Unlike in animals, diets and life style are impossible to control in humans; nevertheless, we must have information on these confounding factors. Furthermore, the blood levels of supplemental vitamins under study, fats, and the immune competency of the host must be monitored at regular intervals. In the absence of a well-designed human intervention study, the results of the efficacy of nutrients in cancer prevention would be inconclusive.

Efforts have been made to test the animal hypothesis on nutrition and cancer in humans by performing classical epidemiological studies. Some studies have supported the hypothesis that there may be an inverse relationship between β-carotene, retinol, α-tocopherol, ascorbic acid, or selenium levels, and the risk of human cancer, whereas others have found no such relationship. Considering the complexities of human epidemiological studies, and considering that each of the nutrients selected for study at physiocological doses may exert only small protective effects, the above conflicting conclusions are not unexpected. Based on the observations that the supplemention of cancer-protective vitamins or minerals is essential for a reduction in chemical- and radiation-induced cancer in the experimental systems and and that the diet contains both cancer-preventive and cancer-causing substances, I propose that a balanced diet, together with a moderate supplement of cancer-protective substances, may be needed for a maximal reduction in cancer incidence among humans. An intervention study can be initiated among the high-risk population to test this hypothesis.

Regarding supplemental nutrition, I must express my deep concern over the flagrant misuse of nutritional supplements by the public. The health-food industries are becoming bolder and bolder in formulating numerous supplements, most of which are based on unscientific principles. Many of them are useless; some of them may even be harmful. For these reasons we must develop an effective program to protect the public against the misuse of supplemental nutrients. This is urgent, since approx 40% of the adult US population is consuming some forms of supplemental nutrients.

We are making rapid progess in our understanking of the molecular mechanisms of immortalization and transformation of normal cells by transfecting them with appropriate vectors carrying well-defined DNA segments of oncogenic viruses. I believe that nutritional oncologists must use these techniques to study and define the molecular mechanisms of action of specific cancer-preventive nutrients. It is very gratifying to note that the Surgeon General's Report on Nutrition and Health has recommeded 10 areas of nutrition and cancer research for investigation and that the molecular biology of nutrition has been given the top priority. It has already been reported that certain vitamins can alter the expression of protooncogenses and the cell signaling systems in mammalian transformed cells. The relevance of these observations to normal cells cannot be evaluated at this time. The availability of immortalized normal cells, which continue to divide and express differentiated functions, should help in elucidating the molecular mechanisms used by vitamins in regulating cellular functions as well as the mechanisms of transformation.

Certain vitamins induce cell differentiation in some well-established cancer cells in culture. They also reduce the action of tumor promoters and initiators. Therefore, the mechanisms of the above effects of vitamins must be investigated.

Over 30 human intervention studies utilizing one or more nutrients are in progress around the world. It should be pointed out that human intervention studies are very complex, costly, and time-consuming, and in the absence of an appropriate experimental design, these results can be inconclusive and misleading. Furthermore, well-controlled cancer prevention studies cannot be performed in humans as they can in animals, because of extreme variations in dietary habits and life styles. However, these variations can be monitored externally, by appropriate questionnaires, and internally, by measuring the biological fluids (blood and urine) and tissues whenever they are available. We have made remarkable progress in refining the questionnaires, which will reflect more accurately the diet and life style factors. The use of such questionnaires may not yield useful results until they are supplemented with the values of biological parameters. During the last five years, we have made remarkable progress in refining methodologic issues, which may reduce the impact of the confounding factors on data interpretation. Laboratory experiments have given us adequate biological rationales for using nutrients in human cancer prevention studies. In the design of any human intervention trials, the issues of methodologies are as important as the issue of biological rationales. Attempts to refine one at the cost of the other may produce inconsistent results.

Cancer Treatment

The role of specific nutrients in the treatment of human cancers has not received adequate attention either from the researchers or the funding agencies, in spite of the fact that some laboratory results that have been published appear encouraging. For example, it appears that certain nutrients, such as β-carotene and vitamins A, C, and E, enhance the effects of radiation and chemotherapy on cancer cells in animal tumor models and on transformed cells in vitro, and protect normal tissue against the adverse effect of tumor-therapeutic agents in animal models. However, I want to emphasize that the efficacy of nutrients in modifying the response to tumor-therapeutic agents depends on the type of nutrients, the kind of tumor-therapeutic agents, and the type of tumor. Hence, it is essential that laboratory experiments are performed to define the interactions between nutrients and therapeutic agents before their use in treating human cancers can be considered.

It is an established concept that when one or more blood elements are depressed during tumor therapy, they are replaced by infusion of new blood elements. Such a concept is not applied when the levels of vital nutrients are decreased during radiation therapy or chemotherapy. Only in acute cases are supplemental nutrients given parenterally. Unfortunately, parenteral nutrition in patients with advanced cancer is considered costly and ineffective. When one examines the formulations of some parenteral nutritions, it appears that they have not taken into account the recent advances made on the role of specific nutrients in the regulation of growth and differentiation of cancer cells. Therefore, new formulations of parenteral nutrition that meet the needs of cancer patients should be developed by a joint collaboration of basic and clinical scientists and appropriate industries.

Conclusion

I believe that new mechanistic results on the effects of nutrients on animal and human carcinogenesis are impressive. I hope that, in the future, new concepts in cancer prevention and treatment will be developed and the old ones will be modified. Many animal and some human studies suggest that certain nutrients, if properly used, may markedly reduce the incidence of human cancer. Furthermore, they may also improve the effectiveness of current treatment modalities. We undoubtedly have a long way to go before our goals of reducing cancer incidence and achieving more effective cancer treatment are reached; however, I believe we have made an excellent beginning.

Mechanisms of Carcinogenesis

Nutrients and Cancer Prevention K. N. Prasad and F. L. Meyskens, Jr., eds. © 1990 The Humana Press

TWO OPERATIONAL MODES OF TRANSMEMBRANE MIGRATION OF CYCLIC GMP SIGNAL PATHWAY

Sharma, Rameshwar K.

Section of Regulatory Biology, Cleveland Clinic

Research Institute, Cleveland, Ohio 44106

ABSTRACT

The transformation of a normal cell into a terminal stage of malignancy is a multiple-step biological process in which the initial signal appears to activate a protooncogene into an active oncogene. In this activation process growth factors, including catecholamines and polypeptide hormones, play an important role in the oncogene expression. The mechanisms by which the extracellular signals, such as those of the growth factors, are translated into biological responses is therefore an important problem in both regulatory and cancer biology. There are at present three recognized signal pathways -- cyclic AMP, phosphatidylinositol, and cyclic GMP -- for the propagation of these receptor-mediated events. In my presentation I will address the most recent developments on the nature and the mechanisms of the generation and regulation of transmembrane migration of receptor-mediated cyclic GMP signals. There appear to be at least two very different (direct and indirect) modes of operation of this signal pathway, suggesting the existence of at least two different types of receptor-coupled guanylate cyclases. To date, only one such guanylate cyclase (ANF-dependent) has been identified, which appears to be bifunctional; it is both an ANF receptor and a guanylate cyclase. But evidence strongly suggests the existence of another type of guanylate cyclase that is indirectly coupled to the guanylate cyclase. Both modes of cyclic GMP operational systems at the membrane level appear to be down regulated by protein kinase C, representing a close interaction of the two major cyclic GMP and protein kinase C signal pathways in the generation and regulation of cyclic GMP signals.

BACKGROUND

Hormones play an important role in both genetic and epigenetic changes that occur during the processes of cellular transformation and expression of the cancer phenotype (1). To fully comprehend the biochemical basis for these transformations and the resultant oncogenic expression processes, it is important first to understand the precise mechanisms of normal cellular regulation.

It is now clear that there are at least three major signal pathways--cyclic AMP, phosphatidylinositol, and cyclic GMP--by which the sensory signals generated at the extracellular surface are translated into appropriate biological responses. In all these three pathways, the first step in signal transduction is the ligand interaction with specific domains of plasma membrane receptors. These receptors are specific and individual for each of the hormones. In the case of cyclic AMP and phosphatidylinositol signal pathways, transmembrane migration of receptor signals is mediated by the activation of a specific protein, termed G-protein, belonging to the family of GTP-binding proteins. These proteins are individualized for each of the signal pathways, and the G-protein for the phosphatidylinositol signal pathway has not been characterized as yet. Interaction of hormone-bound receptor-G-protein results in the stimulation of adenylate cyclase which catalyzes the formation of cyclic AMP in this signal pathway, and the activation of phospholipase C in the phosphatidylinositol signal pathway (reviewed in 2). By contrast, only very recent studies have started to reveal the biochemical nature and physiology of guanylate cyclase and the cyclic GMP system, which is the subject of the present brief review.

Cyclic GMP was discovered in 1963 in rat urine (3). At almost the same time the remarkable discovery of cyclic AMP was made by Sutherland and his associates (4). Pioneered by the initial study of George *et al.* (5) which implicated cyclic GMP as a biologic effector molecule, mediating the effect of acetylcholine through adrenergic receptors, a peak of activity ensued for about 5 years to explore the proposed validity of the "Yin Yang" hypothesis. This hypothesis postulated that the biological regulation of a cell is governed by the opposing biological activities of cyclic AMP and cyclic GMP (6). However, this and the general concept bearing upon the second messenger role of cyclic GMP in receptor-mediated signal transduction processes became seriously compromised because: a) the attempts to demonstrate a hormonally dependent guanylate cyclase failed in every tested system (7); b) in contrast, the guanylate cyclase activity was nonspecifically stimulated by a variety of agents such as polyunsaturated fatty acids, peroxides, hydroperoxides, free radicals, ascorbic acid, sodium nitroprusside, and other agents that presumably affected the oxidation-reduction potential of the biochemical reactions (8); and c) there was a general consensus that cyclic GMP-dependent protein kinase--the effector enzyme of cyclic GMP signal transduction--does not phosphorylate a specific protein clearly distinct from that of the cyclic AMP-dependent protein kinase (9). Despite the fact that the very initial studies had suggested the existence of distinct forms of soluble and particulate guanylate cyclases which could be differentiated from each other by their physical and certain kinetic proprerties (10-13), the mere fact that guanylate cyclase could be nonspecifically stimulated by non-hormonal agents made these original observations on the independent existence of hormonally dependent guanylate cyclase suspect. These observations were then reinterpreted to be artifactually tributable to the "assay conditions, other constituents in crude preparations, or possibly other factors," (8). This view was transformed into a belief with the discovery of a nonspecific form of guanylate cyclase and, at that time, the apparent lack of evidence for the hormonally dependent guanylate cyclase (8).

In direct contrast to the above dominant concept, which completely negated the role of cyclic GMP in hormonal signal transduction, parallel studies with the model cell systems of isolated fasciculata cells of rat adrenal cortex and rat adrenocortical carcinoma from our laboratory supported the mediatory role of cyclic GMP in steroidogenic signal transduction and led to the proposal of a hypothetical working model in which membrane guanylate cyclase was the key enzyme in receptor-mediated cyclic GMP signal pathway (reviewed in 14). Clearly, this concept was completely opposite to the other dominant concept that questioned the second messenger role of cylcic GMP. Which of these two concepts was valid depended, therefore, on one single factor: Is there or is there not a hormonally dependent membrane guanylate cyclase in mammalian cells?

For this reason, the ACTH-dependent guanylate cyclase in rat adrenal cortex is a landmark discovery (15-17). This, for the first time, established the identity of an enzyme that was hormone-specific, was distinct from the nonspecific soluble form, and was linked with cyclic GMP-mediated transmembrane signal transduction. This also provided a catalyst for the scrutiny of other hormone receptor coupled guanylate cyclase systems.

OPERATIONAL MODES OF CYCLIC GMP SIGNAL
TRANSDUCTION

Direct Coupling Mechanism

Purification and characterization of 180-kDa ANF-dependent guanylate cyclase. In order to elucidate the mechanism of cyclic GMP signal transduction, a 180-kDa guanylate cyclase was purified (23) from rat adrenal cortical carcinoma. This protein was found to be not only a guanylate cyclase, but also to contain an additional extraordinary activity of an ANF receptor (24,25). ANF is an atrial peptide hormone that regulates sodium excretion, water balance, blood pressure, and the process of steroidogenesis (18-21). The finding that the second messenger of certain ANF signal transductions is cyclic GMP (22) had a major impact on the culmination of the intense debate that questioned the mediatory role of cyclic GMP in signal transduction. Thus the discovery of a new class of a bifunctional surface receptor protein which was both a guanylate cyclase and an ANF receptor was made.

The same, but tentative, conclusion that ANF binding activity and guanylate cyclase activity reside on a single lung protein was also independently arrived at in another laboratory (26). The basis for this conclusion was that through multiple purification steps, the guanylate cyclase and ANF binding activities were associated with each other on a highly purified, but apparently not a homogeneous 120-kDa protein (26,27). Purity of this protein in this case became an important issue because less than pure protein would not warrant the above conclusion that a single protein contains both the ligand-binding and guanylate cyclase activities. (For a commentary on this important point see references 28,29). Very recent studies from another laboratory challenge the claim that 120-kDa protein is an ANF receptor; the authors contend that the marginal ANF binding associated with the protein could be an associated contaminating protein (30).

The identification of a 130-kDa bifunctional protein containing both guanylate cyclase and ANF receptor in bovine adrenal cortex was subsequently reported from two other laboratories (31,32). How 180-kDa and 130-kDa are biochemically related, or not related, remains to be established. A complementary DNA (cDNA) of a protein from rat brain has now been cloned, and the expression of the cloned cDNA supports the conclusion that ANF receptor and guanylate cyclase are indeed one protein (33). Thus it is established that the ANF receptor is also a guanylate cyclase, representing a new class of surface receptor proteins.

<u>Ubiquity of the bifunctional protein</u>. The 180-kDa mGC is ubiquitous and dominant in rat adrenal glands, testes (rat and mouse), kidney and neural tissues (34-36,25), suggesting its signal transducer role in both endocrine and neuronal regulatory processes.

<u>Coupling of 180-kDa mGC with ANF-dependent cyclic GMP levels</u>. Studies with rat particulate fractions derived from adrenal glands (37), kidney (36) and mouse testes (34) show that ANF-dependent guanylate cyclase activity in each case is inhibited with polyclonal anti-membrane guanylate cyclase antibody, demonstrating the hormonal dependence of the 180-kDa mGC.

<u>Dual regulation of the 180-kDa mGC activity by ANF and protein kinase C (PKC)</u>. Studies with the rat adrenocortical carcinoma and aortic smooth muscle cells indicate that the phorbol ester signal inhibits ANF-dependent cyclic GMP formation (38,39) and both the hormone-dependent cyclic GMP levels and guanylate cyclase activity (38). Because the major phorbol ester receptor is protein kinase C (40), we proposed a hypothetical model in which the two signal pathways, cyclic GMP and phosphatidylinositol, were linked (35). The linkage was such that the activation of protein kinase C caused the negation of the ANF-dependent guanylate cyclase activity. In direct support of this model, the preliminary evidence demonstrating the inhibition of the ANF-dependent guanylate cyclase by protein kinase C in crude rat adrenocortical carcinoma membranes has been presented (35).

Similar to a situation in the rat adrenocortical carcinoma cells, *vide supra*, protein kinase C inhibits ANF-dependent guanylate cyclase in rat testicular particulate fraction (37). In molecular terms the obvious mechanism by which protein kinase C negates the hormone-dependent guanylate cyclase activity is via the process of phosphorylation. Since the 180-kDa membrane guanylate cyclase is ANF-dependent, the logical substrate of protein kinase C would be the 180-kDa guanylate cyclase. Preliminary studies indicate that this indeed is the case. A 180-kDa protein band is phosphorylated by protein kinase C in crude testicular membranes and partially-purified (GTP-affinity fraction) enzyme; the phosphorylation is blocked by the 180-kDa membrane guanylate cyclase antibody (25). This blocking action indicates that the phosphorylated form of the enzyme uncouples the hormonal signal. This suggests a novel "switch on" and "switch off" mechanism of the cyclic GMP signal transduction. The switch is the 180-kDa membrane guanylate cyclase, the dephosphorylated form representing the "switch on" and the phosphorylated form the "switch off" signal. This up-graded model is depicted in Figure 1.

In the up-graded model, there is an intermembrane link between the phosphatidylinositol and cyclic GMP signal pathways. This link suggests that a phosphatidylinositol signal that activates PKC, through the hypothetical phosphorylation of 180-kDa mGC, will result in the inhibition of the ANF signal pathway.

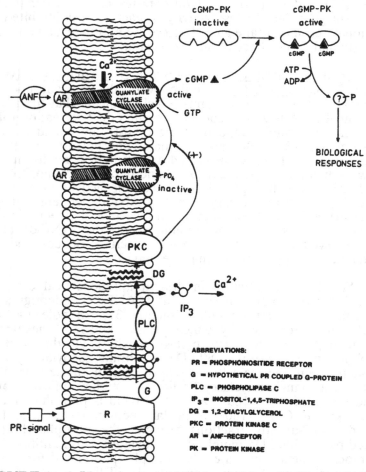

FIGURE 1. A Hypothetical ANF-dependent cGMP signal pathway model depicting its intermembrane-mediated negative regulation by PKC signal (Ref. 37).

It is noted that the model tentatively assumes that guanylate cyclase is a transmembrane protein whose ANF receptor domain is on the outside plasma membrane and the catalytic domain is inside the membrane. It is speculated that ANF dissociates a peptide component, an accessory protein, or alters the architectural configuration of the membrane for the activation of guanylate cyclase. The cyclic GMP thus generated causes a biological response via cyclic GMP-dependent protein kinase.

The membrane guanylate cyclase and PKC interaction raises other interesting points. The two limbs of the phosphatidylinositol signal pathway are turned on by the activation of phospholipase C. This catalyzes the cleavage of phosphatidylinositol 4, 5-biphosphate into inositol triphosphate (IP_3), and 1,2 diacylglycerol, which activates PKC. This means that a signal capable of generating 1, 2-diacylglycerol through PKC will terminate the ANF-dependent cyclic GMP signal. This might be the reason that the vasopressin receptor signal also negatively regulates the ANF-dependent formation of cyclic GMP (39). Although it has not been directly demonstrated, the link between vasopressin and ANF receptor signals might also be through PKC (40A). These results indicate that these transmembrane receptor signals, in which cyclic GMP plays a bona fide "second messenger" role, are intertwined.

Indirect Coupling Mechanism

An intriguing aspect of the above studies is that in contrast to the corresponding cyclic AMP system where receptor and adenylate cyclase components are distinct, one protein appears to contain both the receptor and guanylate cyclase (*vide supra*). This raises an important question. Are all cyclic GMP-mediated transmembrane signaling mechanisms identical?

To answer this question I will briefly discuss our studies with a newly purified and characterized rat adrenocortical carcinoma α_2-receptor subtype that will indicate that this is not the case.

Catecholamines, polypeptide hormones, and neurotransmitters trigger their respective biological responses by interacting with specific domains of plasma membrane receptors. One of the predominant catecholamine receptors is α_2-adrenergic; on the basis of its pharmacological characterization, it is found to be located in the membranes of diverse tissues: rat heart (47), human blood platelets (48-50), digital arteries (51), nerve terminals (52), rat brain

(53), hamster adipocytes (54), salivary gland (55,56), and liver (57,58). Activation of this receptor results in a variety of tissue-specific biological responses, such as platelet aggregation, inhibition of lipolysis, presynaptic feedback inhibition of norepinephrine release from noradrenergic nerve endings, postsynaptic smooth-muscle relaxation in gastrointestinal tract, smooth-muscle contraction in selected vascular beds, inhibition of renin release from juxtaglomerular cells of the kidney, stimulation of water secretion by salivary glands, and inhibition of insulin release from pancreatic islet cells (59,60). These results suggest that the α_2-receptor-mediated signal(s) in one form or the other regulates the activities of entire sympathetic and at least part of the central nervous system. The logical question is, are these multiple physiological activities mediated by a single a_2-receptor hormone signal? The emerging evidence appears to suggest that this may not be the case.

α2-Adrenergic receptor subtypes. Mounting pharmacological (59, 61-63) and very recent biochemical and genetic evidence (61,64,67) indicates the heterogeneity of α_2-adrenergic receptors. Two research groups have suggested the pharmacological subclassification of these receptors into at least two subtypes, α_{2A} and α_{2B} (61,62); the α_{2A} subtype has 30- to 40-fold lower affinity for prazosin (an α_1 antagonist) than does α_{2B}. Based on this criterion, the human platelet receptor belongs to the α_{2A} subtype and the neonatal rat lung receptor to the α_{2B}-subtype. The human platelet receptor has been purified to homogeneity and its gene cloned (64). Southern blot analysis, using a 0.95-kb pst-restricted α_{2A}-cDNA fragment as a probe, revealed the presence of two additional homologous genes in the human genomic library (64). These genetic results support the pharmacological evidence for the distinct subfamily of α_2-adrenergic receptors. Recent biochemical and cloning studies from our laboratory support this contention, and show the presence of one other novel receptor subtype that does not fit into the defined categories of α_{2A} and α_{2B}.

This receptor subtype was discovered as a result of 15 years of investigative research that uncovered a unique α_2-adrenergic receptor-mediated signal transduction system in cloned rat adrenocortical carcinoma cells (14). Among the population of α-adrenergic receptors these cells have an exclusive population of α_2-receptors (66). No α_1-receptors are detectable. These receptors contain a high- and a low-affinity yohimbine-binding site (Kds of 5.4 and 72 nM), and only one high-affinity clonidine-binding site (Kd of 4.63 nM). Most significantly, these receptors have no affinity for prazosin; the receptor-bound yohimbine is not displaced by up to p 10^{-4} M prazosin. (In contrast 5 x 10^{-5} M prazosin displaces 50% of platelet receptor-bound yohimbine.) Pharmacological distinctness of the two α_2-receptors is substantiated by our biochemical results obtained with the homogeneous receptors of the rat carcinoma and human platelets (67). The proteolytic maps reveal the presence of the following fragments in rat carcinoma that are absent in human platelets: 40-kDa tryptic, 30-kDa and 18-kDa chymotryptic, and 40-kDa *S. aureus*-cleaved. On the other hand, the platelets contain 23-kDa and 16-kDa chymotryptic fragments that are not found in the rat carcinoma receptors. These results clearly demonstrate that the tumor α_2-receptor is biochemically and pharmacologically different from the well-characterized human platelet α_{2A}-receptor, and the other pharmacologically characterized α_{2B}-receptor subtype. We provisionally refer to this receptor as α_{2GC}-adrenergic receptor subtype.

$\alpha2GC$-Receptor-second-messenger systems interaction. It is well documented that α_2-receptor signal, through an uncharacterized Gi protein (inhibitory component of the GTP-binding protein), negatively regulates adenylate cyclase (41). This brings us to an important question: Is it the sole mechanism of α_2-receptor signal transduction?

This does not appear to be the case. α_2-Adrenergic receptor-mediated responses such as Na^+/H^+ antiporter, Ca^{2+} channels, and K^+ channels are linked to Gi (as yet uncharacterized) but not to the lowering of cyclic AMP (41). Our studies have shown a fascinating mechanism of the linkage of α_{2GC}-receptor signal to two predominant second-messenger molecules, cyclic AMP and cyclic GMP (42). In this "dual regulation model" the signal positively regulates the guanylate cyclase, causing an increased production of cyclic GMP, and concomitantly negates the β-receptor signal for the production of cyclic AMP by inhibiting adenylate cyclase. Negative adenylate cyclase coupling is beyond the β-adrenergic receptor level because forskolin-dependent cyclic AMP production is also inhibited by the α_{2GC}-receptor signal (42).

There is an intriguing aspect of the coupling of α_{2GC}-receptor signal with guanylate cyclase. It only occurs in an intact cell. No coupling is observed in a cell-free system (38). These results indicate that α_2-receptor-guanylate cyclase coupling is indirect.

Down-regulation of $\alpha2GC$-receptor-coupled guanylate cyclase activity by protein kinase C: The studies with a phorbol ester (phorbol 12-myristate 13-acetate) (PMA), a protein kinase C activator, indicate that α_{2GC}-receptor-mediated cyclic GMP formation is inhibited by the protein kinase C signal in a dose-dependent and time-dependent fashion: the half-maximal inhibitory concentration of PMA is 10^{-10} M with $T_{1/2}$ of 2.5 min (38). A protein kinase C inhibitor, 1-(5-isoquinolinyl-sulfonyl)-2-methyl piperazine (H-7), caused the release of the PMA-dependent attenuation of α_2 agonist (p-aminoclonidine)-stimulated cyclic GMP formation. These results suggest that protein kinase C signal down-regulates the α_{2GC}-receptor-mediated cyclic GMP formation. The mechanism for this is not known. But three attractive possibilities are at the level of 1) the receptor itself; 2) the hypothetical G-protein; and 3) the catalytic subunit of guanylate cyclase.

Similar to the situation in α_{2GC}-receptor-mediated cyclic GMP formation (an indirectly receptor-coupled system), neurotransmitter (muscarinic and histaminic) receptor-mediated cyclic GMP responses occur only in intact neuroblastoma cells (43,44). In these cells phorbol ester also inhibits muscarinic- and histaminic-dependent cyclic GMP formation, suggesting that protein kinase C is the inhibitory mediator. The well-characterized ANF-dependent guanylate cyclase is also down-regulated by protein kinase C (*vide supra*). This guanylate cyclase, in contrast to the α_2-agonist-dependent cyclase, is directly coupled to the receptor-mediated signal. These results suggest a pattern in that all hormonally positively coupled cyclic GMP receptors, regardless of the manner of their coupling (i.e., direct or indirect), are negatively regulated by the protein kinase C receptor signal. Taking into consideration that the α_{2GC}-receptors of the adrenocortical carcinoma negatively regulate hormone-dependent adenylate cyclase (42), these results indicate that a single α_{2GC}-receptor signal exhibits dual transmembrane regulation of cyclic GMP and cyclic AMP signal pathways and in turn is negatively regulated by protein kinase C signal. Remarkably, an altogether opposite pattern of regulation appears to be operating in the regulation of soluble guanylate cyclase, which is stimulated upon phosphorylation by protein kinase C (44A). It is noted that the well characterized ANF-dependent 180-kDa membrane guanylate cyaclase antigenically shows no structural similarity with the soluble guanylate cyclase. Equally interesting is the contrasting regulatory feature of the sea-urchin sperm guanylate cyclase, which, upon phosphorylation, is stimulated in its activity (45,46).

In conclusion, results of these limited studies together have started to unfold a charming story of the nature and the mechanisms

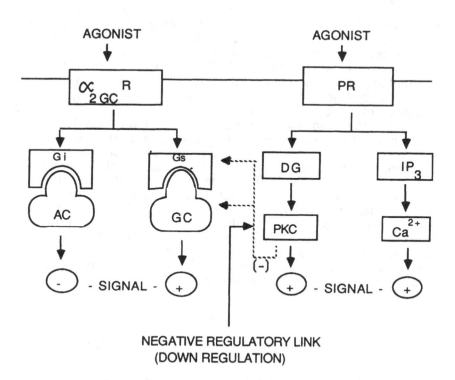

Abbreviations:

$\alpha_{2GC}R$ = guanylate cyclase coupled α_2 receptor
PR = phosphoinositide receptor
Gi = inhibitory G protein
Gs = stimulatory G protein
AC = adenylate cyclase
GC = guanylate cyclase
DG = 1,2-diacyl glycerol
IP_3 = inositol-1,4,5-triphosphate

FIGURE 2. A model for the dual regulation of hypothetical α_{2GC}-receptor coupled guanylate cyclase.

of the generation and regulation of transmembrane migration of receptor-mediated cyclic GMP signals. There appear to be at least two very different (direct and indirect) modes of operation of this signal pathway, suggesting the existence of at least two different types of receptor-coupled guanylate cyclases. To date the identity of only one such guanylate cyclase (ANF-dependent) has been revealed and that appears to be bifunctional; it is both an ANF receptor and a guanylate cyclase (35,37). But evidence strongly suggests the existence of another type of guanylate cyclase that is indirectly coupled to the guanylate cyclase (38). Neither the identity nor the mechanism of its coupling to the receptor signal is known. Some of the possible mechanisms of its regulation are depicted in Figure 2. This model depicts the dual regulation of hypothetical α_{2GC}-receptor coupled guanylate cyclase. This scheme assumes the presence of a pertussis-toxin-sensitive component which positively couples the α_2-receptor-mediated signal. Protein kinase C signal, generated by PR coupled events, down regulates the α_2-receptor signal. Nevertheless, both modes of cyclic GMP operational systems appear to be regulated at the membrane level by protein kinase C. It is anticipated that the future research will contribute to revealing the mechanisms of these regulatory processes.

REFERENCES

1.   Sharma RK Criss WE eds. (1978) In: <u>Endocrine Control in Neoplasia</u>, Raven Press, NY.

2.   Gilman AG (1987) Ann Rev Biochem 56: 615-649.

3.   Ashman DF, Lipton R, Melicow MM, Price TD (1963) Biochem Biophys Res Commun 11: 330-334.

4.   Sutherland EW Rall TW (1960) Pharmacological Reviews 12, 265-299.

5.   George WJ, Polson JB, O'Toole AG, Goldberg ND (1970) Proc Natl Acad Sci USA 66: 398-403.

6.   Goldberg ND, Haddox MK, Nicol SE, Glass DB, Sanford CH, Kuehl FA, Estensen R (1975) Adv Cyclic Nucleotide Res 5, 307-330.

7.   Goldberg ND, Haddox MK (1977) Ann Rev Biochem 46: 823-896.

8.   Murad F, Arnold WP, Mittal CK, Braughler JM (1979) Adv Cyclic Nucleotide Res 11: 175-204.

9.   Gill GN, McCune RW (1979) Curr Top Cell Regul 15: 1-45.

10. Siegel MI, Puca GA, Cuatrecasas P, (1976) Biochim Biophys Acta 438: 310-323.

11. Kimura H, Murad F (1975) Metabolism 24: 439-445.

12. Kimura H, Murad F (1975) J Biol Chem 250: 4810-4817.

13. Nakazawa K, Sano M, Saito T (1976) Biochim Biophys Acta 444: 563-570.

14. Sharma RK (1985) In: Hormonally Responsive Tumors (Hollander VP, ed). Academic Press, New York, pp 185-217.

15. Nambi P, Aiyar NV, Sharma RK (1982) Arch Biochem Biophys 217: 638-646.

16. Nambi P, Sharma RK (1981) Biochem Biophys Res Commun 100: 508-514.

17. Nambi P, Sharma RK (1981) Endocrinology 108: 2025-2027.

18. Atlas SA, Laragh JH (1986) Ann Rev Med 37: 397-414.

19. Cantin M, Genest J (1985) Endocrinol Rev 6: 107-127.

20. deBold AJ (1985) Science 230: 767-770.

21. Schwartz D, Geller DM, Manning PT, Siegel NR, Fok KF, Smith CE, Needleman P (1985) Science 229: 397-400.

22. Waldman SA, Rapport RM, Fiscus RR, Murad F (1985) Biochim Biophys Acta 845: 298-303.

23. Paul AK, Sharma RK (1985) 67th Annual Endocrine Meeting, June 9-12, Abst. #744.

24. Paul AK, Marala RB, Jaiswal RK, Sharma RK (1987) Science 235: 1224-1226.

25. Sharma RK, Marala RB, Duda T (In press) Steroids "Nes Memorial Issue".

26. Kuno T, Andresson W, Kamisaki Y, Waldman SA, Chang LY, Saheki S, Leitman DC, Nakane M, Murad F (1986) J Biol Chem 261: 5817-5823.

27. Waldman SA, Murad F (1987) Pharmacol Rev 39: 163-196.

28. Sharma RK (1988) Science 240: 805-806 (reply).

29. Waldman SA, Leitman DC, Andressen J, Murad F (1988) Science 240: 805-806 (letter).

30. Ishido M, Fujita T, Shimonaka M, Saheki T, Ouchi S, Kume T, Ishigaki I, Hirose S (1989) J Biol Chem 264: 641-645.

31.   Takayanagi KS, Snajdar RM, Imada T, Timura M, Pandey K, Inagami T (1987) Biochem Biophys Res Commun 144: 244-250.

32.   Meloche S, McNicoll N, Liu B, Ong H, DeLean AD (1988) Biochemistry 27, 8151-8158.

33.   Chinkers M, Garbers DL, Chang MS, Lowe DG, Chin H, Goeddel DV, Schulz S (1989) Nature (London) 338: 78-83.

34.   Marala RB, Sharma RK (1988) Biochem J 251: 301-304.

35.   Sharma RK, Jaiswal RK, Duda T (1988) In: UCLA Symposia, Biological and Molecular Aspects of Atrial Factors (Needleman P, ed). Alan R Liss, New York, pp 77-96.

36.   Ballermann BJ, Marala RB, Sharma RK (1988) Biochem Biophys Res Commun 157: 755-761.

37.   Sharma RK, Duda T, Marala RB (In press) In: American Society of Hypertension Series 3: Advances in Biologically Active Atrial Peptides (Brenner BM and Laragh JH, eds).

38.   Jaiswal RK, Jaiswal N, Sharma RK (1988) FEBS Letters 227: 47-50.

39.   Nambi P, Whitman M, Gressner G, Aiyar N, Crooke ST (1986) Proc Natl Acad Sci USA 83: 8492-8495.

40.   Nishizuka Y (1986) Science 233: 305-312.

40A. Nambi P, Whitman M, Aiyar N, Stassen F, Crooke ST (1987) Biochem J 244: 481-484.

41.   Limbird LE (1988) FASEB J 2: 2686-2695.

42.   Jaiswal N, Sharma RK (1986) Arch Biochem Biophys 249: 616-619.

43.   Kanaba S, Kanaba KS, Richelson E (1986) Eur J Pharmacol 125: 155-156.

44.   Lai WS, El-Fakahany E (1987) J Pharmacol Exp Ther 233: 134-140.

44A. Zwiller J, Revel MO, Malviya AN (1985) J Biol Chem 260: 1350-1353.

45.   Ramarao CS, Garbers DL (1988) J Biol Chem 263: 1524-1530.

46.   Ward GE, May GW, Vacquier VD (1986) J Cell Biol 103: 95-101.

47. Guicheney P, Garay RP, Levy-Marchal C, Meyer P (1978) Proc Natl Acad Sci USA 75: 6285-6289.

48. Hoffman BB, Yim S, Tsai BS, Lefkowitz RJ (1981) Biochem Biophys Res Commun 100: 724-731.

49. Lynch CJ, Steer ML (1981) J Biol Chem 256:3298-3303.

50. Sabol SL, Nirenberg M (1979) J Biol Chem 254: 1913-1920.

51. Jauering RA, Moulds RFW, Shaw J (1978) Arch Int Pharmacol 231: 81-89.

52. Berthelsen S, Pettinger WA (1977) Life Sci 21: 596-606.

53. Miach PJ, Dansse JP, Meyer P (1979) Nature 274: 492-494.

54. Pacquery R, Guidicelli Y (1980) FEBS Lett 116: 85-90.

55. Bylund DB, Martinez JR (1977) Physiologist 20: 16.

56. U'Prichard DC, Snyder SH (1979) Life Sci 24: 79-88.

57. Hoffman BB, DeLean A, Wood CL, Schocken DD, Lefkowitz RJ (1979) Life Sci 24: 1739-1746.

58. Hoffman BB, Mulikin-Kilpatrick D, Lefkowitz RJ (1980) J Biol Chem 255: 4645-4652.

59. Graham RM, Lanier SM (1986) In: The Heart and Cardiovascular System, Vol II (Fozzard HM, Haber E, Jennings R, Katz A, Morgan H, eds.), Raven Press, New York pp 1059-1095.

60. Smith EL, Hill RL, Lehman IR, Lefkowitz RJ, Handler P, White A (1983) In: Principles of Biochemistry: Mammalian Biochemistry, 7th ed. Vol 2, McGraw Hill, New York.

61. Bylund DB (1988) Trends Pharmacol Sci 9: 356-361.

62. Cheung Y-D, Barnett DB, Nahorski SR (1982) Eur J Pharmacol 84: 79-85.

63. Dickinson KEJ, McKernan RM, Miles CMM, Leys KS, Sever PS (1986) Eur J Pharmacol 120: 285-293.

64. Kobilka BK, Matsui H, Kobilka TS, Yang-Feng TL, Francke U, Caron MG, Lefkowitz RJ, Regan JW (1987) Science 238: 650-656.

65. Lanier SM, Homcy CJ, Patenaude C, Graham RM (1988) J Biol Chem 263: 14491-14496.

66. Nambi P, Aiyar NV, Sharma RK (1983) J Nutr Growth Cancer 1: 77-84.

67.   Jaiswal RK, Marshak DR, Sharma RK (1989) Molecular Cell Biochem 86: 41-53.

Mechanisms of Action
of Nutrients in Cancer Prevention

Nutrients and Cancer Prevention K. N. Prasad and F. L. Meyskens, Jr., eds. © 1990 The Humana Press

COUNTERACTIONS OF RETINOIC ACID AND PHORBOL ESTER TUMOR

PROMOTER RELATED TO CHANGES IN PROTEIN KINASE ACTIVITIES

W. B. Anderson, C. Liapi, and J. Strasburger

Laboratory of Cellular Oncology, NCI, NIH
Bethesda, MD USA 20892

R. Gopalakrishna

Department of Pathology, UCLA School of
Medicine
Los Angeles, CA USA 90024

A. Plet, F. Raynaud, and D. Evain-Brion

Laboratoire de Physiopathologie du
Developpement, CNRS-ENS, 75230
Paris, Cedex 05, France

ABSTRACT

Retinoids, derivatives of vitamin A, are antagonistic
toward some of the actions of phorbol ester tumor promoters
(TPA) in many cell systems, and may be important as agents
in cancer chemotherapy and prevention. We have been
involved with studies to elucidate the effects and counteractions of retinoic acid (RA) and TPA on two key protein
kinase systems known to play a role in the regulation of
cell growth, differentiation, and malignant transformation:
protein kinase C (PKC) and cyclic AMP-dependent protein
kinase (PKA). Results indicate that RA treatment of cells
causes marked changes in PKA activity, and in the PKA
regulatory subunits RI and RII, and suggest an important
synergism between RA and cyclic AMP to regulate cell growth
and differentiation. Treatment of cells with TPA induces a
rapid activation of PKC at the plasma membrane. Within 10
min TPA also causes an increase in PKA activity, and in RI
and RII, in the cytosol of PYS cells. RA, when added
simultaneously with TPA, negates this TPA effect on PKA.

Further, prolonged TPA treatment of cells results in a loss
of PKC, whereas prolonged RA treatment of some undifferentiated cell types elevates PKC activity in the cytosol.
Thus, RA and TPA can elicit opposite and antagonistic
effects on PKA and PKC. These changes in protein kinase
activities may be involved in the antineoplastic and
therapeutic actions of retinoids.

INTRODUCTION

The regulation of cellular growth and differentiation
is dependent upon the transduction of information from
extracellular signals initially acting at the cell membrane
to, in turn, modulate events in the cytoplasm and at the
nucleus. Among the transduction systems involved in
transmitting signals from extracellular hormones or growth
factors through cell surface receptors to regulate intracellular processes are the adenylate cyclase—cyclic AMP-
dependent protein kinase (PKA) system (1) and the
phosphatidylinositol turnover—protein kinase C (PKC)
system (2). Due to the crucial role of these signaling
systems in mediating cell proliferation, they are potential
targets for oncogene products and carcinogens in tumor
initiation and tumor promotion. Thus, a better understanding of nutritional conditions and factors that may act
to alter these signaling pathways to modulate cell growth
regulation and tumor promotion is important in the
prevention, and possible treatment, of cancer.

Retinoids are biological compounds that have been
shown to modulate the growth and differentiation of
numerous cell types (3,4). The phorbol ester tumor
promoter 12-0-tetradecanoylphorbol 13-acetate (TPA) is
another agent that can produce numerous functional and
biochemical changes closely resembling or mimicking those
induced by growth factors and transforming viruses (5,6).
Further, retinoic acid (RA) has been shown to act as an
antitumor promoter to antagonize some of the effects of TPA
(4). As suggested from these biological responses, RA and
TPA have proven to be extremely useful in elucidating the
properties and interactions of the transmembrane signaling
systems. Here we briefly summarize results of studies
carried out to determine the effects and counteractions of
RA and TPA in altering the signaling protein kinases PKA
and PKC. Such studies provide insight into the
mechanism(s) underlying altered cell growth and
differentiation in malignant cells as well as provide
insight into improved therapies in the control of cancer.

RETINOIC ACID AND PROTEIN KINASE A

Cyclic AMP has been implicated in the regulation of growth and differentiation in a variety of normal and malignant cell types (7,8). Most, if not all, of the biological effects of cyclic AMP are mediated through association with the cyclic AMP-dependent protein kinase (PKA) (1,9). Cyclic AMP exerts its effects by binding to the regulatory subunits of either the type I or type II PKA (1). These enzymes have a common catalytic subunit but differ in their cyclic AMP-binding regulatory subunits RI and RII (1,10). The levels of the RI and RII regulatory subunits, and thus the levels of the protein kinase isozymes, can be measured using the photoaffinity ligand 8-azido[^{32}P]cyclic AMP, which binds covalently to the regulatory subunits (11).

Embryonal carcinoma (EC) cells are highly malignant, undifferentiated stem cells that resemble early embryonic cells. These cells in culture have been used as a model system for studying the process of differentiation, and the conversion from malignant to nonmalignant cell types (12). RA is a potent inducer of the differentiation of murine EC cells (13), and the addition of cyclic AMP analogues during exposure of F9 EC cells to RA enhanced the differentiation of these cells to parietal endoderm (14). These findings indicated that RA treatment sensitizes F9 cells to elevated levels of cyclic AMP to alter cell growth and the onset of differentiation. Our studies revealed that treatment of F9 cells (15) and other EC cell types (16) with RA caused an early increase in both cytosolic and plasma membrane-associated PKA activity. Of particular interest was the rapid (within 2-15 h) preferential increase in the amount of PKA activity associated with the membrane fraction. Cyclic AMP has been observed to potentiate the effects of RA in several other cell types as well, including melanoma (17), myeloid leukemia (18,19), and macrophages (20). Furthermore, RA has been shown to increase the activity of PKA also in melanoma (17,21) and promyelocytic leukemia (22) cells, and in mouse (23) and human (24) breast carcinoma cells.

Since retinoids have been used with limited success to treat the hyperproliferative skin disease psoriasis, studies were carried out to determine if exposure of human psoriatic fibroblasts with RA might sensitize these cells to cyclic AMP. Our initial studies determined that PKA activity is decreased in psoriatic cells, and that the amount of the RII regulatory subunit is significantly decreased, or undetectable, in the cytosol prepared from psoriatic fibroblasts (25). Further, RA treatment of psoriatic fibroblasts was found to induce a pronounced increase in the levels of RI and RII subunits, and in PKA activity (26). In a related study, membranes prepared from erythrocytes obtained from psoriatic patients showed significantly decreased levels of RI when compared to that of normal erythrocyte membranes (27). Of interest is the observation that the RI level found in erythrocyte membranes inversely correlates with the severity of the disease as expressed by the PSAI score. More importantly, oral retinoid treatment of four patients induced an increase in cyclic AMP binding to the RI regulatory subunit of erythrocyte membranes (27).

These results strongly suggest an important inter-relationship among RA, cyclic AMP, and PKA. That the increases noted in cyclic AMP binding protein and PKA activity occur shortly after exposure of the cells to the retinoid indicates that this is a relatively early event in the action of RA to enhance the responsiveness of the treated cells to the cyclic nucleotide. It should be pointed out, however, that not all cell types will respond to retinoids with an increase in PKA activity. Cells that already have sufficient PKA activity to mediate cyclic AMP regulatory functions would not require an increase in PKA activity to promote additional actions of the retinoid, such as altered gene expression. Results to date suggest that it predominantly will be malignant, undifferentiated, rapidly growing cell types that may respond to RA with an increase in PKA activity to sensitize the cells to cyclic AMP modulation of growth and differentiation. Thus, a combination of retinoids along with increased cyclic AMP may be an advisable approach in research and therapeutic treatments.

EFFECTS ON NUCLEAR PROTEIN KINASE ACTIVITY

If retinoids act to modulate signal transduction pathways, it would be expected that they also will alter gene expression and DNA synthesis at the nucleus. The products of proto-oncogenes (the cellular homologues of transforming retroviral oncogenes) appear to function as the regulators of various cellular processes including proliferation and differentiation. Retinoid-induced differentiation of EC cells is accomplished by changes in the expression of various proto-oncogenes (28). However, the mechanism(s) through which RA acts to alter nuclear events remain to be fully elucidated. Chytil and Ong (29) initially reported the presence of specific binding proteins for RA and retinol, designated as cRABP and CRBP, respectively, in the cytosol of various tissues. However, not all RA target cells contain cRABP, which suggests that it apparently is not essential for the actions of RA. It has been proposed that cRABP may play a role in the transport of RA to the nucleus, although results indicate that this binding protein is not required in the regulation of gene expression by retinoids (30).

Recently, two specific nuclear receptors for RA have been identified that appear to belong to a larger family of nuclear receptors that includes the steroid hormone, thyroid hormone, and vitamin D_3 receptors (31-34). These nuclear RA receptors apparently act as transcriptional factors and are likely to play an important role in regulating, both positively and negatively, the transcription of specific genes. These high affinity RA receptor proteins have been shown to be present in the nucleus of EC and F9 cells (35). Certainly, these nuclear RA receptors play a significant role in mediating many of the regulatory effects of retinoids on cellular proliferation and differentiation in normal and neoplastic cells.

Another interesting effect of RA at the nucleus, recently reported by Takahasi and Breitman (36), is the covalent modification of a 55 kDa nuclear protein by retinoylation. However, the identity of the modified protein has not yet been determined. Thus, what role retinoylation may play in the many actions of RA to modulate various biological responses remains to be established.

Nuclear PKA has been implicated in the regulation of gene transcription, although the mechanism of action has yet to be fully elucidated (37). Thus, modulation of nuclear PKA activity by RA could have pronounced effects on cell growth and differentiation. Our recent studies have shown that RA treatment of F9 and PC13 undifferentiated stem cells causes a rapid (within 2 h) and pronounced (~50%) decrease in the RI and RII regulatory subunits, and in PKA activity, at the nucleus (38). As depicted in Fig. 1, this effect of RA on nuclear PKA activity also is observed with PCC4 EC cells, which differentiate into mesenchymal cells in response to RA (39). RA treatment of PCC4 cells induces a rapid (within 4 h) decrease in nuclear PKA activity. Studies also were carried out with a PCC4 stem cell variant (PCC4 • RA) that is resistant to

RA-induced differentiation. This variant lacks the
cytosolic RA binding protein (cRABP). In the PCC4 • RA
variant, nuclear PKA activity is decreased when compared to
the parent stem cells. RA treatment caused only a slight
decrease in PKA activity in these cells at 4 h, with PKA
activity then rising after 18 h of RA treatment (Fig. 1).
The reason for this low level of nuclear PKA, as well as
the small change in nuclear PKA in response to RA addition
to the PCCR • RA variant, is not known. While the lack of
cRABP in these variant cells might suggest a role for this
binding protein in regulating nuclear PKA, additional
studies are required to better elucidate this possibility.
Further, the possible involvement of this altered response
of nuclear PKA to RA in the resistance of these cells to
undergo differentiation also remains to be determined.

These results indicate that the rapid decrease in PKA
activity and in the levels of RI and RII at the nucleus is
an early event of RA treatment of EC stem cells. This
retinoid-induced change in PKA at the nucleus may be
involved in regulating the transcription of specific mRNAs.
Phosphorylation of regulatory nuclear proteins by PKA
(41,42) or the interaction of the RI and RII regulatory
subunits with chromatin (43) are possible mechanisms for
the modulation of gene expression. Early changes induced
by RA treatment in the levels of mRNA (both stimulation as
well as suppression) and changes in the pattern of in vitro
translation have been shown by Omori and Chytil (44).
Similar observations have been reported in EC cells (45).

The involvement of cyclic AMP in the regulation of
gene transcription is further supported by the existence of
a specific DNA sequence, CRE (46), that is common to
promoter regions of genes coding for proteins whose
synthesis is modulated by changes in the intracellular
concentration of cyclic AMP. The retinoid-induced
alteration in PKA at the nucleus may be an underlying event
in mediating cell growth inhibition and the onset of
differentiation in undifferentiated, malignant cells by RA
and cyclic AMP. This suggests that the antineoplastic
effect of RA plus cyclic AMP may, in part, be due to
alterations in aberrant gene transcription in the malignant
cells.

We have carried out several experiments to determine
if tumor promoter (TPA) treatment of differentiated
endodermal cells caused any alteration in PKA activity at
the nucleus, but were unable to demonstrate any consistent
effect on this protein kinase (unpublished results).

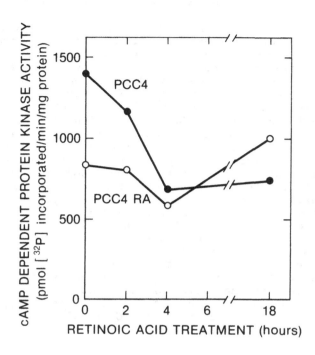

Figure 1. Time course of the effect of RA treatment of PCC4 (●——●) and PCC4 • RA (○——○) cells on PKA activity present in intact purified nuclei. Three dishes of subconfluent parental PCC4 and variant PCC4 • RA cells (kindly provided by Dr. M. Sherman, Hoffman-La Roche Institute) were treated with 0.1 μM all-<u>trans</u> RA for 2-18 h as indicated. The cells then were harvested and nuclei isolated as described previously (38). The purified nuclei were assayed immediately for PKA activity with kemptide as substrate as described by Roskoski (40).

Phorbol ester (TPA) treatment of NIH 3T3 cells, however, does induce rapid (within 20 min) activation (stable association) of PKC at the nucleus (47). Since TPA has been shown to generally have effects opposite to RA in regulating cell growth, differentiation, and tumor promotion (4), these results suggest that TPA and RA may alter nuclear PKC and PKA, respectively, to perhaps differentially modulate gene expression.

RETINOIC ACID AND PROTEIN KINASE C

Since retinoids are antagonistic toward the effects of phorbol ester tumor promoters in many cell systems, studies were carried out to assess possible changes in PKC activity in response to retinoids. RA treatment of F9 cells was found to provoke a time-dependent increase in cytosolic PKC activity (48). In contrast to PKA activity, which is increased within 3-15 h after RA treatment (15), little change is observed in PKC activity 24 h after the addition of RA. A significant increase in PKC activity is noted 5 days after exposure to RA. This time course corresponds to the time required (2-3 days) to observe retinoid-induced differentiation of F9 cells to the endoderm cell type (13,14), and to see RA-induced changes in the hormonal responsiveness of the adenylate cyclase system (49). More recently, Niles and Loewy (50) have reported that treatment of B16 mouse melanoma cells with RA also induces an increase in both the activity and amount of PKC. These authors note an increase in PKC at 24 and 48 h after RA treatment. The results of these time course studies suggest that the induced increase in PKC activity is not an early event in the action of RA to mediate cell proliferation and differentiation. Nonetheless, it is apparent that RA can influence the level of PKC in malignant, rapidly proliferating cell populations.

COUNTERACTION OF RETINOIC ACID TOWARD PHORBOL ESTER TUMOR PROMOTER

Retinoids have been shown to inhibit tumor promotion in vivo and in vitro (51) and to antagonize some of the biological effects of phorbol esters (3,4). For example, RA has been reported to inhibit TPA-induced polyamine accumulation and TPA-induced formation of skin papillomas (52), and to antagonize the TPA-mediated induction of ornithine decarboxylase (53,54). Also, RA has been shown to block TPA-induced anchorage-independent growth of cells (55), and to counteract the TPA-stimulated release of fibronectin from a number of cell types (56,57). Yet, the mechanism(s) by which retinoids inhibit the actions of TPA is unclear. Thus, it is of importance to determine possible counteractions between RA and TPA in altering membrane-associated protein kinase activities.

In addition to the RA- and TPA-mediated changes in the activities and subcellular distribution of PKA and PKC described above, recent studies from our laboratories have shown that exposure of PYS cells to TPA provokes a rapid (within minutes) increase in cytosolic PKA activity, accompanied by a concomitant decrease in PKA activity found with the membrane fraction (58). Likewise, TPA also induced the rapid redistribution of the RI and RII regulatory subunits from the plasma membrane to the cytosol. Byus *et al*. (59) also have observed that TPA treatment of H35 hepatoma and Chinese hamster ovary cells rapidly enhances PKA activation and increases the amount of the free catalytic subunit in the cytosol and nucleus. However, our results indicate a rapid relocation of PKA from the membrane to the cytosol rather than an activation of the enzyme.

Interestingly, when RA is added simultaneously with TPA to the cell culture media, the TPA-induced increase in cytosolic PKA activity, as well as in the levels of RI and RII, is markedly inhibited (58). The addition of RA alone had no effect on PKA at these very early time periods. Further, it was found that RA was effective in counter-acting this effect of TPA on PKA only when added simultaneously with the tumor promoter. When RA was added 25 min prior to TPA, no antagonism was observed. This finding is similar to the antagonistic effects of RA toward other rapid effects of TPA, where the retinoid is effective in inhibiting the TPA response only when added simultaneously along with the phorbol ester (53,57).

One possible mechanism for the RA effect to block the TPA-induced increase in cytosolic PKA activity might be that RA could directly antagonize TPA activation of PKC. However, RA does not block TPA-mediated activation (stabilized association) of PKC at the membrane in PYS cells (unpublished results) nor does it prevent the TPA-induced activation of PKC in 2C5 rat tracheal epithelial cells (60). Further, other studies have shown that retinoids do not directly alter phorbol ester binding to its receptor (PKC) (61,62).

Since the inhibitory effect of RA is so rapid (2-5 min), this response appears to take place at the plasma membrane. The TPA-induced redistribution of PKA from the membrane to the cytosol is likely due to a modification of membrane component(s) mediated through the activation of membrane-associated PKC. RA may counteract this response by transiently altering the component or modulating another activity to, in turn, prevent PKC from having an effect (i.e., *via* phosphorylation or oxidative modification through enhanced generation of superoxide radical), rather

than having a direct effect on PKC itself. The
counterregulation of these protein kinase activities by RA
and PKC is schematically summarized in Fig. 2. The rapid
opposite and antagonistic effects of RA and TPA on the
subcellular localization of PKA suggest that this may be
one of several early events at the plasma membrane in
response to RA that serves to counteract the effects of the
tumor promoter. The physiological significance of this
effect of RA to antagonize early events to TPA action,
particularly as it relates to anticarcinogenic effects of
RA, is not known. However, the inhibition of this TPA-
mediated redistribution of PKA may be important in the
mechanism by which RA antagonizes later effects of TPA.
Certainly, changes in the cellular distribution of these
protein kinases in response to TPA and RA would alter the
intracellular signal transduction pathways.

REGULATION OF PROTEIN KINASES BY OXIDATIVE MODIFICATION

Oxidant species such as superoxide radicals, hydrogen
peroxide, hydroxyl radicals, and lipid peroxides have been
implicated in a number of disease states, including cancer
(63,64). Further, there is substantial evidence to suggest
the involvement of free radicals, particularly those
derived from molecular oxygen, in the process of tumor
promotion (65). As noted above, one mechanism of tumor
promoter action involves the direct binding and activation
of PKC (2,66). A variety of terpenoid promoters including
phorbol diesters, mezerein, and teleocidin act by binding
to, and directly activating, PKC. However, another class
of tumor promoters, the organic peroxides (including
benzoyl peroxide and cumene hydroperoxide) (67,68), do not
bind to PKC. Yet, the actions of these two classes of
tumor promoters result in a similar pattern of altered
biological responses, indicating a common pathway exists
for PKC-activating promoters and the radical-generating
promoters. In this regard, phorbol ester treatment of
cells has been shown to enhance the generation of reactive
oxygen radicals, and this appears to play an important role
in tumor promotion by TPA (69-71). Other studies have
shown that the presence of reactive oxygen eliminating
enzymes, such as superoxide dismutase, scavengers of
reactive oxygen, and antioxidants, all inhibit tumor
promotion induced by TPA (72-74).

In the course of studies to better elucidate the
regulatory properties of PKC, it was observed that this
enzyme is markedly influenced by oxidative modification.

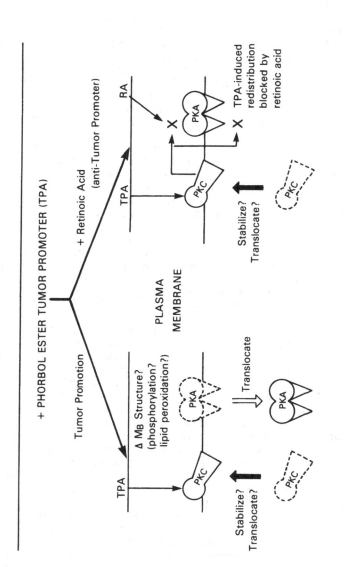

Fig. 2. Hypothetical model for the early (within minutes) alterations in activity and subcellular distribution of PKC and PKA in response to TPA and RA treatment of intact PYS cells.

Under mild conditions, treatment of the isolated enzyme or of intact cells with agents that generate oxygen species leads to direct activation of PKC (75). The treatment of intact C6 glioma and B16 melanoma cells with H_2O_2 causes a time- and temperature-dependent decrease in Ca^{2+}/phospholipid-dependent PKC along with a transient increase in an oxidatively modified isoform of PKC that exhibits activity in the absence of Ca^{2+} and phospholipids. The results indicate that the selective oxidative modification of the regulatory domain may negate the requirement for Ca^{2+} and lipids for activation of PKC. This oxidative activation of PKC may relate to the mechanism of tumor promotion by agents such as benzoyl peroxide and cumene hydroperoxide that do not bind directly to PKC as do the TPA class of tumor promoters, but nonetheless, may activate PKC by enhancing the reactive oxygen species within the cell. In turn, nutritional factors such as RA (76), β-carotene (77,78), and α-tocopherol (79,80) may exhibit antitumor promoter activity through their ability to act as antioxidants. In this way they could act to prevent direct PKC activation by the peroxide tumor promoters and to prevent later steps in the process of tumor promotion by the phorbol ester-type promoters following activation of PKC and subsequent generation of superoxide radical.

With more prolonged and intense exposure to H_2O_2 and hydroxyl radicals, PKC both in the isolated form and in intact cells is susceptible to inactivation (75,81). Prior treatment of cells with TPA to induce the stable association of PKC with the plasma membrane, followed by exposure to H_2O_2, resulted in increased inactivation of PKC. This suggested that membrane-associated PKC is more highly susceptible to oxidative inactivation. The pharmacological action of a number of antineoplastic agents appears to be *via* a free radical mechanism. Protein kinase C might represent a key target in the transmembrane signaling pathways for such anticarcinogenic agents. We have observed that the addition of the antineoplastic agent diaziquone (AZQ) to intact leukemia P388 cells causes the rapid inactivation of membrane-associated PKC (unpublished results). Antioxidants, including RA, protect PKC from AZQ-mediated oxidative inactivation. These results indicate a possible interrelationship between the oxidative modification of PKC and RA to influence cell proliferation and tumor promotion.

SUMMARY

Alterations in membrane signal transduction systems and protein kinase activities have been implicated in the regulation of cell growth, differentiation, and malignant transformation. Here we have summarized the results of studies carried out to better elucidate the effects and counteractions of RA and TPA on two kinase systems known to play a key role in the regulation of these cellular responses: protein kinase C and cyclic AMP-dependent protein kinase.

The studies discussed and reported in this communication concerning the early and late stages of RA action to counteract TPA activation of PKC and to modulate PKA within the cell are schematically summarized in the hypothetical model presented in Fig. 3. As depicted, initial RA actions at the plasma membrane to block TPA-induced effects are very rapid (within minutes) and may be due to the antioxidant effect of RA. In this manner, RA might antagonize such early biological responses induced by TPA as the increase in cytosolic PKA activity and the release of fibronectin from the cell. It should be emphasized, however, that RA does not appear to block direct TPA activation of PKC. Further, the significance of these very rapid effects of RA to antagonize early events of tumor promoter action, particularly as it relates to the anticarcinogenic effect of RA, is unknown.

The next stage of RA action (occurring within 1-2 h after addition to EC cells) is a pronounced decrease in PKA activity and in the levels of RI and RII regulatory subunits at the nucleus accompanied by altered gene expression. RA treatment of F9, PC13, and PCC4 cells (which differentiate into parietal endoderm, visceral endoderm, and mesenchymal cells, respectively) in each case induces a rapid loss in nuclear PKA activity. This appears to suggest that an early effect of RA on PKA at the nucleus may be important in the initiation of differentiation. At later time periods (10-20 h) after RA treatment of F9 cells there is an increase in both cytosolic and membrane-associated PKA activity. This later increase in PKA activity may regulate the direction of this differentiation process. Further, it is not known what role, if any, the well known cellular retinoic acid binding protein (cRABP) (29) or the recently described high affinity nuclear RA receptors (31-34) might play in regulating PKA. Also, it is not known if retinoylation of a 55 kDa nuclear protein (36) might influence PKA activity.

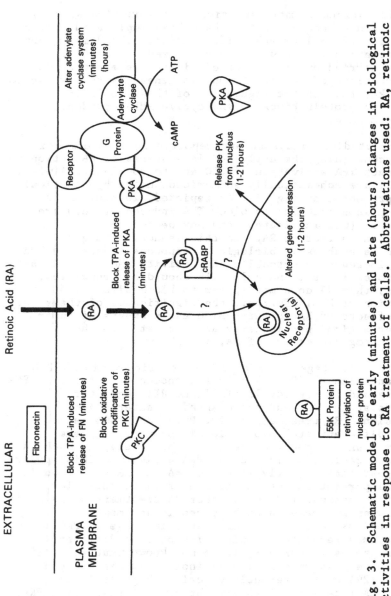

Fig. 3. Schematic model of early (minutes) and late (hours) changes in biological activities in response to RA treatment of cells. Abbreviations used: RA, retinoic acid; TPA, 12-0-tetradecanoylphorbol-13-acetate; FN, fibronectin, PKC, protein kinase C; PKA, cyclic AMP-dependent protein kinase; cRABP; cellular retinoic acid binding protein.

The indication that RA and tumor promoters may exhibit antagonistic effects in altering signal transduction pathways by oxidative modification may be central to a better understanding of the mechanisms of chemical carcinogenesis and tumor promotion. This may provide a common link between oncogene product alteration of signal transduction systems, and chemical carcinogens and tumor promoters that may alter signal transduction by the oxidative modification of phospholipid metabolism and PKC. Elucidation of the regulation of PKC, PKA, and signaling systems by oxidative modification will, in turn, help to identify environmental and nutritional factors that may act by altering the oxidative state of the cell to implement their carcinogenic or anticarcinogenic effects.

REFERENCES

1. Rubin, J., and Rosen, O. (1975) Annu. Rev. Biochem. 44:831-887.
2. Nishizuka, Y. (1984) Nature 308:693-698.
3. Sporn, M., and Roberts, A. (1983) Cancer Res. 43:3034-3040.
4. Jetten, A., and DeLuca, L. (1982) Carcinogenesis 7:513-520.
5. Blumberg, P.M. (1980) Crit. Rev. Toxicol. 8:153-197.
6. Mastro, A.M. (1982) Lymphokines 6:263-313.
7. Pastan, I., Johnson, G.S., and Anderson, W.B. (1975) Annu. Rev. Biochem. 44:492-522.
8. Whitfield, J.F.G., Boynton, A.L., and MacManus, J.P. (1979) Mol. Cell. Biochem. 27:155-179.
9. Cohen, P. (1982) Nature 296:613-620.
10. Nimmo, H.G., and Cohen, P. (1977) Adv. Cyclic Nucleotide Res. 8:146-166.
11. Walter, U., Uno, I., Liu, A.Y.C., and Greengard, P. (1977) J. Biol. Chem. 252:6494-6500.
12. Martin, G. (1980) Science 209:768-776.
13. Strickland, S., and Mahdavi, V. (1978) Cell 15:393-403.
14. Strickland, S., Smith, K., and Marotti, K. (1980) Cell 21:347-355.
15. Plet, A., Evain, D., and Anderson, W.B. (1982) J. Biol. Chem. 257:889-893.
16. Plet, A., Gerbaud, P., Sherman, M.I., Anderson, W.B., and Evain-Brion, D. (1986) J. Cell. Physiol. 127:341-347.
17. Ludwig, K.W., Loewy, B., and Niles, R.M. (1980) J. Biol. Chem. 255:5999-6002.

18. Olsson, I.L., and Breitman, T.R. (1982) Cancer Res. 42:3924-3927.
19. Davies, P.J.A., Murtaugh, M.P., Moore, W.T., Johnson, G.S., and Lucas, D. (1985) J. Biol. Chem. 260:5166-5174.
20. Murtaugh, M.P., Moore, W.T., and Davies, J.A. (1986) J. Biol. Chem. 261:614-621.
21. Rogelj, S., Loewy, B., and Niles, R.M. (1984) Eur. J. Biochem. 139:351-357.
22. Fontana, J.A., Emler, C., Ku, K., McClung, J.K., Butcher, F.R., and Durham, J.P. (1984) J. Cell. Physiol. 120:49-60.
23. Abou-Issa, H., and Duruibe, V. (1986) Biochem. Biophys. Res. Commun. 135:116-123.
24. Abou-Issa, H., and Duruibe, V. (1988) FASEB J. 2:A859.
25. Evain-Brion, D., Raynaud, F., Plet, A., Laurent, P., Leduc, B., and Anderson, W. (1986) Proc. Natl. Acad. Sci. USA 83:5272-5276.
26. Raynaud, F., Leduc, C., Anderson, W.B., and Evain-Brion, D. (1987) J. Invest. Dermatol. 89:105-110.
27. Raynaud, F., Gerbaud, P., Enjolras, O., Gorin, I., Anderson, W.B., and Evain-Brion, D. (1989) Lancet (in press).
28. Sejersen, M., Jin, T., Rahm, P., and Ringertz, N.R. (1989) Environ. Health Perspect. 80:247-275.
29. Chytil, F., and Ong, D.E. (1983) Adv. Nutr. Res. 5:13-30.
30. Jetten, A.M., Anderson, K., Deas, M.A., Kagechika, H., Rearick, J.I., and Shudo, K. (1987) Cancer Res. 47:3523-3530.
31. Petkovich, M., Brand, N.J., Krust, A., and Chambon, P. (1987) Nature 330:444-448.
32. Giguere, V., Ong, E.S., Segui, P., and Evans, R.M. (1987) Nature 330:624-627.
33. Benbrook, D., Lernhardt, E., and Pfahl, M. (1988) Nature 333:669-673.
34. Brand, N., Petkovich, M., Krust, A., Chambon, P., de Thé, H.D., Macchio, A., Tiollais, P., and Dejean, A. (1988) Nature 332:850-854.
35. Daly, A.K., and Redfern, C.P.E. (1987) Eur. J. Biochem. 168:133-137.
36. Takahashi, N., and Breitman, T.R. (1989) J. Biol. Chem. 264:5159-5163.
37. Jungmann, R.A., and Kranias, E.G. (1977) Int. J. Biochem. 8:819-830.
38. Plet, A., Evain-Brion, D., Gerbaud, P., and Anderson, W.B. (1987) Cancer Res. 47:5831-5834.
39. Jetten, A.M., Jetten, M.E.R., and Sherman, M. (1979) Exp. Cell Res. 124:381-385.

40. Roskoski, R. (1983) Methods Enzymol. 99:3-6.
41. Harrison, J.J., Schwoch, G., Schweppe, J.S., and Jungmann, R.A. (1982) J. Biol. Chem. 257:13602-13609.
42. Murdoch, G.H., Rosenfeld, M.G., and Evans, R.H. (1982) Science 28:1315-1317.
43. Glukhov, A.I., Nesterova, M.V., Bukhman, V.L., and Severin, E.S. (1986) Biochemistry (Engl. Trans. Biokhimiya) 51:87-94.
44. Omori, M., and Chytil, F. (1982) J. Biol. Chem. 257:14370-14374.
45. Schindler, J., and Sherman, M. (1984) Differentiation 28:78-85.
46. Montminy, M.R., and Bilezikjian, L.M. (1987) Nature 328:175-178.
47. Thomas, T.P., Talwar, H.S., and Anderson, W.B. (1988) Cancer Res. 48:1910-1919.
48. Kraft, A.S., and Anderson, W.B. (1983) J. Biol. Chem. 258:9178-9183.
49. Evain, D., Binet, E., and Anderson, W.B. (1981) J. Cell. Physiol. 109:453-459.
50. Niles, R.M., and Loewy, B.P. (1989) Cancer Res. 49:4483-4487.
51. Boutwell, R.K. (1974) Crit. Rev. Toxicol. 2:419-443.
52. Verma, A.K., Rice, H.M., Shapas, B.G., and Bontwell, R.K. (1978) Cancer Res. 38:793-801.
53. Paranjpe, M., DeLarco, J., and Todaro, G. (1980) Biochem. Biophys. Res. Commun. 94:586-591.
54. Astrup, E.G., and Paulsen, J.E. (1982) Carcinogenesis 3:313-320.
55. Yuspa, S., Lichti, U., Ben, T., and Hennings, H. (1981) Ann. N.Y. Acad. Sci. 359:260-273.
56. Zerlauth, G., and Wolf, G. (1984) Carcinogenesis 5:863-868.
57. Zerlauth, G., and Wolf, G. (1985) Carcinogenesis 6:531-534.
58. Plet, A., Gerbaud, P., Anderson, W.B., and Evain-Brion, D. (1988) Cancer Res. 48:3993-3997.
59. Byus, C.V., Trevillyan, J.M., Cavit, L.J., and Fletcher, W.H. (1983) Cancer Res. 43:3321-3326.
60. Jetten, A., and Shirley, J. (1986) Exp. Cell Res. 166:519-525.
61. Driedger, P.E., and Blumberg, P.M. (1980) Proc. Natl. Acad. Sci. USA 77:567-571.
62. Shoyab, M., and Todaro, G.J. (1980) Nature 288:451-458.
63. Slater, T.F. (1984) Biochem. J. 222:1-15.
64. Halliwell, B., and Gutteridge, J.M.C. (1984) Biochem. J. 219:1-14.

65. Kensler, T.W., and Taffe, B.G. (1986) Adv. Free
    Radical Biol. Med. 2:347-387.
66. Blumberg, P.M., Jaken, S., Konig, B., Sharkey, N.A.,
    Leach, K., Jeng, A.Y., and Yeh, E. (1984) Biochem.
    Pharmacol. 33:933-940.
67. Slaga, T.J., Klein-Szanto, A.J.P., Triplett, L.L.,
    Yotti, L.P., and Trosko, J.E. (1981) Science 273:1023-
    1025.
68. Bull, A.W., Nigio, N.D., and Marnett, L.J. (1988)
    Cancer Res. 48:1771-1776.
69. Goldstein, B.D., Witz, G., Amoruso, M., Stone, D.S.,
    and Troll, W. (1981) Cancer Lett. 11:257-262.
70. Slaga, T.J., Fischer, S.M., Weeks, C.E., Klein-Szanto,
    A.J.P., and Reinders, J. (1982) J. Cell. Biochem.
    18:99-119.
71. Ames, B.N. (1983) Science 221:1256-1263.
72. Kensler, T., Bush, D.M., and Kazumbo, W.J. (1983)
    Science 221:75-77.
73. Emerit, I., Levy, A., and Cerutti, P.A. (1983) Mutat.
    Res. 110:327-335.
74. Friedman, J., and Cerutti, P.A. (1983) Carcinogenesis
    4:1425-1427.
75. Gopalakrishna, R., and Anderson, W.G. (1989) Proc.
    Natl. Acad. Sci. USA 86:in press.
76. Witz, G., Goldstein, B.D., Amoruso, M., Stone, D.S.,
    and Troll, W. (1980) Biochem. Biophys. Res. Commun.
    97:883-888.
77. Kunert, K.J., and Tappel, A.L. (1983) Lipids 18:271-
    274.
78. Weitberg, A.B., Weitzmann, S.A., Clarke, E.P., and
    Stossel, T.P. (1985) J. Clin. Invest. 75:1835-1841.
79. Tappel, A.L. (1972) Ann. N.Y. Acad. Sci. 203:12-27.
80. McCay, P.B., and King, M.M. (1980) in Vitamin E
    (Machlin, L., ed.) pp. 289-317, Dekkar, New York.
81. Gopalakrishna, R., and Anderson, W.B. (1987) FEBS
    Lett. 225:233-237.

EFFECT OF ALPHA TOCOPHERYL SUCCINATE ON CELL

DIFFERENTIATION AND ADENYLATE CYCLASE SYSTEM

Kedar N. Prasad and Judith Edwards-Prasad
Center for Vitamins and Cancer Research,
Department of Radiology,
School of Medicine,
University of Colorado Health Sciences Center
Denver, Colorado   80262

INTRODUCTION

Increased daily dietary intake of alpha tocopherol (vitamin E) at levels higher than Recommended Dietary Allowance (RDA) reduces the risk of animal cancer induced by tumor initiators and promoters (1-7). Two human epidemiological studies (8-9) have supported the hypothesis that there may be an inverse relationship between the vitamin E level and risk of some cancer. Additional human studies are needed to substantiate this hypothesis. Except for its function as an antioxidant (10-13), the mechanisms of its action remain largely unknown. This may have been due to the fact that the tissue culture models, which are commonly used for mechanistic studies, could not be utilized, because both alpha tocopherol and alpha tocopheryl acetate were inactive in this experimental system. Some of the earlier effects of water soluble alpha tocopherol preparations on neuroblastoma and glioma cells (14) may have been at least in part due to toxicity of solvents (15).

In 1982, we discovered that alpha tocopheryl succinate (α-TS) was the most active form of vitamin E in cell culture (15). Subsequent

studies confirmed the high potency of α-TS on
other criteria.   and in other systems (16-
20).   This review will discuss recent studies on
the effect of α-TS on some transformed cells in
culture on the criteria of cell differentiation,
growth   inhibition   and   adenylate   cyclase
activity.

Effect of Alpha Tocopheryl Succinate (α-TS) on
Cell Differentiation and Growth Inhibition:

        α-TS caused cell differentiation in murine
B-16 melanoma cells in culture as evidenced by
the formation of long bipolar and multipolar
cytoplasmic processes, enlargement of cell size,
parallel arrangement of cells during growth and
increased melanin content (15).   It also reduced
growth and survival of these cells.   α-TS-
induced differentiated phenotype was largely
irreversible; however, cells resistant to α-TS
were present in the culture.   The solvent of α
-TS (ethanol or ethanol plus sodium succinate)
did not affect growth or morphology of melanoma
cells in culture.

        When alpha tocopherol, alpha tocopheryl
acetate and alpha tocopheryl nicotinate were
solubilized in ethanol, and then added to
melanoma cell cultures, they did not affect
growth or morphology (15).   This may be due to
the fact that these forms of vitamin E do not
enter melanoma cells in culture. Indeed, when
these cells were incubated in the presence of
various forms of Vitamin E, extracted and then
measured by HPLC, only α-TS was detected in the
cells (21).

        α-TS treatment also inhibited the growth of
murine and human neuroblastoma (16-17), rat
glioma (17) and human prostate cancer cells (18)
without causing cell differentiation.   Two lipid
soluble antioxidants, butylated hydroxyanisole
and butylated hydroxytoluene, also inhibited
growth of these transformed cells and caused
some morphological changes in melanoma cells
(17).   This   suggests that α-TS-induced   growth

inhibition may in part be due to an antioxidation mechanism. This is further
substantiated by the fact that the higher uptake
of α-TS may increase the intracellular level of
alpha tocopherol which reduces the level of
oxidation reactions that are needed for cell
proliferation. In addition, α-TS may directly
cause alterations in gene expression which
inhibits growth and causes differentiation,
depending upon the cell type.

The specificity of α-TS-induced differentiation in melanoma cells was tested with respect
to other antioxidant vitamins. Results showed
that β-carotene-induced morphological differentiation is similar to that produced by α-TS;
however, unlike α-TS, it did not increase
melanin content (22). Retinol and retinoic acid
inhibited growth without morphological
differentiation and without changing melanin
content.

Combined Affect of Alpha Tocopheryl Succinate
and a cAMP Stimulating Agent:

α-TS doses, which inhibited the growth of
NB (17) and melanoma (15) cells, enhanced the
levels of cAMP-induced differentiation of these
transformed cells (23-24). The mechanisms of
this effect of α-TS are unknown.

Effect of Alpha Tocopheryl Succinate on
Adenylate Cyclase (AC) Activity:

The effect of α-TS on adenylate cyclase
(AC) system was studied because (AC) is a
membrane located enzyme which mediates the
action of agents which regulate cell
proliferation, differentiation and transformation ( ). The AC systems consists of receptor
protein, gunanine nucleotide binding (G)
proteins and catalytic subunit. It has been
reported that α-TS treatment reduces basal and
PGE_1-stimulated AC activity in murine
neuroblastoma (NBP_2) (Figure 1) and fibroblasts
(L-cells) in culture (25); and basal and

melanocyte-stimulating hormone (MSH)-stimulated
AC activity in murine B-16 melanoma cells in
culture (26).   The treatment time of about 24
hours is needed for the above effects. The
addition of α-TS directly into the AC assay
reaction mixture did not alter basal or ligand-
stimulated AC activity, suggesting that there is
no direct interaction between αTS and AC system.

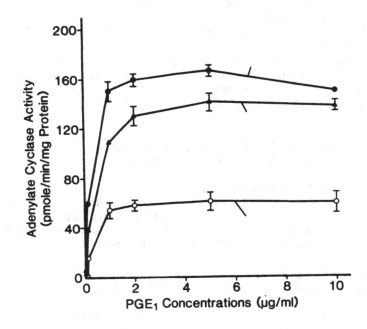

The adenylate cyclase activity was determined in
NB cells 3 days after treatment (25).
o-o-control, o-o vitamin E succinate (6 μg/ml)
      vitamin E succinate (2 μg/ml).

The treatment of cells with alpha tocopherol, alpha tocopheryl acetate or alpha tocopheryl nicotinate did not alter basal or ligand-stimulated AC activity in NB or melanoma cells (25-26). This suggests that α-TS is the most potent form of vitamin E in reducing AC activity in some mammalian transformed cells in culture. To study the specificity of the effect of α-TS with respect to other lipid soluble vitamins, the effects of β-carotene, retinol and retinoic acid (RA) on AC activity of melanoma cells were studied. Results show that the growth inhibitory concentrations of these vitamins also reduce basal and MSH-stimulated AC activity (26). This raised a question as to whether vitamin-induced inhibition of AC activity is related to growth inhibition or to vitamin effect. The former possibility was ruled out by the observations that RO20-1724 [4-(3-butoxy-4-methoxybenzyl-2-imidazolidinone), an inhibitor of cyclic nucleotide phosphodiesterase] and prostaglandin, which induced cell differentiation and growth inhibition in melanoma cells, did not alter basal or MSH-stimulated AC activity (26). Furthermore, butylated hydroxyanisole, a lipid soluble antioxidant, which also inhibited growth, did not alter AC activity (26). These results suggest that vitamin-induced inhibition of AC activity is neither strictly related to growth inhibition nor to the antioxidation mechanism of vitamins.

Since sodium fluoride (NaF) (27-28) and forskolin (29) stimulate AC activity by directly acting on G-proteins and catalytic subunit, respectively; the effect of α-TS on NaF- and forskolin- stimulated AC activity was studied. Results showed that α-TS treatment also reduced NaF- and forskolin-stimulated AC activity in both NB (25) and melanoma cells (26). This suggests that the activities of G-proteins and catalytic subunit of AC are reduced after α-TS treatment. G-proteins consist of Gs (stimulatory) and Gi (inhibitory) subunits. Therefore, α-TS induced reduction in the G-protein activity could be due to an increase in Gi activity or a decrease in Gs activity.

Effect of Tumor Promoters on AC Activity:

Treatment of melanoma cells with a tumor-promoting phorbol ester, phorbol-12-myristate-13-acetate (PMA) (Table 1) and a non-phorbol tumor-promoting compound, mezerein, (Table 2) for a period of 5 minutes to 60 minutes enhances basal and MSH-stimulated AC activity in melanoma cells (30). The addition of PMA directly into AC reaction mixture did not alter AC activity, suggesting that there is no direct interaction between PMA and AC system. Since PMA (31) and mezerein (32) activate protein kinase C (PKC) in several systems, the role of PKC in the regulation of AC activity in melanoma is proposed. The above hypothesis is consistent with the previous studies in which phorbol esters stimulate AC activity in adipocytes (33), S49 lymphoma cells (34), frog erythrocytes (35) and human keratinocytes (37).

Table 1

Effect of a Short PMA Treatment of Melanoma
Cells on Adenylate Cyclase Activity In Vitro

Treatments	Adenylate Cyclase Activity (pmole/min/mg protein)	
	Basal	MSH (1 μM)
Control	$251 \pm 6*$	709 ± 24
DMSO (0.001%)	282 ± 20^a	805 ± 29
PMA 10^{-5}M, 15 min.	$352 \pm 15^{a,b}$	$966 \pm 22^{a,b}$
PMA 10^{-7}M, 15 min.	$431 \pm 8^{a,b}$	$1275 \pm 14^{a,b}$

Cells (0.5×10^6) from older cultures were
plated in 100 mm tissue culture dishes and
phorbol-12-myristate-13-acetate (PMA) was added
4 days after plating. The adenylate cyclase
activity was determined in 16,500 x g pellet.
Each value represents an average of 3 samples.
Each experiment was repeated 3 times and similar
changes were observed.

* = Standard Error of the Mean

a = Significant difference from control at an
0.05 level of significance.

b = Significant difference from solvent
treated control at an 0.05 level of
significance.

Table 2

Effect of a Short Mezerein Treatment of
Melanoma Cells on Adenylate Cyclase
Activity In Vitro

	Adenylate Cyclase Activity (pmole/min/mg protein)	
Treatments	Basal	MSH (1µM)
Control	$92 \pm 4*$	311 ± 4
DMSO (0.001%) 15 min.	95 ± 2	322 ± 14
Mezerein 10^{-8}M 15 min.	92 ± 3	329 ± 11
Mezerein 10^{-7}M 15 min.	$154 \pm 11^{a,b}$	$394 \pm 10^{a,b}$

Cells (0.5×10^6) from younger cultures were
plated in 100 mm tissue culture dishes and
mezerein was added 4 days after plating. The
adenylate cyclase activity was determined in
16,500 x g pellet. Each value represents an
average of 3 samples. Each experiment was
repeated 3 times and similar changes were
observed.

* = Standard Error of the Mean

[a] = Significant difference from control at an
0.05 level of significance.

[b] = Significant difference from solvent
treated control at an 0.05 level of
significance.

Treatment of melanoma cells with α-TS 15 minutes before PMA or simultaneous with PMA did not affect PMA-induced stimulation of AC activity (data not shown). Furthermore, PMA continued to stimulate AC activity in melanoma cells which had been previously treated with α-TS for a period of 3 days. These results suggest that α-TS-induced inhibition and PMA-induced stimulation of AC activity is due to changes of different subunits of AC. Also, there is no direct interaction between α-TS and PMA on the AC system.

CONCLUSION

Alpha-TS provides a new biological tool to study the mechanisms of action of vitamin E in tissue culture. However, it is possible that α-TS may have some unique functions not shared by alpha tocopherol or alpha tocopheryl acetate. Based upon the current view of metabolism of the esterified form of vitamin E, it can be stated that α-TS will be picked up by mammalian cells in vitro where it will be converted to alpha tocopherol, which will then act as an antioxidant. The rate of uptake and conversion of α-TS could be important factors in determining the effect of α-TS in mammalian cells, and may depend upon the status of cells i.e., normal, immortalized, or transformed. Alpha-TS can induce cell differentiation and/or inhibit growth, depending upon the type of tumor cells Alpha-TS inhibits basal and ligand-stimulated AC activity in some transformed cells; this effect of α-TS is not related to growth inhibition or differentiation.

References

1. Jaffe W.   The influence of wheat germ oil
    on the production of tumors in rats by
    methylcholanthrene. Exp Med Surg 4:278-282,
    1946.

2. Haber SL, Wissler, RW. Effect of vitamin E
    on carcinogenicity of methylcholanthrene.
    Proc Soc Exp Biol & Med 111:774-775, 1962.

3. Cook MG, McNamara P.   Effect of dietary
    vitamin E on dimethylhydrazine-induced
    colonic tumors. Cancer Res 40:1311-1329,
    1980.

4. Weerapdist W, Shklar G.   Vitamin E inhibi-
    tion of hamster buccal pouch carcinogenesis.
    Oral Med Oral Path Surg 54:304-312, 1982.

5. Boutwell RK.   Biology and biochemistry of
    the   two-step model of carcinogenesis. In
    Meyskens FL Jr, Prasad KN (eds): "Modulation
    and Mediation of Cancer by Vitamins," Basel,
    Karger, pp 2-9, 1983.

6. Slaga T.J.   Multistage skin carcinogenesis
    and specificity of inhibitors.   In Meyskens
    FL Jr., Prasad, K.N. (eds):   "Modulation
    and Mediation of Cancer by Vitamins," Basel,
    Karger, 1983.

7. Trickler D, Shklar G. Prevention by vitamin
    E of experimental oral carcinogenesis.
    J Natl Cancer Inst 78:165-169, 1987.

8. Wald NJ, Boreham J, Hayward JL, Bulbrook RD.
    Plasma retinol beta-carotene and vitamin E
    levels in relation to the future risk of
    breast cancer. Prospective studies   in-
    volving 5,000 women.   Brit J Cancer   49:
    321-324, 1984.

9. Mankes M, Comstock G.   Vitamin A and E and
    Lung Cancer.   Am J Epidemiology 120:490,
    1986.

10. Dam H, Granados H. Peroxidation of body fat in vitamin E deficiency. Acta Physiol Scand 10:162-171, 1945.

11. McCay PB, King MM. Vitamin E: It's role as a biological free radical scavenger and its relationship to the microsomal mixed-functions oxidase system. In Machlin L (ed): "Vitamin E," New York: Dekker, pp 289-317,1980.

12. Tappel AL. Vitamin E and free radical perioxidation of lipids. Ann NY Acad Sci 203:12-27, 1972.

13. Diplock At, Lucy JA. The biochemical modes of action of vitamin E and selenium: A hypothesis. FEBS Letters 29:205-210, 1973.

14. Prasad KN, Ramamujam S, Gaudreau D. Vitamin E induces morphological differentiation and increases the effect of ionizing radiation on neuroblastoma cells in culture. Proc Soc Exp Biol & Med 16:570-573, 1979.

15. Prasad KN, Edwards-Prasad J. Effect of tocopherol (vitamin E) acid succinate on morphological alterations and growth inhibition in melanoma cells in culture. Cancer Res 42:550-555,1982.

16. Helson L, Verma M, Helson C. Vitamin E and human neuroblastoma. In Meyskens FL Jr., Prasad KN (eds): "Modulation and Mediation of Cancer Cells by Vitamins," New York, Karger Press, pp 258-265, 1983.

17. Rama BN, Prasad KN. Study on the specificity of alpha tocopheryl (vitamin E) acid succinate effects on melanoma, glioma and neuroblastoma cells in culture. Proc Soc Exp Biol & Med 174:302-307, 1983.

18. Ripoll EAP, Rama BN, Webber MM. Vitamin E enhances the chemotherapeutic effects of adriamycin on human prostate carcinoma cells

in vitro. J Urology 136:529-531, 1986.

19. Radner BS, Kennedy AN. Suppression of x-ray induced transformation by vitamin E in mouse $CH_3 10T1/2$ cells. Cancer Letters 32:25-32, 1986.

20. Borek C, Ong A, Mason H, Donahue L, Biaglow JE. Selenium and vitamin E inhibit radiogenic and chemically-induced transformation in vitro via different mechanisms. Proc Natl Acad Sci USA 83:1490-1494, 1986.

21. Prasad KN. Mechanisms of action of vitamin E on mammalian tumor cells in culture. In: Nutrition, Growth, and Cancer, eds. GP Trytiates and KN Prasad, pp. 363-375. Alan R. Liss, N.Y., 1988.

22. Hazuka MB, Edwards-Prasad J, Newman F, Kinzie JJ, and Prasad KN. Beta-carotene induces morphological differentiation and decreases adenylate cyclase activity in melanoma cells in culture. J Am Coll Nutr (In Press).

23. Rama BN, Prasad KN. Effect of dl-alpha tocopheryl succinate in combination with sodium butyrate and cAMP stimulating on neuroblastoma cells in culture. Int J Cancer 34:863-867.

24. Prasad KC, Induction of differentiated phenotypes in melanoma cells by a combination of an adenosive 3^1, 5^1 -cyclic menophosphate stimulating agent and d-alpha tocopheryl succinate. Cancer letters 44: 17-22, 1989.

25. Sahu SN, Prasad JE, Prasad KN (submitted). Vitamin E succinate-induced inhibition of prostaglandin-stimulated adenylate cyclase activity in neuroblastoma cells. J Am Coll Nutr 7:285-294, 1988.

26. Sahu SN, Prasad JE, Prasad KN. Alpha

tocopheryl succinate inhibits melanocyte stimulating hormone (MSH)-sensitive adenylate cyclase activity in melanoma cells. J Cellular Physiol. 133:585-589, 1987.

27. Gilman AG. G-protein and dual control of adenylate cyclase. Cell 36:577-579, 1980.

28. Rodbell M. The role of hormone receptors and GTP-regulatory proteins in membrane transduction. Nature (Lond) 284:17-22, 1980.

29. Seamon KB, Vailancourt R, Edwards M, Daly JW. Binding of ^{3}H-forskolin to rat brain membranes. Proc Natl Acad Sci USA 81:5081-5085, 1984.

30. Prasad KN, Edwards-Prasad J. Effect of anti-tumor promoters and tumor promoters on adenylate cyclase activity in murine β-16 melanoma cells in culture. Proc Am Assoc Cancer Res 30:199, 1989.

31. Nishizuka Y. Perspective on the role of protein kinase C in stimulus-response coupling. J Natl Can Inst. 76:363-370, 1986.

32. Miyake R, Tanaka Y, Tsuda T, Kaikuchi K, Kakawa U, and Nishizuka Y. Activation of protein kinase by non-phorbol tumor promoter mezerein. Biochem Biophys Res Commun. 121:649-656, 1984.

33. Naghshineh S, Noguchi M, Huang K-P, and Londos C. Activation of adipocyte adenylate cyclase by protein kinase C. J Biol Chem 261:14534-14538, 1986.

34. Bell JD, and Brunton L. Enhnacement of adenylate cyclase activity in S49 lymphoma cells by phorbol esters. J Biol Chem 261:12036-12041, 1986.

35. Sibley DR, Jeffs RA, Daniel K, Nambi P, and Lefkowitz RJ. Phorbol diester treatment promotes enhanced adenylate cyclase activity

in frog erythrocytes. Arch Biochem Biophys,
244:373-381, 1986.

36. Choi EJ, and Toscano JWA, Modulation of
    adenylate cyclase in human keratinocytes
    by protein kinase C. J Biol Chem,
    263:17167-17172, 1988.

EFFECT OF NUTRITION ON CARCINOGENESIS: MECHANISMS INVOLVING NITROSAMINES

Chung S. Yang

Department of Chemical Biology & Pharmacognosy, College of Pharmacy, Rutgers University, Piscataway, NJ 08855-0789, U.S.A.

Shih-Hsin Lu

Cancer Institute, Chinese Academy of Medical Sciences, Beijing, China.

INTRODUCTION

Dietary and nutritional factors are widely recognized to be important factors in the genesis of human cancer (1-4). The possible mechanisms involved have been discussed in several review articles (5-7). The high incidence of gastrointestinal cancers in many Third World countries is correlated with the presence of carcinogens, such as aflatoxin and nitrosamines, in the diet (8-10) as well as nutritional deficiencies which are believed to enhance carcinogenesis (7,11). For example, a higher risk for gastric cancer has been shown to be associated with infrequent consumption of fruits and vegetables (3,12-15). Similarly, a high incidence of esophageal cancer is frequently found among individuals who consume low levels of vegetables and fruits and with low plasma levels of vitamins C and E as well as other micronutrients. This chapter explores the possible mechanisms by which constituents in vegetables and fruits inhibit carcinogenesis by blocking the endogenous synthesis of carcinogenic *N*-nitroso compounds. The etiology of esophageal cancer in Linxian, China is discussed in detail to substantiate this possibility.

N-Nitroso compounds, which include *N*-nitrosamines and direct-acting N-nitrosamides, such as N-methyl-N-nitrosourea, are among the most potent carcinogens known in many animal species. These compounds are strong esophageal carcinogens not only in rodents but also in species such as dog, cat, and nonhuman primates (16). Because human cells can metabolize nitrosamines and are subject to genotoxicity similarly to animal tissues, it is expected that human beings are also susceptible to the carcinogenic effect of N-nitroso compounds. As will be discussed in subsequent sections, there is evidence to indicate that individuals living in high esophageal cancer risk areas are exposed to substantial amounts of N-nitroso compounds, some of which are preformed and some are synthesized endogenously. The endogenously formed compounds are believed to be the largest source of exposure to N-nitroso compounds for the general population (17) and probably play a role in carcinogenesis among high risk populations. In the next section, the basic chemistry of the formation and inhibition of N-nitroso compounds will be discussed.

MECHANISMS OF NITROSATION AND ITS INHIBITION

Nitrosation Reactions

The chemistry of the formation of N-nitroso compounds has been reviewed in a number of articles (18-21). The reviews by Archer (18) and Bartsch et al. (19) were used as the principle references for this section. The most common and extensively studied nitrosation reaction is the formation of nitrosamines from nitrite and secondary amines. Nevertheless, neither the nitrite ion nor nitrous acid is an effective nitrosating agent. The actual nitrosating species usually bear the structure NOY which can be considered as carriers of NO+. In strongly acidic solutions, NO+ can exist in free form and can react with secondary amines as described in Equation (1):

$$R_2NH + NO^+ \longrightarrow R_2NNO + H^+ \qquad (1)$$

Under mildly acidic conditions, the nitrosating agent, nitrogen trioxide (N_2O_3 or $NONO_2$), is formed from 2 molecules of nitrous acid and reacts with unprotonated amines to form nitrosamines. The rate of the reaction is proportional to the amine concentration and to the square of nitrous acid concentration. These reactions are shown in Equations

(2), (3), and (4):

$$HNO_2 + HNO_2 \longrightarrow NONO_2 + H_2O \qquad (2)$$

$$R_2NH + NONO_2 \longrightarrow R_2NNO + HNO_2 \qquad (3)$$

$$\text{Rate} = K_1[R_2NH][HNO_2]^2 \qquad (4)$$

It is shown in these equations that the rate of the nitrosation is pH-dependent. A low pH enhances the rate of the reaction by allowing the nitrous acid to exist in the unionized acid form. On the other hand, a decrease in the concentration of unprotonated amine due to lowering of pH would decrease the reaction rate. Therefore, the reaction rate is a bell shaped curve with an optimal rate at pH 2.5 - 3.4. Weak bases are generally more efficiently nitrosated than strong bases. For example, at pH 3 morpholine (pKa = 8.5) has a rate constant 260 times higher than dimethylamine (pKa = 10.7). Amides such as ureas, guanidines, and carbamates are not effectively nitrosated by N_2O_3. However, at pH 2, these compounds readily react with the nitrosonium ion ($NO+$) or its hydrated form (H_2ONO+); thus, the rate of nitrosamide formation is proportional to the concentrations of amide, nitrite, and hydrogen ions. Primary and tertiary amino compounds can also be nitrosated to form *N*-nitroso compounds, but the reaction rates are rather slow and mechanisms more complex. Nitrosation of quaternary ammonium salts or amine oxides requires drastic reaction conditions and is unlikely to take place *in vivo*.

Catalysis of Nitrosation Reactions

Nucleophilic anions can serve as a carrier for $NO+$, forming the active nitrosating species, NOX. The sequence of reactions are illustrated by Equations (5), (6), (7), and (8):

$$HNO_2 + H_3O^+ \longrightarrow H_2ONO^+ + H_2O \qquad (5)$$

$$H_2ONO^+ + X^- \longrightarrow NOX + H_2O \qquad (6)$$

$$R_2NH + NOX \longrightarrow R_2NNO + HX \qquad (7)$$

$$\text{Rate} = k_2[R_2NH][HNO_2][X^-][H^+] \qquad (8)$$

The reaction rate shows a first-order dependency on the concentrations of nitrous acid and the nucleophilic anion. The effectiveness of the catalysis is related to the nucleophilic strength of the catalyst; for example, the rate constants of the nitrosation of morpholine in the presence of thiocyanate, bromide, and chloride occurs at ratios of 15,000 : 30 : 1 (22). This type of catalyzed reaction might be important in the formation of N-nitroso compounds *in vivo.* Thiocyanate is known to be present in human saliva at concentrations of 10-30 mg/dl in nonsmokers and three to four times as much in smokers. Nucleophiles in the diet may also play a role in affecting nitrosation reactions in the stomach. It has been reported that the rate of nitrosation of dipropylamine is increased four-fold in the presence of wheat bran (23). It is not known whether the enhanced rate is due to catalysis by nucleophiles. In general, the nucleophile-enhanced nitrosation rates are greater for weakly basic amines than for strongly basic amines, and are not appreciable for amides.

It has been demonstrated that nitrosamines can be formed under neutral or basic conditions in the presence of carbonyl compounds such as formaldehyde and benzaldehyde (24). The aldehyde is believed to react with secondary amines to form iminium ions which are subject to nucleophilic attack by the nitrite ion to form dialkylamino nitrite esters. The latter then collapses to form nitrosamines. Malondialdehyde which is produced by lipid peroxidation decreases nitrosamine formation at pH 3 but increased it at pH 6-7. *p*-Nitrosophenols, which are known to occur in smoked meats, can also catalyze the nitrosation of pyrrolidine, morphine, and other amines. The catalytic species is probably the O-nitroso derivative of the quinone monoxime. In addition, phenols react readily with nitrous acid to produce nitrosophenols. Therefore, an excess of phenol would inhibit nitrosation reactions. At high nitrite to phenol ratios, however, nitrophenol formation would lead to catalysis.

Enzyme-Mediated Nitrosation

It has been discovered in recent years that the nitrosation reactions can be catalyzed by enzyme systems in bacteria and macrophages. This reaction can take place at neutral pH. Several bacterial strains, including *Neisseria Mucosa, Pseudomonas aeruginosa,* and *Escherichia coli,* isolated from human stomach and infected organs can catalyze the formation of nitrosamines from nitrite and secondary amines (25-27). Human subjects with urinary-tract infections by this type of bacteria had high levels of *N*-nitroso compounds in their urine (28). Urinary bladder infections by *E. coli* in rats caused tumorigenesis when nitrate and secondary amines were administered (29). The macrophage-mediated nitrosation reaction may be of considerable importance in human cancer etiology associated with infection and inflammation. Upon stimulation by interferon and *E. coli* lipopolysaccharide, macrophages can produce nitrite and nitrate from nitrogenous precursors (30), and can form active nitrosating species which react with amines (31). This pathway of nitrosamine formation occur at physiological pH at different sites in the body.

Inhibitors of Nitrosation

Numerous naturally occurring and synthetic compounds have been shown to inhibit *N*-nitrosation reactions (18, 19). A brief summary of these compounds or mixtures are shown in Table 1. In general, these compounds destroy nitrosating agents or reduce them to unreactive products. They act as competitors for the amine substrate and their effectiveness depends on the concentrations of the nitrosating species, the inhibitor, and the amine as well as the relative rates of the competing nitrosation reactions involving the inhibitor and amine substrate. Ascorbic acid and the ascorbate ion inhibit the formation of *N*-nitroso compounds over a wide pH range of 2 - 5 in aqueous solution. The inhibition is accomplished by rapid reduction of nitrous acid to NO and production of dehydroascorbic acid. Because of the hydrophilicity of ascorbic acid, it is not an effective inhibitor of nitrosation in the lipid phase. In a heterogeneous reaction mixture, the NO generated by the reduction of ascorbic acid can migrate to the lipid phase, and upon oxidation it can nitrosate nonprotonated lipophilic amines. α-Tocopherol can also reduce nitrosating agent to NO. Because of its lipophilicity, this vitamin is an effective inhibitor of nitrosation in lipids and emulsions in water.

Many sulfur compounds have been shown to be potent inhibitors of nitrosation reaction. Cysteine and glutathione react with nitrosating species to form *S*-nitrosothiols, thus inhibiting *N*-nitrosation of amines. Methionine, without a free thiol group, is a less effective inhibitor. It should be noted that under certain conditions, *S*-

TABLE I
INHIBITORS OF *N*-NITROSATION[a]

Nutrients
Ascorbic acid
α-Tocopherol
Cysteine
Glutathione
Methionine

Phenolic compounds
Butylated hydroxytoluene
Butylated hydroxyanisole
Caffeic and ferulic acids
Catechol
Cinnamic and chlorogenic acids
Gallic acid
Hydroquinones
Pyrogallol
Tannic acid, tannins
Thymol

Miscellaneous compounds
Alcohols
Azides
Caffeine
Carbohydrates
Hydrazine
Reduced
NAD
Hydroxylamine
Sorbic acid
Sulfur compounds
Unsaturated fatty acids
Urea

Complex mixtures
Alcoholic beverages
Betel-nut extracts
Coffee
Fruit juice
Milk and milk products

Radish juice
Soya products
Tea

[a] Modified from Bartsch *et al.* (19)

nitrosothiols can act as nitrosating agents in transnitrosation reactions. Sulfoxide, bisulfite, and sulfamic acid can reduce nitrous acid to NO, N_2O, or N_2. Therefore, these compounds are strong inhibitors of the nitrosation reaction. Many phenols and phenolic compounds have also been shown to inhibit to formation of *N*-nitroso compounds. Phenolics can usually react readily with nitrite under acidic conditions. Polyphenols such as catechol, pyrogallol, and caffeic acid, inhibit the formation of *N*-nitroso compounds by reducing N_2O_3 to NO. However, certain phenolics such as catechin can form *C*-nitroso derivatives which are powerful nitrosating agents. Such an activity can be seen when the relative concentration of phenolics to nitrite is low. When the phenolics are present in molar excess of nitrite, the nitrosating agent is mostly reduced to NO or converted to *C*-nitroso derivatives, and this results in the inhibition of *N*-nitrosation.

Many other compounds have also been studied for inhibitory action against nitrosation. Urea, hydroxylamine, hydrazine, and azide readily reduce nitrous acid to N_2 or N_2O and inhibit nitrosation reactions. Alcohols and carbohydrates have been shown to inhibit nitrosation of secondary amines by the formation of alkyl nitrites, RONO. However, under certain conditions alkyl nitrites can also be converted to nitrosating agents. Various food and beverages have been shown to inhibit the formation of *N*-nitroso compounds. These include tea, coffee, vegetables, fruit juices, milk, milk products, soya products, alcoholic beverages, and betel-nut extracts. Plant phenolic compounds, such as caffeic acid and ferulic acid, are probably the major nitrosation inhibitors in foods due to their wide occurrence and potency in inhibiting nitrosation reactions. At pH 3, the reactivities of different compounds with nitrite follow the ranking order of caffeic acid > ferulic acid >> α-tocopherol > ascorbic acid >> butylated hydroxyanisole > butylated hydroxytoluene (H. Newmark, personal communications).

Inhibition of Nitrosation in Animals

Ascorbic acid has been shown in many studies to be an effective inhibitor of endogenous nitrosation in animal models with mice, rats, and dogs (19). The end points analyzed include nitrosamines formed in the body as well as hepatotoxicity and carcinogenicity caused by the administration of precursors of nitrosamines. α-Tocopherol, phenolics, plant extracts and fruit extracts have also been found to be effective in inhibiting nitrosation in similar systems.

ENDOGENOUS *N*-NITROSATION IN HUMANS AND ITS INHIBITION

In 1981, a non-invasive method for the assessment of endogenous formation of *N*-nitroso compounds was developed by Ohshima and Bartsch (32). Because proline is nitrosated in the body and the product *N*-nitrosoproline is excreted without further metabolism, the difference between the amount of *N*-nitrosoproline excreted in 24-h urine and the amount ingested in foods was used as an index of daily endogenous nitrosation. This method has been used by many investigators to study the endogenous nitrosation in humans under a variety of situations and the inhibition of such synthesis by ascorbate and other compounds (19). In a typical protocol, 325 mg of nitrate in beet or fruit juice and 500 mg of L-proline were given to the study subject. Under these conditions, the amount of urinary *N*-nitrosoproline excreted was about 15 µg/24 h. However, when 1 g ascorbic acid was given to the individual in the same time period as L-proline and nitrite, the increased *N*-nitroproline excretion due to endogenous nitrosation could be inhibited almost completely. Intake of 500 mg α-tocopherol with the same protocol can inhibit 50% of the endogenous synthesis of *N*-nitrosoproline.

In another protocol, the urinary levels of *N*-nitrosoproline, *N*-nitrosothiazolidine 4-carboxylic acid, and *N*-nitroso-2-methyl-thiazolidine 4-carboxylic acid were measured in volunteers on their normal diet without the intake of L-proline and nitrite. With this approach, it was found that supplementation with 100 mg ascorbate three times per day after each meal significantly inhibited the *in vivo* synthesis of all these *N*-nitrosamino acids. The inhibitory effects of ascorbic acid as well as those of caffeic acid and ferulic acids, coffee and tea, betel-nut extracts have been reported by many investigators and this topic has been reviewed by Bartsch *et al.* (19). In these studies, the inhibitor (e.g. ascorbate) must be present with the nitrosamine precursors in order to be effective. If the ascorbate was taken hours ago, then only the residual amount of this vitamin can serve as an inhibitor of nitrosation.

Wagner *et al.* (33) reported that in healthy volunteers, there was a relatively constant basal urinary excretion of *N*-nitrosoproline in excess of the amount found in the diet. This basal synthesis of NPRO was not inhibited by a daily intake of 2 g of ascorbate or 400 mg of α-tocopherol. However, when ^{15}N-nitrate and proline were also given to the individuals, the ascorbate and α-tocopherol inhibited the ^{15}N-nitrate incorporation into *N*-nitrosoproline by 81% and 59%, respectively. These vitamins also block the synthesis *N*-nitrosothiazolidine 4-carboxylic acid after ingestion of nitrate. These results suggest that urinary excretion of *N*-nitrosoproline as a result of endogenous synthesis is not totally derived from ingested nitrate as its precursor. Garland *et al.* (34) also found that with healthy human volunteers, supplementation with 600 mg of ascorbic acid and 100 mg of α-tocopherol 4 times a day for 3 weeks did not influence the urinary excretion of basal *N*-nitrosoproline and *N*-nitrosodimethylamine. Considerable person-to-person and day-to-day variations were observed for the urinary excretion of both nitrosamines, but the urinary excretion of *N*-nitrosodimethylamine was not correlated with that of *N*-nitrosoproline.

Studies with the urinary *N*-nitrosoproline test have made major contributions to our understanding of the endogenous synthesis of *N*-nitroso compounds. However, there are still questions remaining to be answered concerning this topic: (a) Do the urinary excreted *N*-nitrosamino acids accurately reflect the endogenous formation of carcinogenic *N*-nitroso compounds? (b) How important are the pathways which do not take place in the stomach and cannot be inhibited by ascorbic acid? (c) Does vitamin C nutritional status as reflected in tissue levels, versus that in the stomach, affect the rate of the endogenous nitrosation reactions?

DIET AND NUTRITION OF THE POPULATION IN LINXIAN, A HIGH RISK AREA FOR ESOPHAGEAL CANCER

Linxian, a county in the Henan Province located north of the Yellow River and east of the Taihan Mountain range, is a rural community with an area of about 2,000 km^2 and a population of approximately 800,000. It has a very high esophageal cancer mortality rate of 137.79 per 100,000. Diet and nutrition are believed to be important etiological factors for this cancer.

The people in Linxian traditionally had a monotonous diet consisting mainly of corn, millet, wheat, other grains, and sweet potato (35,36). Consumption of fresh vegetables and fruits was seasonal and generally rather low. The intake of meat, eggs, soybean, and oil was also low, and only account for a small portion of the total caloric intake. A food production survey conducted in 1980 estimated the upper limits of the per-capita food consumption (36). The results indicated that the allowances of caloric food and protein were low, but were probably adequate. Allowances for calcium, riboflavin, and ascorbic acid were clearly inadequate, reaching only 70-85% of the U.S. RDA levels. Considering the significant loss of vitamins during food storage and preparation, lower nutritional status concerning riboflavin and vitamin C of the population was expected from this result.

Biochemical Evidence of Nutritional Deficiency

Biochemical analysis indeed confirmed the deficiencies of several vitamins for the population in Linxian. In a study in September, 1980, over 60% of the subjects (ages 35 - 65 years old) had riboflavin deficiency, showing erythrocyte glutathione reductase activation coefficients larger than 1.4 (36). The plasma ascorbate showed a median value of 440 μg/dl and a mean of 570 μg/dl. About 23% of the individuals surveyed had plasma ascorbate levels lower than 200 μg/dl, i.e. in the vitamin C deficient range (36). In a second study conducted in April 1983, average plasma ascorbate levels of 270 μg/dl were observed with about 50% of the subjects in the deficient range (37). In August of the same year, mean plasma ascorbate levels increased to 720 μg/dl and only 5% of the subjects were deficient (37). The results reflect a dramatic seasonal variation in vitamin C nutritional status of this rural population. In August, vegetables and fruits are more plentiful; whereas in April at the beginning of the growing season, the peasants exhausted the vegetables and fruits stored from the previous year and had few dietary sources for vitamin C.

Lower nutritional status of vitamin E was also observed in the study in 1983 (38). The average plasma α-tocopherol level in April was 720 μg/dl with about half of the subjects having levels lower than 700 μg/dl, i.e., in either low or deficient vitamin E nutritional status. In August, the average plasma α-tocopherol level was 790 μg/dl with about 30% of the subjects having levels lower than 700 µg/dl. Low plasma levels of retinol and β-carotene were also observed in the same study (38).

N-Nitroso Compounds and Their Precursors in the Diet

An extensive search for nitrosamines in the environment has been conducted in Linxian (8, 39). *N*-Nitrosodimethylamine, *N*-nitrosodiethylamine, *N*-nitrososarcosine have been detected in food samples by thin layer chromatography in earlier studies. Previous work also indicated that the contents of nitrosamine precursors, i.e., secondary amines and nitrite (or nitrate), in food and water samples were higher in Linxian than in Fanxian, a low-incidence county 150 km away in the Shangdong Province (8, 35). Within Linxian, the esophageal cancer incidence rate was reported to be correlated with the use of water containing high concentrations of nitrite, nitrate, and organic nitrogenous compounds. Contamination of water in pond or in home storage jars by organic materials and microorganisms might be responsible for the production of these nitrogenous compounds. Moldy food, especially grains are believed to be a major source of secondary amines. A new nitrosamine, *N*-1-methylacetonyl-*N*-3-methylbutylnitrosamine, and other nitrosamines were formed in corn meals after being infested with *Fusarium moniliforme* and subsequently nitrosated with nitrite (8).

In recent studies, *N*-nitrosomethylbenzylamine, and *N*-nitrosodiethylamine have been found to be present in many cooked food samples at levels over 100 ppb as determined by gas chromatography - thermal energy analyzer (Lu *et al.*, unpublished results). These two nitrosamines are known to induce esophageal cancer in animals. *N*-Nitrosomethylbenzylamine, in particular, is a very potent and specific esophageal carcinogen in rats. Additional work is in progress to confirm these results, to identify the sources of these nitrosamines, and to assess the dosages of human exposure to these carcinogens. In recent studies, it was found that 70 - 90% of human gastric juice samples collected from several hundred individuals from Linxian contained appreciable amounts of *N*-nitrosodimethylamine, *N*-nitrosodiethylamine, *and* *N*-nitrosomethylbenzylamine (39).

NUTRITIONAL INTERVENTION AND ENDOGENOUS NITROSATION

Urinary Excretion of N-Nitrosamino ACids as Affected by Ascorbate Supplementation

In order to study the etiology of esophageal cancer, urinary excretion of *N*-nitrosamino acids by individuals in a high incidence area, Linxian, and a low incidence area, Fanxian, were compared by Lu *et al.* (40). As an index of exposure to *N*-nitroso compounds or their precursors, the levels of *N*-nitrosoproline, *N*-nitrosothiazolidine 4-carboxylic acid, *N*-nitrososarcosine, and *N*-nitroso-2-methylthiazolidine 4-carboxylic acid were measured. The urinary levels of nitrate and the first three *N*-nitrosamino acids were significantly higher in individuals in Linxian than those in Fanxian. Ingestion of proline resulted in a marked increase in urinary *N*-nitrosoproline levels in subjects from both areas. Intake of 100 mg ascorbic acid, three times per day 1 h after each meal by the subjects in Linxian, effectively reduced the urinary levels of *N*-nitrosoproline and *N*-nitrosothiazolidine 4-carboxylic acid by more than 60%. These results suggest that the high risk population in Linxian is exposed to higher levels of *N*-nitroso compounds and their precursors, and that ascorbic acid can lower the body burden of this group of compounds.

Effect of Nutritional Levels of Ascorbic Acid on Urinary Excretion of N-Nitrosamino Acids

In order to test whether the nutritional status of vitamin C affects the endogenous synthesis of *N*-nitroso compounds, the urinary excretion of *N*-nitrosamino acid was measured after supplementation was stopped for 1, 2, and 3 days (Lu and Yang, unpublished). This experiment was designed to examine the role of vitamin C in tissues, versus that in the stomach, on endogenous nitrosation. Healthy volunteers (ages 40-65 years old) from Linxian were divided into three groups: Group I consisting of 42 subjects took a daily dose of 100 mg ascorbic acid (in one tablet), Group II consisting of 57 subjects took the same dose of ascorbic acid plus a daily dose of 50 mg of α–tocopherol, and Group III consisting of 52 subjects took placebo tablets. The supplementation period was for 30 days. On the 31st, 32nd, and 33rd days (the first, second, and third days without the supplement) blood and urine samples were collected for the determination of plasma ascorbic acid and urinary *N*-nitrosamino acids, respectively. Preliminary analysis of the samples collected on the 31st day reveals the following: (a) The vitamin supplemented groups, Group I and II, had plasma ascorbate levels of 1.02 ± 0.25 and 1.05 ± 0.28 µg/dl, respectively, which was much higher than those in the placebo group, 0.25 ± 0.16 µg/dl. (b) The urinary excretion of *N*-nitrosoproline and of total *N*-nitrosamino acids by subjects in Group I was much lower than that in the placebo group. (c) The supplementation of vitamin E did not produce an additional lowering effect on the *N*-nitrosamino acids. Experiments are in progress to confirm these results. This study is expected to answer the question whether tissue levels of ascorbic acid play a role in inhibiting endogenous nitrosation reactions.

Effects of Nutritional Intervention on Urinary Excretion of N-Nitrosamino Acids

In order to understand the effects of nutrition on endogenous synthesis of *N*-nitroso compounds, we have also utilized ongoing U.S. - China collaborative intervention studies on esophageal cancer in Linxian (41). In one study, 3300 subjects (ages 40-69 years old) with cytologically - demonstrated dysplasia were divided into two groups: In the treatment group, the individuals took daily tablets containing 180 mg of ascorbic acid, 40 mg of α-tocopherol, and 1 to 4 times the U.S. RDA levels of many other vitamins and minerals, similar to the Centrum tablets, from the Lederle Laboratories Inc. The individuals from the control group took placebo tablets. The trial was initiated in May, 1985. In November 1987, 500 subjects were called back for endoscopic examinations and other intermediate endpoint examinations. Urinary samples were also collected, stored, and analyzed for the contents of *N*-nitrosamino acids. About half of the samples have been analyzed and preliminary analysis of the results is underway. Gastric juice samples were also collected and will be analyzed. In this intervention study, we shall have the unique opportunity to analyze the relationships among nutrition, endogenous synthesis of *N*-nitroso compounds, and the eventual end point, cancer incidence. Because multiple nutrients were included in the supplement, the experiment will not reveal the effect of each single nutrient. A second intervention study with the general population (ages 40-69 years old) in Linxian is also ongoing. This trial which started in March, 1986 enrolled 30,000 subjects in a factorial design of 8 groups as follows:

| Placebo | AB | AC | AD |
| BC | BD | CD | ABCD |

where nutrient group Group A contained retinol and zinc, Group B contained riboflavin and niacin, Group C contained ascorbic acid and molybdenum, and Group D contained α-tocopherol, β-carotene, and selenium. In this study, the separated and combined effects of ascorbic acid and α-tocopherol on endogenous nitrosation can be tested by analyzing different treatment groups.

CONCLUDING REMARKS

There is increasing information pointing to the importance of *N*-nitroso compounds in the causation of human cancers. In addition to the results discussed in previous sections, there are also correlation studies suggesting the involvement of *N*-nitroso compounds in the etiology of esophageal cancer in China. In a recent study conducted in eight counties in north China, using the county as a unit, the levels of urinary excretion of *N*-nitrosamino acids were positively correlated with esophageal cancer mortality rates (39). In a second study involving 1035 subjects in 26 rural counties in China, mortality rates of esophageal cancer were found to be associated positively with endogenous nitrosation and negatively with the ascorbic level in the plasma (42).

In a recent study in Northern Japan, subjects living in a high incidence area were found to have greater endogenous nitrosation of proline, which could be inhibited by taking 100 mg ascorbic acid after each meal. However, subjects living in low-risk areas did not show increased nitrosation after a proline dose and ascorbic acid had no inhibitory effect (43). It is possible that individuals in the low-risk area had a sufficient intake of nitrosation inhibitors in their diet. These individuals also had higher urinary nitrate levels than those in high risk areas, reflecting a higher intake of vegetables by the former groups. Nitrate which can be reduced to nitrite, has been considered as a risk factor in some studies. However, in this case the inhibitory effect of vegetables appears to outweigh the contribution of nitrate in endogenous nitrosation reactions. Although ascorbic acid has received greater attention in cancer cause and prevention, other chemicals in vegetables and fruits may be even more important in the inhibition of endogenous nitrosation reactions. Of special importance are phenolics such as caffeic acid and chlorogenic acid which are widely distributed in fresh fruits and vegetables and are potent inhibitors of nitrosation reactions. In addition the plant phenolics may inhibit carcinogenesis by other mechanisms (44, 45). To study the dietary intake of these phenolics is of great importance in our effort to understand the etiology of human cancer and its possible prevention.

Acknowledgements

The authors thank Professor Harold Newmark for stimulating discussions, Mrs. Dorothy Wong for excellent secretarial assistant, and Ms. Diana Lim for assistance in the preparation of this manuscript. This work was supported by U.S. NIH grants ES03646 and CA37037.

REFERENCES

1. Doll, R. and Peto, R. (1981) *J. Natl. Cancer Inst.,* 66, 1191-1308.
2. Byers, T. and Graham, S. (1984) *Adv. Cancer Res.,* 41, 1-69.
3. Weisburger, J.H., Wynder, E.L., and Horn, C.L. (1982) *Cancer,* 50, 2541-2549.
4. Reddy, B.S., Cohen, L.A., McCoy, G.D., Hill, P., Weisburger, J.H., and Wynder, E.L. (1980) *Adv. Cancer Res.,* 32, 327-345.
5. Ames, B.N. (1983) *Science,* 221, 1256-1264.
6. Fiala, E.S., Reddy, B.S., and Weisburger, J.H. (1985) *Ann. Rev. Nutr.,* 5, 295-321.
7. Yang, C.S. and Newmark, H.L. (1987) *CRC Critical Reviews in Oncology/Hematology,* 7, 267-287.
8. Yang, C.S. (1982) in: *Nitrosamines and Human Cancer,* Banbury Rep. No. 12, P.N., Magee, (Ed.), Cold Spring Harbor Laboratory, New York, 487-501.
9. Charnley, G., Tannenbaum, S.R., and Correa, P. (1982) in: *Nitrosamines and Huamn Cancer,* Banbury Rep. No. 12, P.N., Magee, (Ed.), Cold Spring Harbor Laboratory, New York., 503-522.
10. Yeh, F.S., Yu, M.C., Mo, C.C., Luo, S., Tong, M.J., and Henderson,

B.E. (1989) *Cancer Res.,* 49, 2506-2509.

11. Yang, C.S.   (1984) in: *Environmental Mutagenesis, Carcinogenesis, and Teratogenesis,* E.H.Y. Chu, and W.M., Generoso, (Ed.), Plenum Press, New York, 465.

12. Kolonel, L.N., Nomura, A.M.Y., Hinde, M.W., Hirohata, T., Hankin, J.H., and Lee, J. (1983) *Cancer Res.,* 43, 2397S-2402S.

13. Hirayama, T. (1981) *Gann Monogr.* , 3, 15-27.

14. Haenszel, W. and Correa P. (1975) *Cancer Res.,* 35, 3452-3459.

15. Choi, N.W., Miller A.B., Fodor, J.G., Jain, M., Howe, G.R., Rish, H.A. and Ruder A.M. (1987) in: *Relevance of N-Nitroso Compounds to Human Cancer: Exposure and Mechanisms,* H. Bartsch, R. Schulte-Hermann and I.K. O'Neil (Eds.), IARC Sci. Pub. No. 84, International Agency for Research on Cancer, Lyon, pp.   492-496.

16. Yang, C.S., Chung, R. and Ding, I. (1989) in: *Thoracic Oncology* J.A., Roth, J.C., Ruckdeschel, and T.H. Weisenburger, (Eds.) Saunders Co. Philadelphia, pp. 305-315.

17. National Research Council (1981) *The Health Effects of Nitrate, Nitrite and NN-Nitroso Compounds (Part 1 of a 2-part study),*National Academy Press,   Washington DC.

18. Archer, M.C.   (1984) in: *N-Nitroso Compounds: Occurrence, Biological Effects and Relevance to Human Cancer,* I.K. O'Neill, R.C. von Borstel, C.T. Miller, J. Long and H. Bartsch (Eds.), IARC Sci. Publ. No. 57, International Agency for Research on Cancer, Lyon, pp.   263-274.

19. Bartsch, H. Ohshima, H. and Pignatelli, B. (1988) *Mutation Research,*   202, 307-324.

20. Williams, D.L.H. (1983) *Adv. Phys. Org. Chem.,* 19, 381-429.

21. Mirvish, S.S. (1975) *Toxicol. Appl. Pharmacol.,* 31, 325-351.

22. Fan, T.Y. and Tannenbaum, S.R. (1973) *J. Agric Food Chem.,* 21, 237-240.

23. Wishnok, J.S. and Richardson, D.P. (1979) *J. Agric Food Chem.,* 27, 1132-2234.

24. Keefer, L.K., and Roller, P.P. (1973) *Science,* 181, 1245-1247.

25. Calmels, S., Ohshima, H., Crespi, M., Leclerc, H., Cattoen, C., and Bartsch, H. (1987) in: *Relevance of N-Nitroso Compounds to Human Cancer: Exposure and Mechanisms,* H. Bartsch, R.

Schulte-Hermann and I.K. O'Neil (Eds.), IARC Sci. Pub. No. 84, International Agency for Research on Cancer, Lyon, pp. 391-395.

26. Leach, S.A., Cook, A.R., Challis, B.C., Hill, M.J., and Thompson, M.H. (1987) in: *Relevance of N-Nitroso Compounds to Human Cancer: Exposure and Mechanisms,* H. Bartsch, R. Schulte-Hermann and I.K. O'Neil (Eds.), IARC Sci. Pub. No. 84, International Agency for Research on Cancer, Lyon, pp. 396-399.

27. O'Donnell, C.M., Edwards, C., Corcoran, G.D., Ware, J. and Edwards, P.R. (1987) in: *Relevance of N-Nitroso Compounds to Human Cancer: Exposure and Mechanisms,* H. Bartsch, R. Schulte-Hermann and I.K. O'Neil (Eds.), IARC Sci. Pub. No. 84, International Agency for Research on Cancer, Lyon, pp. 400-403.

28. Ohshima, H., Calmels, S., Pignatelli, B., Vincent, P. and Bartsch, H. (1987) in: *Relevance of N-Nitroso Compounds to Human Cancer: Exposure and Mechanisms,* H. Bartsch, R. Schulte-Hermann and I.K. O'Neil (Eds.), IARC Sci. Pub. No. 84, International Agency for Research on Cancer, Lyon, pp. 384-390.

29. Higgy, N.A., Verma, A.K., Erturk, E., Oberly, T.D., El-Aaser, A.A., El-Merzabani, M.M. and Bryan, G.T. (1987) in: *Relevance of N-Nitroso Compounds to Human Cancer: Exposure and Mechanisms,* H. Bartsch, R. Schulte-Hermann and I.K. O'Neil (Eds.), IARC Sci. Pub. No. 84, International Agency for Research on Cancer, Lyon, pp. 380-383.

30. Stuehr, D.J. and Marletta, M.A. (1987) in: *Relevance of N-Nitroso Compounds to Human Cancer: Exposure and Mechanisms,* H. Bartsch, R. Schulte-Hermann and I.K. O'Neil (Eds.), IARC Sci. Pub. No. 84, International Agency for Research on Cancer, Lyon, pp. 335-339.

31. Miwa, M., Stuehr, D.J., Marletta, M.A., Wishnok, J.S. and Tannenbaum, S.R. (1987) in: *Relevance of N-Nitroso Compounds to Human Cancer: Exposure and Mechanisms,* H. Bartsch, R. Schulte-Hermann and I.K. O'Neil (Eds.), IARC Sci. Pub. No. 84, International Agency for Research on Cancer, Lyon, pp. 340-344.

32. Ohshima, H. and Bartsch, H. (1981) *Cancer Res.,* 41, 3658-3662.

33. Wagner, D.A., Shuker, D.E.G., Bilmazes, C., Obiedzinski, M., Baker, I., Young, V.R. and Tannenbaum, S.R. (1985) *Cancer Res.,* 45, 6519-6522.

34. Garland, W.A., Kuenzig, W., Rubio, F., Kornychuk, H., Norkus, E.P. and Conney, A.H. (1986) *Cancer Res.* 46, 5392-5400.

35. Yang, C.S. (1980) *Cancer Res.,* 40, 2633-2644.

36. Yang, C.S., Miao, J., Yang, W., Huang, M., Wang, T., Xue, H., You, S., Lu, J. and Wu, J. (1982) *Nutrition anc Cancer,* 4, 154-164.

37. Ershow, A.G., Zheng, S.F., Li, G.Y., Li, J.Y., Yang, C.S. and Blot, W.J. (1984) *J. Natl. Cancer Inst.,* 73, 1477-1481.

38. Yang, C.S., Sun, Y., Yang, A., Miller, K., Li, G., Zheng, S.-F., Ershow, A.G., Blot, W.J. and Li, J. (1984) *J. Natl. Cancer Inst.* 73, 1449-1453.

39. Lu, S.H., Yang, W.X., Guo, L.P., Li, F.M., Wang, G.J., Zhang, J.S. and Li, P.Z. (1987) in: *Relevance of N-Nitroso Compounds to Human Cancer: Exposure and Mechanisms,* H. Bartsch, R. Schulte-Hermann and I.K. O'Neill (Eds.), IARC Scie. Publ. No. 84, International Agency for Research on Cancer, Lyon, pp. 538-543.

40. Lu, S.-H., Ohshima, H. Fu, H.-M., Tian, Y., Li, F.-M., Blettner, M., Wahrendorf, J. and Bartsch, H. (1986) *Cancer Res.,* 46, 1485-1491.

41. Li, J. Taylor, P.R., Li, G., Blot, W., Yu, Y., Ershow, A.G., Sun, Y., Yang, C.S., Yang, Q., Tangrea, J.A., Zheng, S., Greenwald, P. and Cahill, J. (1986) *J. Nutr. Growth Cancer,* 3, 199-206.

42. Chen, J., Ohshima, H., Yang, H., Li, J., Campbell, T.C., Peto, R. and Bartsch, H. (1987) in: *Relevance of N-Nitroso Compounds to Human Cancer: Exposure and Mechanisms,* H. Bartsch, R. Schulte-Hermann and I.K. O'Neill (Eds.), IARC Sci. Publ. No. 84, International Agency for Research on Cancer, Lyon, pp. 503-506.

43. Kamiyama, S., Ohshima, H., Shimada, A., Saito, N., Bourgade, M.-C., Ziegler, P. and Bartsch, H. (1987) in: *Relevance of N-Nitroso Compounds to Human Cancer: Exposure and Mechanisms,* H. Bartsch, R. Schulte-Hermann and I.K. O'Neil (Eds.), IARC Sci. Pub. No. 84, International Agency for Research on Cancer, Lyon, pp. 497-502.

44. Newmark H.L. (1986) *J. Physiol. Pharmacol.,* 65, 461-466.

45. Bartsch, D.H., and Fox, C.C. (1988) *Cancer Res.,* 48, 7088-1092.

Nutrients and Cancer Prevention K. N. Prasad and F. L. Meyskens, Jr., eds. © 1990 The Humana Press

MECHANISMS IN CANCER PREVENTION BY DIETARY ANTIXODIANTS

Carmia Borek
Center for Radiological Research
Columbia University
New York, New York 10032

INTRODUCTION

Epidemiological studies and data from experiments in vivo and in vitro support the notion that cancer is a multistep process in that a series of specific events is required to transform a normal cell into a malignant one (1,2).

The multistep model of carcinogenesis involves initiation in which irreversible genetic alterations take place and promotion, in which clonal population of initiated cells are expanded and ultimately progress to a malignancy (1,2).

Within the past decade we have witnessed changes in our understanding of the molecular origins of cancer. Much of this progress stems from the discovery of specific genes, the oncogenes, which are present in the genomes of a variety of tumor cells and are responsible for specifying many of the malignant traits of the cells (3,4). A number of oncogenes found in tumor cells or in cells transformed in vivo or in vitro, play a central role in carcinogenesis. This has been underscored by the ability of these genes to confer a malignant state on normal cells when introduced into the normal cells by means of transfection (3,4).

While DNA is the target in carcinogenesis the ultimate course and frequency of the neoplastic processes are determined by an interplay of endogenous and exogeneous factors (1,2). These included permissive factors such as thyroid hormone (5) which may act as cotransforming agents and potentiate carcinogenesis (5). The permissive factors are balanced, under normal conditions, by cellular protective factors which suppress the carcinogenic process at its various stages and antagonize the action of the permissive factors (1,2,6).

Work in our laboratory has focussed on cell transformation by radiation and chemicals using cells cultures (10,11). These systems of human and rodent cells afford the opportunity to study genetic changes associated with transformation, under conditions free from host mediated effects. They also enable us to characterize factors which potentiate or inhibit transformation at a cellular and molecular level.

Antioxidants as Protective Factors in Transformation

The interaction of cells with radiation, both X-ray and ultraviolet (UV) light, as well as with a variety of chemicals, results in an enhanced generation of free oxygen species and free radical intermediates (6,7). The result is a loss in the optimal cellular balance between the oxidative challenge, a source of DNA damage, and in the inherent mechanisms that protect the cell from excess oxidative stress. These protectors include enzymes (SOD, catalase, peroxidases, transferases) and thiols. Also included are a variety of nutrients that directly or indirectly prevent peroxidation and autoxidation of proteins and lipids in cell membranes as well as in the nucleus. These are vitamin A, B-carotens, vitamin C, selenium, and vitamin E (8,9).

In recent years, increasing evidence has implicated free radical mechanisms in the initiation and promotion of malignant transformation in vivo and in vitro. Much of the evidence has come from the fact that the agents that scavenge free radicals directly or that interfere with the generation of free radical-mediated events inhibit the neoplastic process. We have shown in hamster embryo cells that SOD inhibits transformation by radiation and bleomycin and suppresses the promoting actin of TPA (10). Catalase had no effect as an inhibitory agent in this cell system, perhaps because of the inherent high level of the enzyme in the hamster cells (10). SOD had a more dramatic inhibitory effect when maintained on the cells throughout the experiment suggesting that later stages in the transformation process are influenced by free radicals (10).

Selenium and Vitamin E

Agents which qualify as important antioxidants are various examples of nutrients which are critical in controlling free radical damage viz. selenium, a component of glutathione peroxidase, and vitamin E, a powerful antioxidant and a component of the cell membrane (8). We examined the single and combined effects of selenium and vitamin E on cell trans-formation induced in C3H/10T-1/2 cells by X-rays, benzo(a)pyrene, or tryptophan pyrolysate and on the levels of cellular scavenging systems and peroxide destruction. Incubation of C3H/10T-1/2 cells with 2.5 μM Na_2SeO_3 (selenium) or with 7 μM alpha-tocopherol succinate (vitamin E) 24h prior to exposure to X-rays or the chemical carcinogens resulted in an inhibition of transformation by each of the antioxidants with an additive-inhibitor action when the two nutrients were combined (Fig. 1). Cellular pretreatment with selenium resulted in increased levels of cellular glutathione peroxidase, catalase, and non-protein thiols (gluta-thione) and in an enhanced destruction of hydrogen peroxide (8). Cells pretreated with vitamin E did not show these biochemical effects, and the combined pre-treatment with vitamin E and selenium did not augment the effect of selenium on these parameters. The results supported our earlier studies showing that free radical-mediated events play a role in radiation and chemically induced transformation. They indicate that selenium and vitamin E act alone and in additive fashion as radioprotecting and chemopreventing agents. Selenium confers protection in part by inducing or activating cellular free-radical scavenging systems and by enhancing peroxide breakdown. Thus enhancing the capacity of the cell to cope with oxidant stress. Vitamin E acts as a chain breaking antioxidant by lowering peroxidation products (7).

Selenium and vitamin E are a true protectors. Time course experiments indicate that the addition of selenium at various exposures to X-rays results in a suppressive action which diminishes with time (11). Similar results are found with vitamin E.

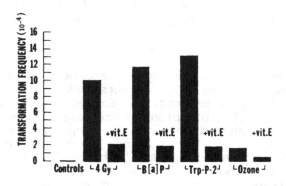

Fig. 1   Inhibition of radiation and chemically induced
          transformation by vitamin E.

An important determinant in the efficiency of
cellular protection by inherent antioxidants lies in
the interaction among various factors. The metabolic
function of vitamin E and selenium are interrelated and
selenium plays a role in the storage of vitamin E (8).

Vitamin E Inhibits Transformation By Specific Oncogenes

Cell transformation by specific cancer genes (oncogenes) require adequate permissive physiological
factors (4). Cells transformed by these genes are
converted to malignancy (3,4).

We tested the ability of vitamin E to inhibit
transformation by oncogenes which are activated
following exposure of cells to radiation in vitro (4).
We found that vitamin E dramatically inhibited transformation by radiation induced activated oncogens
indicating that processes of oxidation may be involved
(Borek et al., submitted). Vitamin E may do so by
virtue of its antioxidant properties or by another
function yet unknown.

Our findings also indicate that vitamin E is a
powerful inhibitor of transformation induced by
ultraviolet light (Borek et al., in preparation).

Vitamin E also inhibited transformation by the air pollutant ozone (12) (Fig. 1) and suppressed the enhancement of transformation by the tumor promoter TPA (Borek et al., submitted).

Vitamin E appears to acts as an anticarcinogen in part by modifying the production of lipid peroxidation products in the cell (7). It is therefore a powerful non-toxic anticarcinogen which suppresses both initiation as well as promotion of carcinogenesis.

Interaction of Vitamin E and Vitamin C

The synergistic interaction between vitamin E and C as antioxidants are known (12,13). Vitamin C spares vitamin E by reducing the vitamin E radical to regenerate vitamin E. Vitamin E scavenges lipid peroxyl radical (LOO˙) to interfere with the chain propagation. The resulting vitamin E radical is reduced by ascorbate to regenerate vitamin E (12,13).

The lipid peroxyl radicals in the membrane are scavenged exclusively by vitamin E. The vitamin E radical formed may undergo several competing reactions. It may savenge another peroxyl radical to give stable product, react with another vitamin E radical to give a dimer, or interact with vitamin C to regenerate vitamin E. The lower the peroxyl radical concentration, the higher the efficiency of vitamin E regeneration.

Since vitamin C is in the aqueous phage of the cell it cannot scavenge free radicals in the membrane. Thus its action complements that of vitamin E which acts in the lipid phase but does not substitute for it.

We conducted studies to test if vitamin E and vitamin C were synergistic in their capacity to prevent transformation. We pretreated cells with vitamin E 7μM and vitmin C (0.1 μg/ml) alone or in combination. We found a synegistic interaction between vitamin C and vitamin E (7) (Fig. 2).

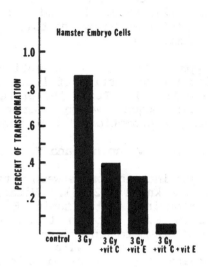

Fig. 2   Inhibition of radiogenic transformation by vitamin E and vitamin C

It must be emphasized that different organs vary in their content of inherent antioxidants and these may vary from one species to another as well as from one individual to another.   Thus, tissues and cells will vary in their response to oxidant stress.   Adding external antioxidants may be effective in helping some cells mount a protective response while being ineffective in helping some cells mount a protective response while being ineffective in others.

CONCLUSIONS

One of the basic conundrums in carcinogenesis evolves from our ability toe unequivocally distinguish primary events associated with initiation of malignant transformation from those which function as secondary events.   Thus the role of oncogenes, mutations, gene rearrangements, amplification and other DNA alterations in transformation is yet unclear.   The changes which take place give rise to abnormal expression of cellular genes.

We must always be cognizant of the fact that a variety of factors may modify the neoplastic process at its various stages of development. These constitute physiological permissive or protective factors. When permissive factors prevail, such as genetic susceptibility, optimal stage in the cell cycle, optimal hormonal control or a particular stage in differentiation, initiation of transformation will take place. By contrast if these permissive factors do not prevail, protective factors such as free radical scavengers will inhibit to varying degrees, the onset and progression of the neoplastic process. These may be inherent cellular factors or those added externally by dietary means acting as anticarcinogens. Thus, the interplay between inherent genetic and physiological factors and lifestyle influences which either enhance or inhibit the neoplastic process, are critical determinants in the process of multistage carcinogenesis and in establishing the incidence of cancer.

ACKNOWLEDGEMENTS

This work was supported by Grant No. CA-12536 from the National Cancer Institute, and by a contract from the National Foundation for Cancer Research.

REFERENCES

1. C. Borek, The induction and control of radiogenic transformation in vitro: Cellular and molecular mechanisms, in: D. Grunberger and S. Goff (eds.), Mechanisms of Cellular Transformation by Carcinogenic Agents, Pergamon Press, New York, 1987, pp. 151-195.
2. C. Borek, Permissive and protective factors in malignant transformation of cells in culture, in: H. Greim et al. (eds.), The Biochemical Basis of Chemical Carcinogenesis, Raven Press, New York, 1984, pp. 175-188.
3. B.Z. Shilo and R.A. Weinberg, Unique transforming gene in carcinogen-transformed mouse cells, Nature, 289 (1981) 607-609.
4. C. Borek, A. Ong, and H. Mason, Distinctive transforming genes in X-ray transformed mammalian cells, Proc. Natl. Acad. Sci. USA, 84 (1987) 794-798.

5. C. Borek, D.L. Guernsey, A. Ong, and I.S. Edelman, Critical role played by thyroid hormone in induction of neoplastic transformation by chemical carcinogens in tissue culture, Proc. Natl. Acad. Sci. USA, 80 (1983) 5749–5752.

6. C. Borek, Oncogenes, hormones and free radical processes in malignant transformation in vitro. Ann. N.Y. Acad. of Sci., 551 (1989) 95–102.

7. C. Borek, The role of free radicals and antioxidants in cellular and molecular carcinogenesis in vitro, in: O. Hayaishi, E. Niki, M. Kondo, T. Yoshikawa (eds.), Medical, Biochemical and Chemical Aspects of Free Radicals, Elsevier Science Publishing Co., The Netherlands, 1461–1469.

8. C. Borek, A. Ong, H. Mason, L. Donahue, and J.E. Biaglow. Selenium and vitamin E inhibit radiogenic and chemically induced transformation in vitro via different mechanisms of action, Proc. Acad. Sci. USA, 83 (1986) 1490–1494.

9. R. Doll and R. Peto, The causes of cancer: quantitative estimates of avoidable risks of cancer in the United States, J. Natn. Cancer Inst., 66 (1981) 1191–1308.

10. C. Borek and W. Troll, Modifiers of free radicals inhibit in vitro the oncogenic actions of X-rays, bleomycin and the tumor promoter 12-0-tetradecanoylphorpbol 13-acetate, Proc. Natl. Acad. Sci. USA, 80 (1983) 1304–1307.

11. C. Borek, Radiation and chemically induced transformation: Free radicals, antioxidants and cancer, Br. J. Cancer, 55 (1987) 74–76.

12. L. Packer, T.F. Slater, and R.L. Willson, Direct observation of a free radical interaction between vitamin E and vitamin C, Nature, 278 (1979) 737–738.

13. E. Niki, T. Saito, A. Kawakami, and Y. Kamiya, Inhibition of oxidation of methyl linoleate in solution by vitamin E and vitamin C, J. Biol. Chem., 259 (1984) 4177–4182.

Effects of Protease Inhibitors and Vitamin E
in the Prevention of Cancer

Ann R. Kennedy
Department of Radiation Oncology
University of Pennsylvania School of Medicine
Philadelphia, PA   U.S.A.   19104

SUMMARY

Protease inhibitors and Vitamin E have been the most effective of the potential human cancer chemopreventive agents we have studied in the ability to suppress radiation-induced malignant transformation in vitro. Although neither of these agents affect malignant cells, they appear to be working by different mechanisms to suppress the conversion of a cell to the malignant state, as their in vitro effects are markedly different. The effects of Vitamin E are reversible; if the compound is removed from cultures destined to produce transformed foci, transformed cells arise. The effects of protease inhibitors are irreversible in that these agents need to be present in cultures for only short periods of time to reverse the carcinogenic process (1). Protease inhibitors have their suppressive effect on carcinogenesis when present while cells are actively proliferating (1); vitamin E is effective when cells are in the confluent, stationary phase of growth (2). Relatively large concentrations of vitamin E (at nearly toxic levels) are necessary to inhibit transformation in vitro, while very low concentrations of protease inhibitor (nanomolar-picomolar ranges) are capable of suppressing the transformation process (1,2).

Protease inhibitors have proven to be so effective in our studies on the prevention of radiation transformation <u>in vitro</u> that we have now performed many other studies to determine the effects of these agents in animal model carcinogenesis systems. Studies with the soybean-derived Bowman-Birk inhibitor have shown that this protease inhibitor is capable of suppressing dimethylhydrazine-induced colon (3,4) and liver (4) carcinogenesis in mice, 7, 12 dimethylbenz(a)anthracene-induced oral carcinogenesis in hamsters (5) and 3-methylcholanthrene-induced lung tumorigenesis in mice (Witschi and Kennedy, unpublished data). Studies on the mechanism of the protease inhibitor suppression of carcinogenesis have suggested that these agents may act by suppressing oncogene expression or specific proteases involved in the conversion of a cell to the malignant state.

INTRODUCTION

Many different types of agents have been shown to affect transformation in vitro, as has been reviewed (6). While many agents suppress transformation, the degree to which they can suppress the process involved is markedly different. We have observed that various different protease inhibitors (6-17) and Vitamin E (2,15) are particularly effective at suppressing transformation in vitro; some of our studies with these agents will be presented and discussed in this report.

Other dietary agents are also potential chemopreventive agents for cancer in human populations. Our studies with some of these agents, specifically onion and garlic oils, vitamin D and selenium, will also be presented here.

MATERIALS AND METHODS

Two different in vitro transformation systems were utilized for the studies reported here; the C3H10T1/2 cell system, which has been used extensively in our previous studies (1,2,6-17) and cells derived from Balb/c3T3 clone A31 [#163, ATCC, Rockville, MD), as originally described by Kakunaga (18)].

Details of experimental techniques for radiation transformation experiments using C3H10T1/2 cells have been described elsewhere (1,2,6-17). Stock cultures were maintained in 60-mm Petri dishes and were passed by subculturing at a 1:20 dilution every 7 days. The cells used were in passages 9-14. They were grown in a humidified 5% CO_2 atmosphere at 37°C in Eagle's basal medium supplemented with 10% heat-inactivated fetal bovine serum and gentamycin. Cells were exposed to X-radiation   24 h after seeding. Plating efficiencies were determined from 3 plates seeded with a cell density one fifth that of the plates used for the transformation assay; these cultures were terminated at 10 days. The various treatment toxicities were considered in the design of the experiments such that all dishes used for the transformation assay contained approximately 300 viable cells per dish. Types 2 and 3 foci were scored as transformants.

The characteristics of the 3T3 cell assay system have been previously described in detail for both chemical and radiation induced transformation in vitro (14,18-21). These cells were subcloned to select for populations with low yields of spontaneous transformants. The number of passages subsequent to subcloning did not exceed ten at the initiation of any experiment. Cells were routinely grown in Eagle's Minimum Essential Medium with Earle's salts (Gibco) supplemented with 10% heat inactivated (56° for 30 min) fetal bovine serum (Gibco) and maintained in a humidified atmosphere of 95% air, 5% CO_2. Stock cultures were maintained at subconfluence and passaged at weekly intervals. Details of the in vitro transformation assay have been published elsewhere (14,21).

RESULTS

The results of C3H10T1/2 cell transformation experiments utilizing onion oil #1 (Mexican), onion oil #2 (Dutch) and garlic oil are shown in Table 1. All compounds were kindly supplied by Dr. Sidney Belman (New York University Institute of Environmental Medicine). All of the oils were dissolved in acetone and used in the cultures at a concentration of 1.0 μg/ml, a concentration shown in preliminary toxicity studies to be the highest (possible) non-toxic concentration. [Concentrations of the oils which inhibit 50% of highly purified soybean lipoxygenase (I_{50}) are as follows: onion oil #1 - 1 µg/ml; onion oil #2 - 2 µg/ml; garlic oil - 15 µg/ml. (Personal communication - Dr. Sidney Belman)] The oils were added to the cell cultures once per week throughout the 6-week assay period, beginning immediately post-irradiation. As can be observed in Table 1, at the concentration utilized, none of the oils suppressed radiation transformation in a statistically significant fashion.

The effects of selenium on radiation transformation in C3H10T1/2 cells are shown in Table 2. 3×10^{-6} M selenium was studied since, in preliminary toxicity studies, this was the concentration of selenium found to be the highest non-toxic concentration. To study the effects of selenium, the compound needed to be added to the cultures in serum-free medium. At all medium changes (two times per week for six weeks), selenium was added in serum-free medium (BME); 24 hours later serum was added to the culture media. Selenium treatment began immediately after X-irradiation. As can be observed in the Table, this non-toxic concentration of selenium led to a significant decrease in the yield of transformed foci, reducing the fraction of dishes containing transformants by approximately 1/2.

The effects of 1,25-Dihydroxyvitamin D3 on radiation transformation in C3H10T1/2 cells are shown in Table 3. Although there was not a statistically significant effect, some inhibition of transformation by this compound was observed when it was utilized at 10^{-9} M; at 10^{-10} M, there was no effect of 1,25-Dihydroxyvitamin D3 on radiation transformation. For these experiments, 1,25-Dihydroxyvitamin D3 was initially dissolved in ethanol.

Results of C3H10T1/2 cell transformation experiments utillizing DMSO (0.05%) or Vitamin E (5 µg/ml) and subculture of some of the dishes are shown in Table 4.

The vitamin E experiments were performed with d-
α tocopherol acid succinate Type IV, initially dissolved in
ethanol (0.25%), as this form was shown previously to
affect radiation transformation in vitro (2). In the
experiments involving subculture, irradiated cells were
maintained for the entire six week assay period (which
involves a two week proliferative period followed by 4
weeks in confluence) before the cells were trypsinized
and reseeded at low cell density (300 viable cells per
dish), as both Vitamin E and DMSO have been shown
previously to have their suppressive effects on
transformation when present during confluence (2,22).
In these studies, it can be observed that both DMSO and
Vitamin E suppressed radiation transformation when
present for the usual 6 week assay period (Table 4,
groups 3 vs 6 and 3 vs 9). When Vitamin E and DMSO
were removed from the irradiated cultures at 6 weeks,
and the irradiated cells then reseeded and maintained for
an additional 6 weeks, the suppressive effects of the
compounds were not maintained. The fraction of dishes
containing transformed foci in the irradiated cultures was
not significantly different from that observed for
irradiated cultures previously exposed to DMSO or
Vitamin E (and from which DMSO or Vitamin E were
removed after subculturing, with or without subsequent
TPA treatment). These results suggest that the DMSO and
Vitamin E effects on radiation transformation are
reversible.

We have previously reported that protease
inhibitors are highly effective at suppressing radiation
transformation in vitro (6-17).The pure Bowman-Birk
inhibitor (BBI) from soybeans, as well as a soybean
extract containing BBI, have been studied in several
different transformation systems (11-14). A summary of
data showing that the crude extract containing BBI
prevents transformation in vitro induced by a physical
carcinogen (radiation), a chemical carcinogen requiring

metabolism (benzo (a) pyrene) and a direct acting chemical carcinogen (b- propiolactone), both with and without cocarcinogenesis by pyrene, are shown in Figs. 1-3. As can be observed in Figs. 1-3, treatment with the extract containing BBI reduced transformation yields to background levels in all carcinogen treatment groups. Thus, protease inhibitor treatment was equally effective at suppressing transformation induced by different doses of various carcinogens, both with and without simultaneous treatment with a cocarcinogen. These studies are described in greater detail elsewhere (14).

DISCUSSION

The results of studies to determine the effects of several different dietary compounds on carcinogen induced transformation in vitro are reported here. The most effective anticarcinogenic dietary agents in our studies have been the protease inhibitors. As can be observed in Figs. 1-3, the soybean extract containing BBI is capable of essentially abolishing in vitro transformation induced by a variety of carcinogenic agents, both with and without cocarcinogenesis induced by pyrene. The suppression of transformation in vitro by BBI is not related to carcinogen dose. In these studies, higher doses of carcinogen led to higher yields of transformants, yet the extract containing BBI reduced transformation to background levels in each case.

Other potentially anticarcinogenic dietary agents we have studied, such as 1,25-dihydroxyvitamin D_3, Vitamin E, and selenium have been able to suppress the yield of radiation induced transformants by approximately 1/2 when assayed under "optimal" conditions. The compounds studied in this report were assayed at the highest non-toxic concentrations in C3H10T1/2 cells for their ability to suppress transformation. Other specific assay conditions for these compounds involved studying the effects of selenium given in serum-free medium, and studying vitamin E in the particular form (the acid succinate form) shown previously to have the ability to suppress radiation induced transformation in vitro (2).

It has been observed previously that onion and garlic oils suppress promotion in vivo (Personal Communication, Dr. Sidney Belman) presumably due to their ability to inhibit fatty acid oxygenases (23). Unfortunately, these agents did not have a significant suppressive effect on radiation induced transformation in our studies. Other dietary agents studied here, however, did have a suppressive effect on radiation transformation.

1,25-dihydroxyvitamin D3 is known to regulate Ca levels in blood (24) and is the active form of vitamin D3. Sequential hydroxylation of vitamin D3 in the liver and then the kidney produce this hormonally active form of vitamin D3 (24).Both enhancing and suppressing effects of this conpound on carcinogenesis have been reported (25-28). 1 ,25-dihydroxyvitamin D3 was shown to be a promoter for in vitro transformation in Balb/3T3 cells (25), and was initially studied in the system on the basis of its known effects in other cell systems being similar to those observed for the tumor promoting agent, TPA (25). In other studies, however, 1,25-dihydroxyvitamin D3 has been shown to inhibit carcinogenesis (26-28). These studies support the results reported here on the inhibiton of radiation induced transformation in vitro by 1,25-dihyroxyvitamin D3.

Selenium has been shown previously to inhibit radiation induced transformation in vivo (29), and we have confirmed those initial studies in this report. We observed that the presense of selenium reduced radiation induced transformation by approximately 1/2 in our studies. It is of interest that most investigators studying the effect of selenium in in vivo carcinogenesis studies have observed that the tumor incidence was reduced by approximately 1/2 in the selenium-treated animals compared to the appropriate control animals (reviewed in reference 30). Similarly, vitamin E has the ability to reduce radiation transformation in vitro by approximately 1/2, as reported here; a similar reduction factor has been observed for several in vitro carcinogenesis studies (reviewed in reference 30).

As discussed above, protease inhibitors such as BBI are capable of suppressing transformation in vitro completely. These agents appear to be reducing transformation in vitro by a different mechanism than the other potential chemopreventive agents for cancer studied here. We have observed that vitamin E and DMSO have a reversible effect on radiation induced transformation in vitro. When these compounds are removed from irradiated cultures, transformed cells arise. Transformed cells do not arise from irradiated cultures treated with protease inhibitors under similar conditions, as previously reported (1). Thus, protease inhibitors have a reversible effect on the transformation process (1, 9,10).

As protease inhibitors have been so effective in our studies on the prevention of radiation induced transformation in vitro, we have performed many studies on their possible mechanisms of action, as reported elsewhere (31-35). Our studies on the prevention of in vivo carcinogenesis with the protease inhibitors (3-5) suggest that these agents are highly promising as human cancer chemopreventive agents.

Acknowledgements
The research discussed in this report has been supported by NIH Grants CA 22704, CA 34680, and CA 46496.

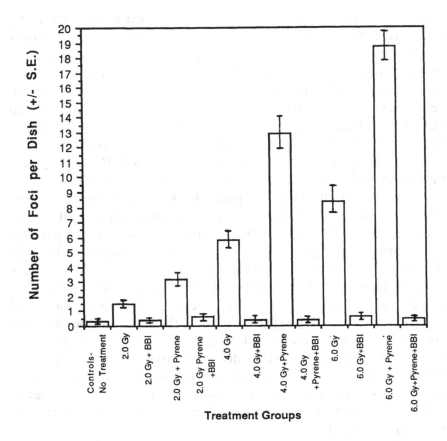

Fig. 1   Suppressing effect of soybean extract
           containing BBI on radiation induced
           transformation in vitro in Balb/c3T3
           Clone A31 cells. Details of these studies
           can be found in reference 14.

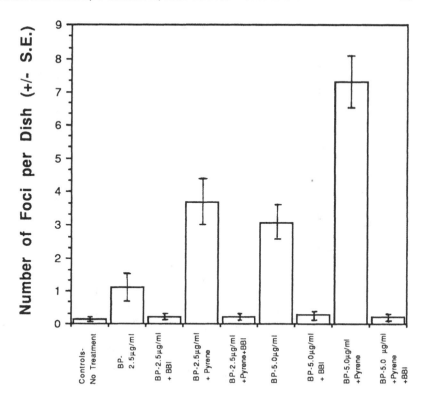

Treatment Groups

Fig. 2   Suppressing effect of soybean extract containing BBI on transformation in Balb/c3T3 cells induced by benzo(a)pyrene. Details of these studies are given in reference 14.

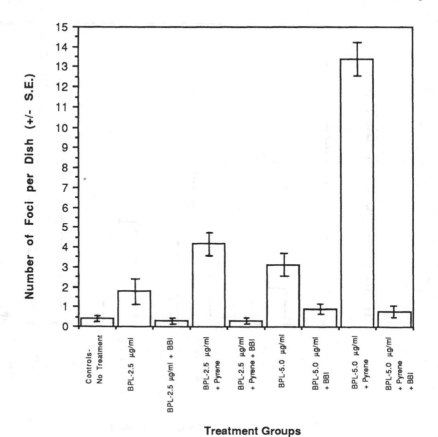

Treatment Groups

Fig. 3   Suppressing effect of soybean extract containing BBI on transformation in Balb/c3T3 cells induced by β-propiolactone. Details of these studies are given in reference 14.

Table 1   Effects of Onion Oil and Garlic Oil on Radiation Transformation In Vitro

Treatment	Plating Efficiency (%)	Number of Viable Cells	Total Number of Foci	Fraction of Dishes Containing Transformed Foci	
				Type 3	Types 2 & 3[1]
1. Controls- No Treatment	45.8	5496	0	0/12	0/12
2. 6.0 Gy	3.4	8160	17	2/24	13/23=0.54
3. 6.0 Gy+ onion oil (Mexican) (1.0 ug/ml)	2.8	6720	33	3/24	16/24=0.67
4. 6.0 Gy+ onion oil (Dutch) (1.0 ug/ml)	3.1	5580	22	6/18	13/18=0.72
5. 6.0 Gy + garlic oil (1.0 ug/ml)	1.5	3150	28	7/21	11/21=0.52

1. Statistical Analysis (Chi-Square): Groups 2 vs. 3,4,5, $p>0.05$.

Table 2   Effects of Selenium on Radiation Transformation In Vitro

Treatment	Experiment Number	Plating Efficiency (%)	Total Number of Viable Cells	Total Number of Foci (Types 2&3)	Fraction of Dishes Containing Transformed Foci		
					Type 3	Types 2&3	Total[1]
1. Controls- No Treatment	1	915	33.9	0	0/3	0/3	
	2	2672	22.3	0	0/8	0/8	0/11
2. Selenium (3x10^-6 M)	1	2880	40.0	0	0/8	0/8	0/8
3. 6.0 Gy	1	6460	3.8	10	5/17=0.29	10/17=0.59	
	2	7590	2.3	9	6/22=0.27	8/22=0.36	18/39=0.46
4. 6.0 Gy + Selenium (3x10^-6 M)	1	6120	3.6	4	2/17=0.12	4/17=0.24	
	2	5700	1.9	4	1/20=0.05	4/20=0.20	8/38=0.21

1 Statistical Analysis (Chi Square): Groups 1 vs. 2, $p > 0.05$; Groups 3 vs. 4, $p < 0.02$.

Table 3 Effects of 1,25-Dihydroxyvitamin D_3 (Vitamin D) on Radiation Transformation *In Vitro*

Treatment[1]	Exp. No.	Plating Efficiency (%)	Number of Viable Cells	Total Number of Foci (Types 2&3)	Fraction of Dishes Containing Transformed Foci — Type 3	Types 2 & 3	Total[2]
1. Controls- No treatment	1	38.7	4176	0	0/12	0/12	0/23
	2	39.0	3861	0	0/11	0/11	
2. Vit.D; 10^{-10}M	2	37.3	3693	0	0/11	0/11	0/22
Vit. D; 10^{-9}M	2	32.3	3198	0	0/11	0/11	
3. 6.0 Gy	1	4.8	10560	5	2/22=.09	5/22=0.23	13/42=0.31
	2	2.3	4600	8	5/20=.25	8/20=0.40	
4. 6.0 Gy + Vitamin D (10^{-10}M)	1	4.9	10780	4	0/22	2/22=0.09	7/43=0.16
	2	2.6	5460	7	1/21=.05	5/21=0.24	
5. 6.0 Gy + Vitamin D (10^{-9} M)	2	3.8	4998	8	6/21=.29	6/21=0.29	6/21=0.29

1 Vitamin D was present in cultures at the concentrations indicated for 5 days; treatment was started immediately after the radiation exposure.
2 Statistical Analysis (Chi-Square): Groups 3 vs 4, $p < 0.20$.

TABLE 4
EXPERIMENTS DESIGNED TO DETERMINE WHETHER
THE EFFECTS OF DMSO AND VITAMIN E ON RADIATION
TRANSFORMATION ARE REVERSIBLE

Treatment	Fraction of Dishes Containing Transformed Foci (Types II and III)[1]
1. Controls- No Treatment	0/26
2. Controls-Subcultured Dishes	0/27
3. 6.0 Gy	23/59=0.39
4. 6.0 Gy-Subcultured	15/50=0.30
5. 6.0 Gy-Subcultured + TPA	30/51=0.59
6. 6.0 Gy + Vitamin E throughout transformation assay period	6/45=0.13
7. 6.0 Gy + Vitamin E-subcultured; Vitamin E removed after subculture	12/47=0.26
8. 6.0 Gy + Vitamin E-subcultured; Vitamin E removed after subculture, TPA added after subculture	22/45=0.49
9. 6.0 Gy + DMSO throughout transformation assay period	3/25=0.12
10. 6.0 Gy + DMSO-subcultured; DMSO removed after subculture	5/22=0.23
11. 6.0 Gy + DMSO-subcultured; DMSO removed after subculture,TPA added after subculture	11/22=0.50

1. Statistical Analysis (Chi-Square): Group 3 vs 6, $p<0.05$; 3 vs 7, 3 vs 8, $p>0.05$; 3 vs 9, $p<0.05$; 3 vs 10, 3 vs 11, $p>0.05$.

REFERENCES

1.   Kennedy, A.R.   The conditions for the modification of radiation transformation *in vitro* by a tumor promoter and protease inhibitors.   Carcinogenesis 6: 1441-1446, 1985.

2.   Radner, B.S. and Kennedy, A.R.   Suppression of x-ray induced transformation by Vitamin E in mouse C3H/10T1/2 cells. Cancer Letters 32: 25-32, 1986.

3.   Weed, H., McGandy, R.B. and Kennedy, A.R.   Protection against dimethylhydrazine induced adenomatous tumors of the mouse colon by the dietary addition of an extract of soybeans containing the Bowman-Birk protease inhibitor.   Carcinogenesis 6: 1239-1241, 1985.

4.   St. Clair, W., Billings, P., Carew, J., Keller-McGandy, C., Newberne, P. and Kennedy, A.R.   Suppression of DMH-induced carcinogenesis in mice by dietary addition of the Bowman-Birk protease inhibitor. (submitted)

5.   Messadi, P.V., Billings, P., Shklar, G. and Kennedy, A.R. Inhibition of oral carcinogenesis by a protease inhibitor.   J. Natl. Cancer Inst. 76: 447-452, 1986.

6.   Kennedy, A.R.   Promotion and other interactions between agents in the induction of transformation *in vitro* in fibroblasts. In: Mechanisms of Tumor Promotion, Vol. III, "Tumor Promotion and Carcinogenesis In Vitro" edited by T.J. Slaga, CRC Press, Inc., Chapter 2, pp. 13-55, 1984.

7.   Kennedy, A.R. and Little, J.B.   Protease inhibitors suppress radiation induced malignant transformation *in vitro*.   Nature 276: 825-826, 1978.

8.   Kennedy, A.R. and Weichselbaum, R.R.   Effects of 17-B-estradiol on radiation transformation *in vitro*; inhibition of effects by protease inhibitors.   Carcinogenesis 2: 67-69. 1981.

9.   Kennedy, A.R. and Little, J.B.   Effects of protease inhibitors on radiation transformation *in vitro*.   Cancer Res. 41: 2103-2108, 1981.

10.   Kennedy, A.R.   Antipain, but not cycloheximide, suppresses radiation transformation when present for only one day at five days post-irradiation.   Carcinogenesis 3: 1093-1095, 1982.

11.   Yavelow, J., Finlay, T.H., Kennedy, A.R. and Troll, W. Bowman-Birk soybean protease inhibitor as an anticarcinogen. Cancer Res. 43: 2454-2459, 1983.

12.   Kennedy,   A.R.   Prevention   of   Radiation-Induced Transformation In Vitro. In: Vitamins. Nutrition and Cancer (ed. K.N. Prasad), S. Karger, A.G. Basel, pp. 166-179, 1984.

13.   Yavelow, J., Collins, M., Birk, Y., Troll, W. and Kennedy, A.R. Nanomolar   concentrations   of   Bowman-Birk   soybean   protease inhibitor suppress X-ray induced transformation in vitro. Proc. Natl. Acad. Sci. USA 82: 5395-5399, 1985.

14   Baturay,   N.Z.   and   Kennedy,   A.R.   Pyrene   acts   as   a cocarcinogen   with   the   carcinogens,   benzo(a)pyrene,   B-propiolactone   and   radiation   in   the   induction   of   malignant transformation   of   cultured   mouse   fibroblasts;   soybean   extract containing   the   Bowman-Birk   inhibitor   acts   as   an anticarcinogen. Cell Biol Toxicol. 2: 21-32, 1986.

15.   Kennedy,   A.R.   Implications   for   mechanisms   of   tumor promotion and its inhibition by various agents from studies of in vitro transformation. In: Tumor Promoters.   Biological Approaches for Mechanistic Studies and Assay Systems. (Editors: Langenbach, R., Barrett, J.C. and Elmore, E.), Raven Press, New York, pp. 201-212, 1988.

16.   Billings, P.C., St. Clair, W., Ryan, C.A. and Kennedy, A.R. Inhibition   of   radiation-induced   transformation   of   C3H/10T1/2 cells by chymotrypsin inhibitor 1 from potatoes.   Carcinogenesis 8: 809-812, 1987.

17.   Kennedy, A.R. and Billings, P.C.   Anticarcinogenic actions of protease inhibitors. Proceedings of the 2nd International Conference on "Anticarcinogenesis and Radiation Protection," Cerutti, P.A., Nygaard, O.F.and Simic, M.G., editors), Plenum Press, New York, pp. 285-295,1987.

18.   Kakunaga,   T.   A quantitative system for assay of malignant transformation   by   chemical   carcinogens   using   a   clone   derived from BALB/3T3.   Int. J. Cancer 12:463-473, 1973.

19.   Little, J.B.   Quantitative studies of radiation transformation with the A31-11 mouse BALB/3T3 cell line.   Cancer Res. 39:1474-1480, 1979.

20.   Cortese, E., Saffiotti, U., Donovan, P.J., Rice, J.M. and Kakunaga, T. Dose-response studies on neoplastic transformation of Balb/3T3 clone A31-11 cells by Aflatoxin B, Benzidine, Benzo(a)pyrene, 3-Methylcholanthrene and N-methyl-N[1]-nitro-N-nitroso-guanidine.   Teratogenesis,   Carcinogenesis, Mutagenesis 3:101-110, 1983.

21.   Baturay, N.Z., Targovnik, H.S., Reynolds, R.J. and Kennedy, A.R.   Induction of in vitro transformation by near UV light and

its interaction with Beta-propiolactone. Carcinogenesis 6:465-468, 1985.

22.   Symons, M.C.R. and Kennedy, A.R. " Water structure" versus "radical scavenger" theories as explanations for the suppressive effects of DMSO and related compounds on radiation-induced transformation in vitro. Carcinogenesis 8: 683-688, 1987.

23.   Vanderhoek, J.Y., Makheja, A.M., and Bailey, J.M. Inhibition of fatty acid oxygenases by onion and garlic oils. Biochemical Pharmacology 29: 3169-3173, 1980.

24.   De Luca, H.F. and Schnoes, H.K. Metabolism and mechanism of action of vitamin D. Ann. Rev. Biochem. 45: 631-642, 1976.

25.   Kuroki, T., Sasaki, K., Kazuhiro, C., Abe, E. and Suda, T. 1a,25-Dihydroxyvitamin D$_3$ markedly enhances chemically-induced transformation in Balb 3T3 cells. Gann 74: 611-614, 1983.

26.   Eisman, J.A., Barkla, D.H., and Tutton, P.J.M. Suppression of in vivo growth of human cancer solid tumor xenografts by 1,25-dihydroxyvitamin D$_3$. Cancer Research 47: 21-25, 1987.

27.   Frampton, R.J., Omond, S.A., and Eisman, J.A. Inhibition of human cancer growth by 1,25-dihydroxyvitamin D$_3$ metabolites. Cancer Research. 43: 4443-4447, 1983.

28.   Colston, D, Colston, M.J., and Feldman, M. 1,25-Dihydroxyvitamin D$_3$ and malignant melanoma: the presence of receptors and inhibition of cell growth in culture. Endocrinology 108: 1083-1086, 1981.

29.   Borek, C., Ong, A., Mason, H., Donahue, L., and Biaglow, J. Selenium and vitamin E inhibit radiogenic and chemically induced transformation in vitro via different mechanisms. Proc. Natl. Acad. Sci. 83: 1490- 1494, 1986.

30.   Grobstein, C. (Chairman of Committee). Diet, Nutrition and Cancer.Committee On Diet, Nutrition and Cancer, National Acadamy of Sciences, National Acadamy Press, Washington, D.C.,1982.

31.   Chang, J.D. Billings, P. and Kennedy, A.R. C-myc expression is reduced in antipain-treated proliferating CH10T1/2 cells. Biochem.Biophys. Res Comm. 133: 830-835, 1985.

32.   Billings, P.C., Carew, J.A., Keller-McGandy, C.E., Goldberg, A., and Kennedy, A.R. A serine protease activity in C3H10T1/2 cells that is inhibited by anticarcinogenic protease inhibitors. Proc. Natl.Acad. Sci. 84: 4801-4805, 1987.

33.   Chang, J.D. and Kennedy, A.R. Cell cycle progression of
C3H10T1/2 cells and 3T3 cells in the absense of a transient
increase in c-myc RNA levels. Carcinogenesis 9: 17-20, 1988.

34.   Billings, P.C., St. Clair, W., Owen, A.J. and Kennedy, A.R.
Potential intracellular target proteins of the anticarcinogenic
Bowman-Birk protease inhibitor identified by affinity
chromatography. Cancer Res. 48: 1798-1802, 1988.

35.   Caggana, M and A.R. Kennedy. C-fos mRNA levels are
reduced in the presence of antipain and the Bowman-Birk
inhibitor. Carcinogenesis (in press).

CAROTENOIDS INHIBIT CHEMICALLY- AND PHYSICALLY-INDUCED NEOPLASTIC TRANSFORMATION DURING THE POST-INITIATION PHASE OF CARCINOGENESIS.[1,2]

J.S. Bertram, J.E. Rundhaug, and A. Pung

Basic Science Program, Cancer Research Center of Hawaii, University of Hawaii

1236 Lauhala Street, Honolulu, Hawaii, USA

ABSTRACT

Diets rich in carotenoids have been strongly implicated as protecting against cancer development at several anatomic sites, however it is unclear whether protection is due to the carotenoid itself or to products of its bioconversion to retinoids. Both Beta-carotene (β-C), a carotenoid with, and canthaxanthin (CTX) a carotenoid without pro-vitamin A activity, have been found to inhibit methylcholanthrene induced neoplastic transformation in 10T1/2 cells. Activity was observed when these compounds were added 7 days after carcinogen exposure and was reversible upon removal of carotenoid. When tested against X-ray induced transformation, carotenoids were ineffective when present during irradiation but, as before, strongly protected when added after carcinogen exposure. Effective doses were not cytotoxic. In both chemical and

[1]Supported by grant CA 39947 and a grant in aid from the National Dairy Council
[2]Abbreviations: β-C: Beta-carotene; CTX: canthaxanthin; MCA: 3-methylcholanthrene; ID50: dose for 50% inhibition of transformation; PE: plating efficiency; PBS: phosphate-buffered saline; HPLC: high performance liquid chromatography; TF: transformation frequency.

physical carcinogensis protocols, CTX was significantly more potent than β-C in inhibiting transformation. Using ^{14}C-β-C no conversion to expected retinoids was detected after incubation with 10T1/2 cells. Thus carotenoids appear to possess intrinsic cancer chemopreventive activity in 10T1/2 cells.

INTRODUCTION

Epidemiologic evidence provides strong evidence for the protective effects of vitamin A and vitamin A precursors of plant origin (carotenoids) on human cancer incidence. However, in many studies, dietary intake of β-C, the carotenoid with the highest provitamin A activity, rather than intake of the vitamin itself, seems best correlated with decreased cancer incidence (for review see 1). It is at present unclear whether risk reduction is due to β-C itself or to the vitamin A produced by its metabolism (2). Animal models have so far not been able to distinguish between these possibilities because of the conversion of β-C to retinoids. Vitamin A and its derivatives are known to be strongly anti-carcinogenic, this has been demonstrated in model in vitro systems, in experimental animals and in human pre-neoplasia (1).

Relatively few studies have examined the activity of β-C. It has been shown to lower tumor incidence and to reduce the growth of transplanted tumors (3, 4). Both β-C and CTX increase immune responsiveness in rats (5). In the only human study of β-C and CTX, β-C but not CTX was shown to be capable of reducing the abnormal pathology in the oral cavity of betel nut/tobacco chewers. Vitamin A was also effective in this study, implying the requirement for conversion of β-C to vitamin A (6).

Because fibroblasts would not be expected to convert β-C to retinoids, we have utilized the C3H/10T1/2 mouse fibroblast line to determine if β-C has intrinsic biological activity as a chemopreventive agent against chemically and physically-induced neoplastic transformation. Extensive studies with this cell line have shown it to respond in a quantitative manner to

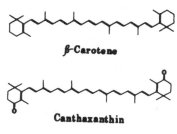

β-Carotene

Canthaxanthin

Figure 1

chemically- or physically-induced carcinogenesis (7,8), and to be sensitive to the chemopreventive action of retinoids (9,10) and other modulators of carcinogenesis (11). We have also examined the effects of CTX, the 4,4' diketo derivative of β-C, which is not capable of being converted to retinoids in mammalian cells (12), yet which possesses similar antioxidant properties to β-C (13) (Fig.1). Our results demonstrate that both carotenoids can reversibly inhibit the development of neoplastically transformed foci without obvious cytotoxic effects on normal, initiated or transformed cells (14).

To formally exclude the possibility of bioconversion of β-C, we have examined the metabolism of ^{14}C-labeled β-C by 10T1/2 cells, and have also examined the metabolic fate of retinal, the expected immediate derivative of β-C conversion to retinoids. We found no evidence that 10T1/2 cells can convert β-C to active retinoids (15). These results clearly indicate that carotenoids possess intrinsic chemopreventive activity in 10T1/2 cells.

MATERIALS AND METHODS

Chemical Transformation

C3H/10T1/2 cells were cultured, and neoplastic transformation quantitated as previously described (14). Briefly, 10T1/2 cells were seeded at 1000 cells/60 mm culture dish and treated 24 h later with 1 µg/ml methylcholanthrene. This was removed after 24 hr. After an additional 7 days, cultures were treated

with the indicated concentration of carotenoid prepared
from the beadlet formulation of Hoffmann-La Roche, or
with an equivalent solution of control beadlets.
Cultures were re-fed and re-treated weekly. In most
cases, cultures were evaluated for neoplastic
transformation after 4 weeks of treatment.

X-ray Transformation

X-irradiation was performed in mass cultures of
late logarithmic growth phase 10T1/2 cells which were
subsequently re-plated at lower cell densities. 10T1/2
cell cultures in 100 mm dishes were irradiated with 6 Gy
X-rays (1.4 Gy/min, 300 KVP, 20 mA, 2 mm Cu) from a
General Electric Maxitron 300 unit. Twenty-four hours
after irradiation, cultures were trypsinized and seeded
at 5000 cells/100 mm dish. For experiments designed to
study carotenoid effects on initiating events, cell
cultures were exposed to β-C or CTX 24 h prior to and 1
h after irradiation. For the study of events during the
progression phase of carcinogenesis, carotenoids were
added 7 days after irradiation and cultures were
re-treated weekly as in the chemical transformation
studies. For both protocols, cells were cultured in
medium containing 10% fetal calf serum until 7 days
after irradiation when it was reduced to 5% serum as in
the chemical transformation experiments. For
determination of X-ray induced cytotoxicity, cells from
irradiated or control cultures, treated with carotenoids
or with vehicle control, were seeded at 400 or 200
cells/60 mm Petri dish respectively. Surviving colonies
were counted after 8 days incubation.

RESULTS

Chemically-induced Transformation

Addition of either β-C or CTX to 10T1/2 cultures
treated 8 days previously with MCA, resulted in a
dose-dependent decrease in transformation frequency. As
shown in Fig. 2, the ID_{50} for β-C was about 9x 10^{-7} M,
while for CTX it was 2 x 10^{-7} M. The consistent shift
in response curves seen over the entire dose range,
demonstrates the greater potency of CTX over β-C as an
inhibitor of MCA-induced transformation. These

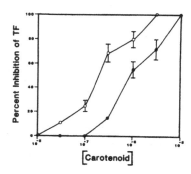

Figure 2. Effects of carotenoids on neoplastic transformation of 10T1/2 cells. β-C (•-•) or canthaxanthin (o-o) were added 7 days after treatment of 10T1/2 cells with methylcholanthrene and maintained in cultures by weekly re-treatment. After 4 weeks, cultures were fixed and stained, the number of transformed foci quantitated and the transformation frequency (TF) calculated. (For experimental details, see 14.)

differences were statistically significant (P < 0.01) over the dose range 10^{-7} - 10^{-6} M. The control beadlet preparation did not significantly alter the transformation frequency observed in carcinogen-only treated cultures.

In Figure 3 is shown the appearance of culture dishes treated with MCA followed by β-C, CTX or with control beadlets. The lack of transformed foci in the carotenoid-treated cultures is readily apparent.

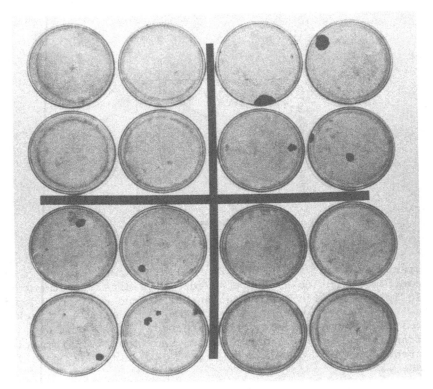

Figure 3. 10T1/2 cells growing in 60 mm culture dishes were exposed to MCA for 24 hr, or acetone as control. After 7 days cultures were treated with canthaxanthin or vehicle control for the duration of the experiment. Clockwise from top left: Acetone 0.5% control; MCA 1 μg/ml; MCA then canthaxanthin 3x10-6 M; MCA then vehicle control.

Reversibility Studies

In our previous work on the retinoids, we reported that their inhibitory effects were reversible upon drug withdrawal, but only after a prolonged latent period (9). We therefore conducted similar studies with β-C or CTX in MCA treated cultures. As shown in Fig. 3, removal of the β-C and CTX after 4 weeks of treatment

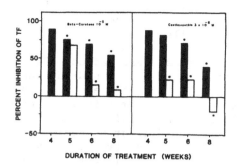

Figure 4. Effects of removal of carotenoids from carcinogen-treated cultures. After 4 weeks of carotenoid treatment as in Figure 2 replicate cultures were either maintained with carotenoid, or had treatment withdrawn. The development of transformed foci was quantitated with time. Solid bars, continuous treatment; open bars, treatment withdrawn. (For experimental details see ref. 14.)

allowed the development of foci. Frequencies within 20% of control carcinogen-only values were attained 2 weeks after removal. In cultures maintained in the presence of carotenoids over this time period, a slow increase in focus formation occurred, indicating that the block of transformation is not absolute. Taken together, these results demonstrate that carotenoids are not selectively cytotoxic to initiated cells but slow their progression to cells having the transformed phenotype.

X-Ray Transformation

Studies with MCA had demonstrated an inhibitory action of β-C and CTX when present during the promotional phase of transformation. To study effects on initiation we chose to use X-rays as initiator to avoid interpretational problems associated with concurrent exposure of cells to multiple lipophilic agents (MCA, β-C or CTX, or other components of the beadlets). These studies were also extended to examine effects of carotenoids on the promotional phase of X-ray transformation, and on the ability of carotenoids to prevent the expression of transformaion of established transformed cells when seeded on a confluent background of normal 10T1/2 cells.

When carotenoids were added 24 hr prior to irradiation and were maintained during and immediately after radiation, the subsequent development of transformation was only marginally reduced indicating little influence on initiating events. In contrast survival of carotenoid-treated cells was increased by approximately 50%. When treatment was delayed until 7 days after the carcinogenic insult and maintained for an additional 4 weeks, as in the experiments with MCA, transformation was inhibited as efficiently as was observed previously (Fig. 5).

Potential Effects on Expression of the Transformed Phenotype. To examine potential effects on the expression of transformation when in contact with 10T1/2 cells, two transformed lines were plated onto confluent

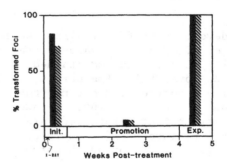

Figure 5.   Effects of carotenoids when administered during the initiation, promotion or expression phase of carcinogenesis. 10T1/2 cultures received 6 Gy of X-rays, and β-C (solid bars) or CTX (hatched bars) at 10^{-5} M and 3×10^{-6} M respectively: Init; 24 hr prior to and during irradiation; promotion, 7 days post-irradiation and continuously thereafter; Exp., carotenoids were applied to cultures of confluent 10T1/2 cells overlayed with transformed cells. Results represent numbers of transformed foci as a percent of vehicle treated controls.

monolayers of 10T1/2 cells and treated 24 hrs later withgraded doses of carotenoids. When these cultures were fixed and quantitated after 7 d treatment, the numbers of transformed foci and their size was not reduced by concentrations of β-C and CTX (Fig. 5) causing virtually complete inhibition of transformation. Similar results were seen with a second clone of transformed cells (data not shown). Therefore, carotenoids do not influence the ability of established transformed cells to form foci on a background of non-transformed cells. This again indicates that carotenoids are active on the post-initiation, pre-expression phase of carcinogenesis. This action duplicates in many respects the action of retinoids in 10T1/2 cells (9).

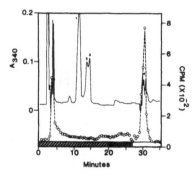

Figure 6. HPLC profile of [^{14}C] β-C-treated culture medium. Confluent cultures of 10T1/2 cells were treated with 10^{-5} M [^{14}C] β-C for 24 hr, then spiked with 10^{-6} M retinol and retinoic acid, and the medium extracted for retinoids. The extract (100 μl) was injected into the Spherisorb ODS-2 column and eluted with 85:15 acetonitrile/1% ammonium acetate at 1.0 ml/min (hatched bar), then 100% acetonitrile (solid bar) and 100% methylene chloride (open bar) at 2.0 ml/min. The solid line, UV absorption profile; the circles and dashed line, ^{14}C profile. Peak 1, all-trans retinoic acid; peak 2, probably a cis-retinol; peak 3, all-trans retinol; peak 4, β-C and the methylene chloride peak. All-trans retinal would elute at ~18-20 min in this system.

Metabolism of ^{14}C-β-carotene

Addition of ^{14}C-β-C (gift from Hoffmann-La Roche) to confluent cultures of 10T1/2 cells, followed by incubation for 1 or 7 days, failed to reveal any conversion of labeled β-C to the expected products of bioconversion to active retinoids (i.e. retinal, retinol or retinoic acid) (Fig. 6). Furthermore, loss of β-C from culture medium occurred no faster in medium overlaying cells than it did from medium contained in otherwise empty dishes, indicating that little or no metabolism of β-C occurs in cultured 10T1/2 cells (15). These observations lead to the conclusion that carotenoids have intrinsic activity as chemopreventive agents in 10T1/2 cells.

DISCUSSION

Our results demonstrate that both β-C and CTX are capable of inhibiting the transformation of chemically- and physically-initiated 10T1/2 cells during the promotional phase of carcinogenesis of these cells. Drug treatment is effective long after carcinogen exposure or removal, and thus cannot be attributed to an inhibition of either free radical production from the carcinogenic stimulus or inhibition of the reaction of chemical or radiation-induced reactive species with DNA. Indeed these drugs did not influence radiation carcinogenesis when present at a time such reactions could be inhibited (Figure 5). When added to proliferating cultures of parental 10T1/2 cells, β-C and CTX caused small reductions in growth rates but did not reduce the colony size of cells treated under conditions comparable to those employed in transformation experiments (14). Neither did these drugs inhibit the growth of established transformed cells on monolayers of 10T1/2 cells (Fig. 5). The reversible nature of the inhibition of transformation upon drug withdrawal (Fig. 3) also indicates a lack of toxicity against latent initiated cells. This type of chemopreventive activity is essentially identical to that previously described for retinoids in 10T1/2 cells (9). Yet, there is no evidence that either carotenoid can yield active retinoids in 10T1/2 cells. Since the chemopreventive activity of retinoids in the 10T1/2 systems is highly correlated with their activities as vitamin A analogs (10), assessed by their ability to inhibit squamous differentiation, and since carotenoids have no known intrinsic vitamin A activity (12), it appears probable that carotenoids and retinoids must have distinct mechanisms of action as inhibitors of transformation of 10T1/2 cells.

The results reported here are the first to demonstrate that carotenoids have intrinsic cancer chemopreventive activity in systems other than those involving photocarcinogenesis in which they may act as sun screens. One activity shared by both β-C and CTX is the ability to inhibit the peroxidation of unsaturated lipids (16) and we suggest that this shared activity could be responsible for the chemopreventive action demonstrated here. Lipid peroxidation can be expected to have severe consequences to the cell such as the release of many biologically active factors, including prostaglandins. Furthermore many promoting agents induce lipid peroxidation (for review see 17). It follows that drugs which inhibit lipid peroxidation should have properties similar to those noted for β-C and CTX.

REFERENCES

1. Bertram J.S., Kolonel, L.N. and Meyskens F.L., Jr. Rationale and strategies for chemoprevention of cancer in humans. Cancer Res., 47:3012-3031, 1987.

2. Peto, R., Doll, R., Buckley, J.D. and Sporn, M.B. Can dietary beta-carotene materially reduce human cancer rates? Nature, 290:201-208, 1981.

3. Rettura, G., Stratford, F., Levenson, S.M. and Seifter, E. Prophylactic and therapeutic actions of supplemental β-carotene in mice inoculated with C3HBA adenocarcinoma cells: lack of therapeutic action of supplemental ascorbic acid. J. Natl. Cancer Inst., 69:73-77, 1982.

4.   Seifter,   E.,   Rettura,   G.,   Padawer,   J.   and
Levenson, S.M.   Moloney murine sarcoma virus tumors in
CBA/J mice: chemopreventive and chemotherapeutic actions
of   supplemental β-carotene.   J.   Natl.   Cancer   Inst.,
68:835-840, 1982.

5.   Bendich,   A.   and   Shapiro,   S.S.   Effect   of
β-carotene and canthaxanthin on the immune responses of
the rat. J.Nutr. 116:2254-2262, 1986.

6.   Stich,   H.F.,   Stich, W., Rosin, M.P. and Vallejera,
M.O.   Use of the micronucleus test to monitor   the   effect
of   vitamin   A, β-carotene and canthaxanthin on the buccal
mucosa of betel   nut/tobacco   chewers.   Int.   J.   Cancer,
34:745-750, 1984.

7.   Reznikoff,   C.A.,   Bertram,   J.S.,   Brankow, D.W. and
Heidelberger, C.   Quantitative and qualitative studies
of   chemical   transformation   of   cloned   C3H mouse embryo
cells   sensitive   to   postconfluence   inhibition   of   cell
division.   Cancer Res.,33:3239-3249, 1973.

8.   Terzaghi, M., Little, J.B.   X-radiation induction
of transformation in a C3H mouse embryo-derived cell
line. Cancer Res., 36:1367-1374, 1976.

9.   Merriman,   R.L.   and   Bertram,   J.S.   Reversible
inhibition   by   retinoids   of 3-methylcholanthrene-induced
neoplastic transformation in C3H/10T1/2 Clone 8 cells.
Cancer Res., 39, 1661-1666.

10.   Bertram,   J.S.   Structure-activity relationships
among various   retinoids   and   their   ability   to   inhibit
neoplastic   transformation   and   to increase cell adhesion
in the C3H/10T1/2 CL8 cell line. Cancer Res., 40,
3141-3146.

11.   Bertram, J.S.   Neoplastic transformation in cell
cultures: in   vitro/in   vivo correlations. In: Kakunaga,
T. and Yamasaki, H. (eds.), Transformation Assay of
Established   Cell   Lines: Mechanisms   and   Application.
IARC Scientific Publication No. 67. IARC, Lyon, pp.
77-91, 1985.

12. Underwood, B.A. Vitamin A in animal and human nutrition. In: Sporn, M.B., Roberts, A.B. and Goodman, D.S. (eds.), The Retinoids. Academic Press, N.Y., Vol. 1, pp. 281-392, 1984.

13. Anderson, S.M. and Krinsky, N.I. Protective action of carotenoid pigments against photodynamic damage to liposomes. Photochem. Photobiol., 18:403-408, 1973.

14. Pung, A., Rundhaug, J.E., Yoshizawa, C.N. and Bertram, J.S. β-carotene and canthaxanthin inhibit chemically- and physically-induced neoplastic transformation in 10T1/2 cells. Carcinogenesis, 9:1533-1539, 1988.

15. Rundhaug, J.E., Pung, A., Read, C.M. and Bertram, J.S. Uptake and metabolism of β-carotene and retinal by C3H/10T1/2 cells. Carcinogenesis, 9:1541-1565, 1988.

16. Burton, G.W. and Ingold, K.U. β-carotene: An usual type of lipid antioxidant. Science, 224:569-573, 1984.

17. Cerutti, P.A. Prooxidant states and tumor promotion. Science, 227:375-381, 1985.

Nutrients and Cancer Prevention K. N. Prasad and F. L. Meyskens, Jr., eds. © 1990 The Humana Press

FATTY ACIDS THAT INHIBIT CANCER: CONJUGATED DIENOIC

DERIVATIVES OF LINOLEIC ACID

Michael W. Pariza and Yeong L. Ha

Food Research Institute

Department of Food Microbiology and Toxicology

University of Wisconsin-Madison

1925 Willow Drive, Madison, WI 53706

ABSTRACT

Evidence for the anticarcinogenic activity of the conjugated dienoic derivatives of linoleic acid (CLA) is reviewed. CLA is present in grilled beef, cheese, and related foods. It is also generated endogenously via carbon centered free radical oxidation of linoleic acid. New findings indicate that CLA is a potent antioxidant. CLA may provide a previously unrecognized in situ defense mechanism against membrane attack by oxygen radicals.

INTRODUCTION

In the quest to control cancer, the search for safe and effective anticarcinogens is an important endeavor. Many potential anticarcinogens have been identified in food, most notably (but not limited to) foods of plant origin. This paper will review the data on a newly recognized cancer inhibitor isolated from an unexpected food source: grilled hamburger.

BACKGROUND

In earlier work on mutagen formation in food during cooking we observed that extracts of fried ground beef contained a mutagenic inhibitory activity (6). The inhibitory activity seemed to act selectively, at the stage of metabolic activation. Mutagenesis mediated by normal rat liver S-9 was inhibited whereas S-9 from the livers of rats treated with Aroclor 1254 appeared resistant to inhibition.

Partially-purified mutagenic inhibitory activity was tested for its effect on the mutagenic activity of two mutagens: 2-amino-3-methylimidazo[4,5-f]quinoline (IQ) and 2-aminofluorene (8). Different effects were observed depending on the mutagen and the type of rat liver S-9 (from normal, phenobarbital-treated, or Aroclor-treated animals) that was utilized. For IQ, the inhibitor produced inhibition irrespective of the type of liver S-9 used although as with previous experiments the Aroclor S-9 was more 'resistant' to the inhibitory effects. By contrast with 2-aminofluorene, mutagenesis mediated by normal rat liver S-9 was inhibited, but that mediated by liver S-9 from Aroclor treated rats was enhanced. When liver S-9 from phenobarbital-treated rats was used the inhibitor had no effect. Based on these findings, we suggested referring to the inhibitory activity as a mutagenesis modulating activity (8).

ANTICARCINOGENIC ACTIVITY OF CLA

The mutagenesis modulator was investigated as a potential anticarcinogen in animals (7). Initial experiments involved the well-studied 2-stage mouse epidermal carcinogenesis system and the carcinogen 7,12-dimethylbenz[a]anthracene. It was found that a partially purified preparation of mutagenesis modulator from grilled beef reduced both the number of papillomas per mouse and the number of mice with papillomas.

An anticarcinogenic principal was then isolated from the extracts and identified as a mixture of conjugated dienoic isomers of the essential fatty acid, linoleic acid (3). The isomers are referred to collectively by the acronym CLA (for conjugated linoleic acid). The observation that CLA is derived from linoleic acid is of interest in that linoleic acid is the only fatty acid that has been proved to enhance carcinogenesis in experimental animals (5).

We have found that CLA is also effective in inhibiting benzo[a]pyrene-induced forestomach neoplasia in mice (unpublished), using methods described in (1). Each week for 4 weeks mice were given CLA by stomach tube prior to administration of the carcinogen. Twenty weeks after the last treatment the animals were sacrificed and the number of forestomach neoplasms determined. In several experiments it was found that CLA administration reduced forestomach neoplasia by 46%-67% relative to controls (animals given linoleic acid or olive oil).

In other experiments we have studied the disposition of CLA in the body following administration by stomach tube (manuscript submitted). CLA is readily incorporated into body fat stores (triglycerides) and cell membranes (phospholipids). All the CLA isomers are found in triglycerides whereas over 95% of the CLA in phospholipid is in the form of just one isomer, c-9, t-11-octadecadienoic acid. This was so even though a mixture of nine CLA isomers had been administered (4).

SOURCES OF CLA

CLA is present in cheese as well as grilled beef (4). The amount varies considerably among products but one cheese spread contained as much CLA as grilled hamburger, when normalized for fat content. We have estimated that CLA consumption in the U.S. may be one gram per person per day (3, 4).

While dietary sources may be important, the major source of CLA may be endogenous synthesis. There is good evidence (2) that CLA is produced within the human body via carbon-centered free radical oxidation of linoleic acid. Additionally, certain serum proteins may mediate this reaction (2).

With regard to endogenous synthesis, the CLA content
of human blood appears to be modulated by oxidative
stress. For example, it is elevated in the blood of
alcoholics and decreases during periods of abstinence (2).

Our working hypothesis is that the modulation of CLA
generation in the body by oxidative stress is more than
just a consequence of oxidative stress. We propose that
the generation of CLA is in fact the key to a feedback
mechanism that helps protect cells from the damaging
effects of oxygen radicals.

ANTIOXIDANT ACTIVITY OF CLA

We have established that CLA is an effective
antioxidant (manuscript submitted). Using a water/ethanol
system involving incubation for 14 days under air (9), CLA
reduced the oxidation of linoleic acid by 86%. Under the
same conditions α-tocopherol reduced oxidation by only 63%
whereas butylated hydroxytoluene (BHT) reduced oxidation
by 92%. Hence, under the test conditions (where the ratio
of linoleic acid to CLA or other test antioxidant was 1000
to 1) CLA was more potent than α-tocopherol, and almost as
effective as BHT.

These observations lend support to the proposal that
the in vivo formation and action of CLA may represent a
feedback loop which serves to protect the cell from
oxidative damage. Dietary CLA may also play a role in
this regard.

REFERENCES

1. Benjamin, H., Storkson, J., Tallas, P.G., and Pariza,
   M.W. (1988) Reduction of benzo[a]pyrene-induced
   forestomach neoplasms in mice given nitrite and
   dietary soy sauce. Fd. Chem. Toxic. 26:671-678.

2. Dormandy, T.L. and Wickens, D.G. (1987) The
   experimental and clinical pathology of diene
   conjugation. Chem. Phys. Lipids 45:353-364.

3. Ha, Y.L., Grimm, N.K., and Pariza, M.W. (1987) Anticarcinogens from fried ground beef: heat-altered derivatives of linoleic acid. Carcinogenesis 8:1881-1887.

4. Ha, Y.L., Grimm, N.K., and Pariza, M.W. (1989) Newly recognized anticarcinogenic fatty acids: Identification and quantification in natural and processed cheeses. J. Agric. Fed. Chem. 37:75-81.

5. Pariza, M.W. (1988) Dietary fat and cancer risk: evidence and research needs. Annu. Rev. Nutr. 8:167-183.

6. Pariza, M.W., Ashoor, S.H., Chu, F.S., and Lund, D.B. (1979) Effects of time and temperature on mutagen formation in pan fried hamburger. Cancer Lett. 7:63-69.

7. Pariza, M.W., and Hargraves, W.A. (1985) A beef-derived mutagenesis modulator inhibits initiation of mouse epidermal tumors by 7,12-dimethylbenz[a]anthracene. Carcinogenesis 6:591-593.

8. Pariza, M.W., Loretz, L.J., Storkson, J.M., and Holland, N.C. (1983) Mutagens and modulator on mutagenesis in fried ground beef. Cancer Res. (Suppl.) 43:2444s-2446s.

9. Ramarathnam, N., Osawa, T., Namiki, M., and Kawakishi, S. (1988) Chemical studies on novel rice hull antioxidants. 1. Isolation, fractionation, and partial characterization. J. Agric. Fd. Chem. 36:732-737.

Nutrients and Cancer Prevention K. N. Prasad and F. L. Meyskens, Jr., eds. © 1990 The Humana Press

THE USEFULNESS OF *IN VITRO* ASSAYS AND ANIMAL EXPERIMENTS IN

THE DESIGN OF CHEMOPREVENTIVE PROTOCOLS WITH BETA-CAROTENE

AND VITAMIN A ON TOBACCO CHEWERS

H.F. Stich, S.S. Tsang, B. Palcic

British Columbia Cancer Research Centre
601 West 10th Avenue
Vancouver, B.C. V5Z 1L3, Canada

B. Mathew, R. Sankaranarayanan, M.K. Nair

Regional Cancer Centre
Medical College P.O.
Trivandrum 695011, India

INTRODUCTION

The design of chemopreventive treatments and the selection of protective agents for the control of pre-cancerous lesions or cancers should be based on well-documented scientific data. This approach would require the cooperation of many laboratories with different areas of expertise. Results from studies ranging from molecular biology on the response of oncogenes to the administration of chemopreventive agents to those on the reaction of humans towards dietary supplementation would be required. Such comprehensive information is currently not available for most of the promising chemopreventive agents, including beta-carotene and retinoids. In this paper, we report experiments on cultured cells, animal models, and human populations, which may reveal results required in the decision making process for chemopreventive trials.

WHAT CAN WE LEARN FROM STUDIES OF *IN VITRO* SYSTEMS?

As a rule, the resolution powers of epidemiological methods are not sufficient to uncover particular carcinogens in the complex mixtures of compounds to which man is exposed. Only the introduction of microbiological and tissue culture assays has permitted the rapid detection of chemicals with genotoxic and, by implication, carcinogenic properties. More recently, short-term *in vitro* assays have been designed to identify compounds with a capacity for tumour promotion (Mizuno *et al.*, 1983; Tsang and Stich, 1988; Tsang *et al.*, 1989). The application of assays for chromatid breakage, micronucleus frequencies and cell transformation by bovine papillomavirus (BPV) (Stich and Tsang, 1989) exemplifies such an approach for the detection of compounds involved in carcinogenesis of the oral cavity. Table 1 shows active genotoxic chemicals

Table 1
Induction of chromatid aberrations in CHO cells exposed to various betel quid ingredients for 3 hr

Betel Quid Compounds	Dose	Percent Metaphases with Chromatid Aberrations[a]
Areca nut[b]	3 mg/ml	37.4
Arecoline	400 µg/ml	13.9
Eugenol	200 µg/ml	2.0
Catechin	0.4 mg/ml	21.3
Slaked lime(mollusc shells)	25 mg/ml	0.2
Betel leaf[b]	3 mg/ml	4.0
Tobacco I (India)	12 mg/ml	22.9
Tobacco II (India)	4 mg/ml	29.4
Arecoline + eugenol eugenol	400 µg/ml 200 µg/ml	75.0
Arecoline + chlorogenic acid	400 µg/ml 200 µg/ml	53.1
None(control)		0.3

[a]Chromatid aberrations include breaks and exchanges.

[b]Aqueous extracts from dried areca nut shavings and fresh betel leaf.

found in ingredients of a tobacco-areca nut chewing mixture (Stich *et al.*, 1983; Stich and Rosin, 1985). These tests can also be used to examine enhancing effects when chemicals are applied in pairs (Table 1) (Stich *et al.*, 1981). Furthermore, the BPV transformation assay revealed a relatively strong promoting activity of aqueous areca nut extracts and arecoline, which is the main alkaloid in areca nuts (Fig. 1). It is of interest to note that all the examined compounds appear in the saliva of betel quid chewers (Stich *et al.*, 1983; Stich, 1986a,b), and could thus penetrate directly into the oral mucosa. The application of these bioassays represents only the first step in tracing the chemical nature of the reactive compounds or their metabolites (IARC, 1985).

The *in vitro* bioassays are also suitable for detecting the action of antimutagenic, anticarcinogenic, or antipromoting agents. For example, studies on the inhibitory effect of beta-carotene on chromatid exchanges and micronuclei induced in Chinese hamster ovary (CHO) cells by a 3-hr exposure to methyl methanesulfonate (MMS) has provided results with potentially practical implications (Fig. 2): (a) the dose of beta-carotene used $(3.5 \times 10^{-8}M)$ exerted an inhibitory effect only over a

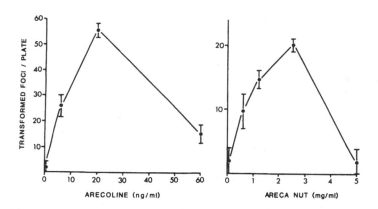

Fig. 1. Enhancement of BPV DNA-induced cell transformation by arecoline and an aqueous extract of areca nut (for experimental outline, see Stich and Tsang, 1989).

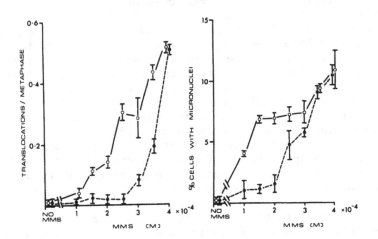

Fig. 2. Frequency of CHO cells with chromatid translo-
cations or micronuclei following exposure to MMS (3 hr)
(o-o) and to MMS plus beta-carotene (3.5 x 10^{-8}M) (o-o)
(for details, see Stich and Dunn, 1986).

restricted range of MMS concentrations; (b) no protective
effect of beta-carotene was obtained at higher doses of
MMS; and (c) the use of different endpoints (chromatid
translocation versus micronuclei) influenced the results
and conclusions (Stich and Dunn, 1986). These results
indicate the importance of using a wide dose range of
chemopreventive agents, which becomes particularly
necessary if the dose range of carcinogens to which man is
exposed is unknown. Results from chemopreventive experiments which are based on only one dose can easily lead to
erroneous conclusions.

Detailed investigations of the action of tumour
promoters which would be difficult to carry out on human
population groups can be performed using the new *in vitro*
assays for promoters (Mizuno *et al.*, 1983; Ohigashi *et
al.*, 1986; Stich and Tsang, 1989; Tsang *et al.*, 1989).
For example, retinol inhibited the formation of foci
transformed by BPV DNA (promoter-independent transformation) as well as those transformed by the combined action
of BPV DNA plus chemical promoter (promoter-dependent
transformation), but it required an approximately tenfold
higher concentration of retinol to obtain this latter

inhibitory effect. If such *in vitro* results are trans-
ferable to human population groups, then an effective
chemopreventive dose should depend on those factors that
initiate and promote carcinogenesis. The second results
of possible interest to clinical trials deal with the
gradual reduction of BPV DNA copies from transformed foci
following treatment with retinoic acid (Tsang *et al.*, 1988;
Li *et al.*, 1988). A "cure" of the transformed phenotype
was obtained only when the BPV DNA copies were eliminated
from the cell. Such cells did not express transformed
properties when retinoic acid treatment was withdrawn.
If the reduction of BPV DNA from the cell population was
only partial, cells that contained BPV DNA formed transformed foci after retinoic acid treatment was terminated.
These results appear to be worth bearing in mind when
retinoids are applied as chemopreventive agents to prevent
the formation or progression of papillomavirus DNA-carrying
human tissues.

USEFULNESS OF ANIMAL MODELS

Extrapolations from *in vitro* systems have been
criticized because of the absence of interplay between
different cell types which may control their behaviour
within a differentiated tissue, and the lack of protective
mechanisms that operate in an organism. In addition, each
tissue and organ may have specific metabolic activation or
inactivation systems for carcinogens, tumour promoters,
anticarcinogens and antipromoters. It therefore appears
prudent to assess the protective as well as the harmful
effects of chemopreventive agents in animal models prior to
their application to human population groups. The
necessity of this approach becomes evident when chromosome
aberrations and necrosis are used as endpoints and hepatocytes of rats as targets for carcinogens and chemopreventive agents (Yee, 1986). Vitamin A-deficient rats (liver
retinol levels less than 43±19 ng/g tissue) showed an
increased sensitivity towards the cytotoxic and genotoxic
action of dimethylnitrosamine (DMN) as compared to control
rats (liver retinol levels of 5.465±2459 ng/g tissue)
(Table 2). This elevated sensitivity was abolished by
supplementation of the vitamin A-deficient diet with vitamin
A (2 mg/kg diet) prior to DMN exposure. However, vitamin A
feeding at higher doses (16 mg/kg diet; supplementation II
in Table 2), which led to an excessive accumulation of

Table 2
Protective and enhancing effects of dietary vitamin A supplementation on the genotoxic
and toxic action of DMN in the livers of vitamin A-deficient rats

DMN (mg/kg)	Number of Rats	Control	Vitamin A Deficiency	Vitamin A Deficiency + Supplementation I[a]	Vitamin A Deficiency + Supplementation II[a]
		Percentage of Hepatocytes with Chromatid Bridges and Fragments			
35	18	10.3±2.1	23.7±5.4	9.3±2.6	29.8±6.6
		Percentage of Necrotic Areas in the Liver			
35	18	0	0.2±0.4	0	3.3±4.3

[a]Supplementation I: vitamin A, 2 mg/kg diet; supplementation II: vitamin A, 16 mg/kg diet. All liver samples were taken after partial hepatectomy.

retinol in the liver (more than 25,000 ng/g tissue),
resulted in an accentuation of the necrotic and genotoxic
action of DMN. These results again show the great
influence of the applied doses of a chemopreventive agent
on the outcome of the experiment. Many of the contradictory results described, which claim either a positive
inhibitory effect of retinoids, no detectable effect, or
even an enhancing action on carcinogenesis, could be due
simply to the use of different doses leading to different
retinoid-carcinogen ratios.

HUMAN POPULATION GROUPS AT ELEVATED RISK FOR ORAL CANCER

Four population groups at elevated risk for oral
cancer were included in the exploratory pilot intervention
trials. They included chewers of tobacco-areca nut mixtures
in Luzon (Philippines) and Kerala (India), snuff dippers
in the Northwest Territories (Canada), and reverse smokers
in Mindoro (Philippines) and Orissa (India). These
particular groups were selected since the cancer-causing
habits were known, tobacco-specific nitrosamines (TSNA)
(Hoffmann and Hecht, 1985) and areca nut-related nitrosamines (Wenke *et al.*, 1984; Nair *et al.*, 1985) can be
measured in the saliva of chewers and snuff dippers
(Brunnemann *et al.*, 1987) and inverted smokers (Stich *et
al.*, unpublished data), the total amount of TSNA carcinogens kept in the oral cavity before the development of oral
leukoplakias and cancer can be calculated, areca nut-
related cancer promoters are becoming known (Stich and
Tsang, 1989), large numbers of chewers, snuff dippers and
inverted smokers are available, oral leukoplakia can be
readily identified and examined during a trial period
(Stich *et al.*, 1984, 1988a,b), and exfoliated mucosal cells
can be repeatedly sampled by non-invasive procedures.

To follow in detail the response of the oral mucosa to
the administration of beta-carotene or vitamin A, a search
for intermediate endpoints was initiated. Micronuclei in
exfoliated cells from different areas of the buccal mucosa,
palate, tongue and gingival groove proved to be an out-
standing marker (Stich, 1987). Based on micronucleated
oral mucosal cells as an intermediate endpoint, the short-
term intervention trials on population groups at elevated
risk for cancer yielded several results of general interest
(Table 3): (a) The frequency of micronucleated mucosal

Table 3
Response of micronucleated buccal mucosal cells of individuals at elevated risk for oral cancer to the administration of vitamin A and beta-carotene for 3 months

Treatment	Dose	Participants (number)	Location	Habit	Cells with Micronuclei (%)	
					Before Treatment[a]	After Treatment
Vitamin A	200,000 IU/wk	Filipinos (24)	Luzon	Betel quid chewers	4.10±0.26	1.59±0.18
Beta-carotene	180 mg/wk	Filipinos (22)	Luzon	Betel quid chewers	3.50±0.26	0.92±0.14
Beta-carotene	180 mg/wk	Indians (26)	Kerala	Betel quid chewers	4.35±0.27	0.86±0.08
Beta-carotene	180 mg/wk	Inuit (23)	Northwest Territories	Snuff dippers	1.97±0.20	0.72±0.09
Beta-carotene + vitamin A	180 mg/wk 150,000 IU/wk	Filipinos (24)	Mindoro	Inverted smokers	2.42±0.16	2.32±0.13
Beta-carotene + vitamin A	180 mg/wk 100,000 IU/wk	Indians (40)	Kerala	Betel quid chewers	4.18±0.22	1.00±0.11
Vitamin A followed by	150,000 IU/wk (14 days) 150,000 IU/mth (2½ mths)	Filipinos (22)	Luzon	Betel quid chewers	4.01±0.19	3.95±0.20

[a]Non-chewers of tobacco and non-smokers (n=120) showed approximately 0.5% of micronucleated oral mucosal cells.

cells was elevated in the oral cavity of individuals engaged in various oral habits, including tobacco-areca nut chewers from the Philippines and India, Inuit snuff dippers, and inverted smokers from the Philippines and India; (b) the twice weekly administration of vitamin A (150,000 or 200,000 IU/week) or beta-carotene (180 mg/week) significantly reduced the frequency of micronucleated cells, whereas vitamin A given for 14 days at a dose of 150,000 IU per week and for an additional $2\frac{1}{2}$ months at a dose of 150,000 IU per month conveyed no protective effect; (c) the administration of beta-carotene (180 mg/week) plus vitamin A (150,000 IU/week) to inverted smokers did not improve the frequency of micronucleated oral mucosal cells, although the same treatment produced a considerable reduction among tobacco-areca nut chewers; and (d) after termination of vitamin A or beta-carotene treatment, the frequency of micronucleated cells gradually rose again, indicating the disappearance of the protective effect. The observation that the same treatment protocol conveyed protection against the formation of micronuclei in the oral mucosa of tobacco-areca nut chewers and snuff dippers (Stich *et al.*, 1985), but failed to have any detectable effect on the oral mucosa of inverted smokers, points to the difficulty of drawing generally applicable conclusions.

Changes in the texture of cell nuclei, which could play a crucial role in the regulation of gene function (Pienta *et al.*, 1989), are worth exploring as possible intermediate markers suitable for following a chemo-preventive treatment (Stich *et al.*, 1989b, 1990). The particular advantage of image analysis of nuclear textures lies in the numerous parameters which can be precisely quantitated. For example, the chromatin distribution pattern of oral mucosal cells was analyzed in tobacco-areca nut chewers prior to and after the administration of vitamin A (200,000 IU/week for 6 months) (Fig. 3). The results shown in Figure 4 exemplify the changes in the variance of intensity. The wide spread in the histogram of chewers (16-1) was greatly reduced (16-2) after administration of vitamin A for 6 months. In the post-treatment period, nuclei with condensed chromatin started to reappear. Four months after withdrawal of vitamin A, the oral mucosa contained nuclei with "normal" textures (16-4A in Fig. 4) and nuclei with a wide spectrum of variance of intensity (16-4B in Fig. 4). Since the formation of nuclei

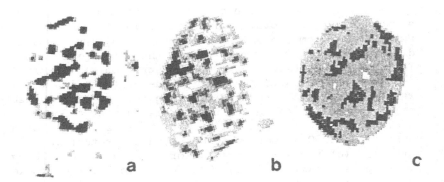

Fig. 3. Digital images of chromatin distribution patterns
in nuclei of an oral leukoplakia of a tobacco-areca nut
chewer prior to (a and b) and after (c) treatment with
vitamin A for 6 months (200,000 IU/week).

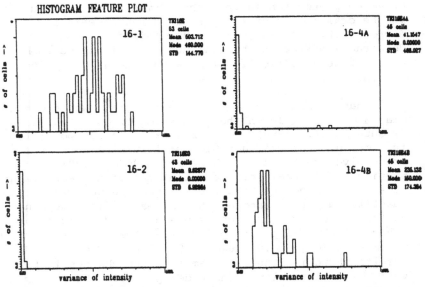

Fig. 4. Histograms showing distribution pattern of
variance of intensity in nuclei of an oral leukoplakia of a
tobacco-areca nut chewer before (16-1) and after (16-2)
treatment with vitamin A for 6 months (200,000 IU/week),
and 4 months post-treatment (16-4A and 16-4B).

with condensed chromatin precedes the development of oral leukoplakia, they could conceivably be used to predict preneoplastic changes.

Oral leukoplakia was our third precancerous endpoint. This lesion appears in various forms and is frequently associated with dysplasia. Since its changes in size and appearance cannot be readily measured, we only recorded its presence and complete remission (Stich *et al.*, 1984, 1988a,b, 1989a). A positive chemoprotective effect could be seen when remission of established leukoplakia was examined, or when the formation of new leukoplakia was counted during the trial period (Table 4). The high frequency of remission is particularly noteworthy since the trial participants continued to chew and were thus continuously exposed to the carcinogens and promoters released by the chewing mixture. The results are comparable to those of Hong *et al.* (1986), who obtained the regression of oral leukoplakias with 13-*cis*-retinoic acid in patients who, at the time of treatment, were not exposed to any known carcinogens or cancer promoters.

Table 4
Response of oral leukoplakias of tobacco-areca nut chewers (Kerala, India) to the administration of chemopreventive agents for 6 months

Treatment	Number of Participants	Individuals with	
		Remission	New Leukoplakia
Placebo	33	1(3.0%)	7(21.2%)
Beta-carotene (180 mg/wk)	27	4(14.8%)	4(14.8%)
Vitamin A (100,000 IU/wk) + beta-carotene (180 mg/wk)	51	14(27.5%)	4(7.8%)
Vitamin A (200,000 IU/wk)	21	12(57.1%)	0(0.0%)

OUTLOOK

Studies on different test systems may contribute to our understanding of issues which cannot be readily analyzed through clinical trials on human population groups, but which could be of paramount importance in the design of chemopreventive protocols. Currently, there is a tendency to administer relatively high doses of retinoids which produce undesirable side-effects. On the other hand, epidemiological evidence points to the protective effect of low dietary doses of beta-carotene or vitamin A. This discrepancy is probably due to numerous, still unknown factors that can influence the efficacy of a chemopreventive agent. For example, the *in vitro* experiments demonstrated a protective effect of beta-carotene over a restricted dose range of a genotoxic carcinogenic agent. Thus in the human situation, any search for a protective dose must take into account exposure levels to carcinogens or promoters. In addition, the type of carcinogenic agents to which an individual is exposed must be considered. Beta-carotene proved to be protective against MMS, but did not exert any detectable inhibitory effect against the free radical forming tannic acid, gallic acid and H_2O_2 (Stich and Dunn, 1986). Studies using the BPV DNA transformation assay revealed a suppressing effect of retinoids on BPV DNA-induced formation of transformed colonies. However, an approximately tenfold higher dose was required to achieve a comparable suppression of transformation when BPV DNA plus chemical promoter were used as inducing agents. Moreover, the degree of sensitivity of cell cultures towards the inhibitory effect of retinoids depended on the time after transfection with BPV DNA (Tsang and Stich, 1988). These results again point to the necessity of knowing those factors which are involved in the cancer-causing events before a treatment protocol can be placed on a scientific basis. Considering the large number of factors influencing the protective dose levels, it may be that a chemopreventive protocol must be designed for each human group at risk for a particular cancer and exposed to particular cancer-causing agents.

ACKNOWLEDGEMENTS

These studies were supported by grants from the National Cancer Institute of Canada. Dr H.F. Stich is a Terry Fox Cancer Research Scientist of the National Cancer Institute of Canada. Dr S.S. Tsang is a Research Scholar of the Medical Research Council of Canada.

REFERENCES

Brunnemann, K.D., Hornby, A.P. & Stich, H.F. Tobacco-specific nitrosamines in the saliva of Inuit snuff dippers in the Northwest Territories of Canada. Cancer Lett. 37: 7-16 (1987).

Hoffmann, D. & Hecht, S.S. Nicotine-derived N-nitrosamines and tobacco-related cancer: current status and future directions. Cancer Res. 45: 935-944 (1985).

Hong, W.K., Endicott, J., Itri, L.M., Doos, W., Batsakis, J.G., Bell, R., Fofonoff, S., Byers, R., Atkinson, E.N., Vaughan, C., Toth, B.B., Kramer, A., Dimery, I.W., Skipper, P. & Strong, S. 13-*cis*-Retinoic acid in the treatment of oral leukoplakia. New Engl. J. Med. 315: 1501-1505 (1986).

IARC. Monographs on the Evaluation of the Carcinogenic Risk of Chemicals to Humans, Vol. 37, Tobacco Habits Other than Smoking; Betel-Nut and Areca-Nut Chewing; and Some Related Nitrosamines, International Agency for Research on Cancer, Lyon (1985).

Li, G., Tsang, S.S. & Stich, H.F. Changes in DNA copy numbers of bovine papillomavirus type 1 after termination of retinoic acid treatment. J. Natl. Cancer Inst. 80: 1567-1570 (1988).

Mizuno, F., Koizumi, S., Osato, T., Kokwaro, J.O. & Ito, Y. Chinese and African *Euphorbiaceae* plant extracts: markedly enhancing effect on Epstein-Barr virus-induced transformation. Cancer Lett. 19: 199-205 (1983).

Nair, J., Ohshima, H., Friesen, M., Croisy, A., Bhide, S.V. & Bartsch, H. Tobacco-specific and betel nut-specific N-nitroso compounds: occurrence in saliva and urine of betel quid chewers and formation *in vitro* by nitrosation of betel quid. Carcinogenesis 6: 295-303 (1985).

Ohigashi, H., Takamura, H., Koshimizu, K., Tokuda, H. & Ito, Y. Search for possible antitumor promoters by inhibition of 12-O-tetradecanoylphorbol-13-acetate-induced Epstein-Barr virus activation; ursolic acid and oleanolic acid from an anti-inflammatory Chinese medicinal plant, *Glechoma hederaceae L.* Cancer Lett. 30: 143-151 (1986).

Pienta, K.J., Partin, A.W. & Coffey, D.S. Cancer as a disease of DNA organization and dynamic cell structure. Cancer Res. 49: 2525-2532 (1989).

Stich, H.F. The use of micronuclei in tracing the genotoxic damage in the oral mucosa of tobacco users. In: Mechanisms in Tobacco Carcinogenesis, D. Hoffmann & C.C. Harris (eds), Banbury Report 23, Cold Spring Harbor Laboratory, Cold Spring Harbor, N.Y., pp. 99-111 (1986a).

Stich, H.F. Reducing the genotoxic damage in the oral mucosa of betel quid/tobacco chewers. In: Antimutagenesis and Anticarcinogenesis Mechanisms, D.M. Shankel, P.E. Hartman, T. Kada & A. Hollaender (eds), Plenum Press, New York, pp. 381-391 (1986b).

Stich, H.F. Micronucleated exfoliated cells as indicators for genotoxic damage and as markers in chemoprevention trials. J. Nutrit. Growth Cancer 4: 9-18 (1987).

Stich, H.F. & Dunn, B.P. Relationship between cellular levels of beta-carotene and sensitivity to genotoxic agents. Int. J. Cancer 38: 713-717 (1986).

Stich, H.F. & Rosin, M.P. Towards a more comprehensive evaluation of a genotoxic hazard in man. Mutation Res. 150: 43-50 (1985).

Stich, H.F. & Tsang, S.S. Promoting activity of betel quid ingredients and their inhibition by retinol. Cancer Lett. 45: 71-77 (1989).

Stich, H.F., Stich, W. & Lam, P.P.S. Potentiation of genotoxicity by concurrent application of compounds found in betel quid: arecoline, eugenol, quercetin, chlorogenic acid and Mn^{++}. Mutation Res. 90: 355-363 (1981).

Stich, H.F., Bohm, B.A., Chatterjee, K. & Sailo, J.L. The role of saliva-borne mutagens and carcinogens in the etiology of oral and esophageal carcinomas of betel nut and tobacco chewers. In: Carcinogens and Mutagens in the Environment, Vol. III, Naturally Occurring Compounds: Epidemiology and Distribution, H.F. Stich (ed.), CRC Press, Boca Raton, FL, pp. 43-58 (1983).

Stich, H.F., Stich, W., Rosin, M.P. & Vallejera, M.O. Use of the micronucleus test to monitor the effect of vitamin A, beta-carotene and canthaxanthin on the buccal mucosa of betel nut/tobacco chewers. Int. J. Cancer 34: 745-750 (1984).

Stich, H.F., Hornby, A.P. & Dunn, B.P. A pilot beta-carotene intervention trial with Inuits using smokeless tobacco. Int. J. Cancer 36: 321-327 (1985).

Stich, H.F., Hornby, A.P., Mathew, B., Sankaranarayanan, R. & Krishnan Nair, M. Response of oral leukoplakias to the administration of vitamin A. Cancer Lett. 40: 93-101 (1988a).

Stich, H.F., Rosin, M.P., Hornby, A.P., Mathew, B., Sankaranarayanan, R. & Krishnan Nair, M. Remission of oral leukoplakias and micronuclei in tobacco/betel quid chewers treated with beta-carotene and with beta-carotene plus vitamin A. Int. J. Cancer 42: 195-199 (1988b).

Stich, H.F., Mathew, B., Sankaranarayanan, R. & Krishnan Nair, M. Remission of oral precancerous lesions of tobacco/areca nut chewers following administration of beta-carotene or vitamin A, and maintenance of the protective effect. Cancer Detect. Prev., in press (1989a).

Stich, H.F., Acton, A.B. & Palcic, B. Towards an automated micronucleus assay as an internal dosimeter for carcinogen-exposed human population groups. Recent Results Cancer Res., in press (1989b).

Stich, H.F., Palcic, B., Sankaranarayanan, R., Mathew, B. & Krishnan Nair, M. Quantitation of chromatin patterns by image analysis as a predictive tool in chemopreventive trials with vitamin A. In: Experimental and Epidemiologic Applications to Risk Assessment of Complex Mixtures, IARC Sci. Publ., International Agency for Research on Cancer, Lyon, in press (1990).

Tsang, S.S. & Stich, H.F. Enhancement of bovine papillomavirus-induced cell transformation by tumour promoters. Cancer Lett. 43: 93-98 (1988).

Tsang, S.S., Li, G. & Stich, H.F. Effect of retinoic acid on bovine papillomavirus (BPV) DNA-induced transformation and number of BPV DNA copies. Int. J. Cancer 42: 94-98 (1988).

Tsang, S.S., Stich, H.F. & Fujiki, H. Cell transformation induced by bovine papillomavirus DNA as an assay for tumour promoters and chemopreventive agents. Cancer Detect. Prev., in press (1989).

Wenke, G., Brunnemann, K.D., Hoffmann, D. & Bhide, S.V.
A study of betel quid carcinogenesis. IV. Analysis of
the saliva of betel chewers: a preliminary report.
J. Cancer Res. Clin. Oncol. 108: 110-113 (1984).

Yee, G.A. The protective effect of beta-carotene and
vitamin A on genotoxicity and cytotoxicity of dimethylnitrosamine in vitamin A-deficient rats. M.Sc. Thesis,
The University of British Columbia, Vancouver, B.C.
(1986).

Nutrients and Cancer Prevention K. N. Prasad and F. L. Meyskens, Jr., eds. © 1990 The Humana Press

DIETARY MODULATION OF TOBACCO-SPECIFIC CARCINOGEN

ACTIVATION

Castonguay, A., Pepin, P., Alaoui-Jamali, M.A.
and Rossignol, G.
Laboratory of Cancer Etiology and Chemoprevention
School of Pharmacy, Laval University, Quebec
City, G1K 7P4, Canada

INTRODUCTION

More than 85% of all lung cancer cases are associated
to cigarette smoking (1). Among the 3800 different compounds present in cigarette smoke, 50 of them have been identified as animal carcinogens (2). The N-nitrosamine, 4-
(methylnitrosamino)-1-(3-pyridyl)-1-butanone (NNK) derived
from nicotine during the curing and burning of tobacco is
abundant in cigarette smoke (3). This N-nitrosamine has a
remarkable organospecificity for lung tissues. Lung tumors are induced by this N-nitrosamine in rodents whether
it is injected s. c., applied topically or by swabbing the
oral mucosa (3). These results suggest that NNK could be a
tobacco component involved in human pulmonary carcinogenesis. In chemoprevention studies, this N-nitrosamine provides not only an excellent model of lung carcinogenesis,
but it is also a carcinogen ubiquitous in the human environment. Numerous epidemiological studies have concluded
that vegetable consumption was associated with reduced
lung cancer risk (4). The aim of our research program is
to investigate how vegetables and fruits nutrients can inhibit pulmonary carcinogenesis induced by NNK in experimental animals.

135

MATERIALS AND METHODS

Chemicals

NNK was synthesized as previously described and was more than 98.5% pure (5). Canadian food grade 2(3)-tert-butyl-4-hydroxyanisole (BHA) (TENOX) was a generous gift from Dr Frank Iverson (Health and Welfare Canada, Ottawa, Ont. Canada). TENOX contains 93.3% 3-BHA, 6.5% 2-BHA and 0.1% tert-butyl-1,4dimethoxybenzene.

Diets

Powdered AIN-76A diet was purchased from ICN Biochemicals (Cleveland, OH) and was used within 8 weeks of shipment. Mixtures of diet and chemopreventive agents were prepared every week.

Mutagenicity assay

Mutagenicity was assayed with exponentially growing His⁻ *Salmonella Typhimurium* TA 1535, using the standard plate incorporation assay (6). The activating system was prepared by 9000 g centrifugation of F344 rat liver homogenate. The NADPH generating system was prepared and the pH adjusted to 6.5 as described (7). The liquid phase S9 mix (0.85 ml) was preincubated with NNK (18.8 nM) and with DMSO or inhibitors dissolved in DMSO, for 30 min. and then mixed with 2ml of top agar before pouring it onto minimal agar plates (100 x 20 mm). Revertants were counted after incubation at 37° for 48 hours. The numbers of revertants with and without inhibitors were compared with Student't test.

Culture of lung explants and assay of NNK metabolites and DNA methylation.

Syrian golden hamsters were sacrificed by CO_2 asphyxiation and lung explants were excised and cultured as described previously (8,9). The explants were cultured in Minimum Essential Medium for 20 hours with or without ellagic acid (EA) (100 μM). Media were then replaced with media containing EA (100 μM) and [5-^{3}H] NNK (3.7 μM) or [5-^{3}H] NNK alone. Media and explants were harvested after 3 hours of culture. NNK and its metabolites were separated by reverse phase HPLC as described previously (10). More than 90% of the radioactivity added to the culture medium as [5-^{3}H] NNK was recovered after explant culture. All the radioactivity injected onto the chromatographic column was recovered. Amounts of protein in the lung explants were assayed according to the method of Lowry et al. (11). The effects of ellagic acid on methylation of DNA was assayed as follow. Sixty-four lung explants were cultured with or without EA (100 μM) in 4 ml of medium (16 explants/dish) for 20 hours. The explants were then cultured with [CH$_3$-^{3}H] NNK (20.6 μM, 1.2 Ci/mmol) and EA (100 μM) for 3 hours. DNA was extracted as described previously (9,12). The DNA sample was dissolved in 200 ml of 0.9% NaCl and combined with a mixture of 3-methyladenine (9.6 μg), 7-methylguanine (3.0 μg), and O^6-methylguanine (200 μg) dissolved in 580 μl of water. After adding 79 μl of 1N HCl, the mixture was incubated at 70o for 30 min. Then, the mixture was cooled to 0o and the pH was adjusted to 4.5 with 1N NaOH (~ 80 μl). A 500 μl aliquot was injected onto a μBondapak-C$_{18}$ column and eluted as described by Milligan et al. (13). Fractions of one ml were collected and radioactivity measured by liquid scintillation. The retention times were 10.2 (guanine), 19.3 (7-methylguanine) and 24.4 min (O^6-methylguanine).

Lung adenoma assay in A/J mice

Female A/J mice (6 to 7 weeks old) were caged in groups of 5. They were fed powdered AIN-76A diet *ad libitum* starting 2 weeks before carcinogen treatment and throughout the experiment. Diet consumption and wasting was monitored five times before carcinogen treatment. Stock solutions of NNK were prepared in distilled water (11 mg/ml) and diluted in tap water. The initial concentration of NNK was 62.4 μg/ml. It was thereafter adjusted for each cage according to water consumption. During carcinogen treatment, water consumption was monitored twice a week. Details of the treatment with NNK and with the chemopreventive agents are included in Table 4. The first group (negative control) received the diet without chemopreventive agent or NNK and was given tap water, *ad libitum*.

The second group received NNK only. The four other groups were given NNK and the chemopreventive agents. A similar profile of NNK administration was obtained by adjusting the concentrations of NNK in the drinking water. All mice were sacrificed by CO_2 asphyxiation and necropsied 16 weeks after the end of carcinogen treatment. Liver specimen were frozen and ten µ sections were stained with Sudan 4. The lungs and major organs were fixed in Tellyksniczky's fluid for 7 days before counting the number of surface adenomas under a dissecting microscope. Statistical evaluation of the multiplicities was achieved by analysis of variance, logarithmic transformations of the values and Fisher test. Incidences of tumors were compared with Chi square test.

Isolation and culture of hepatocytes

Male F344 rats, 6 to 8 weeks old were anaesthesized with ether and hepatocytes were isolated by a two step collagenase perfusion and then purified by Percoll gradient centrifugation as described previously (14). A viability of more than 90% was observed, as measured by trypan blue exclusion. The hepatocytes were washed once with α−minimum essential medium to remove dead cells before exposure to the chemicals. Freshly isolated hepatocytes (2×10^6) were suspended in 2 ml of α−minimum essential medium containing [5-^{3}H] NNK (5 µCi/ml) and incubated under an atmosphere of 5% CO_2 and 95% air. Incubations were carried out in 60 x 15 mm culture dishes. Cells were pelleted by centrifugation (9000 g, 10 min.) and the supernatants were removed. Cells treated with boiling water prior to incubation with [5-^{3}H] NNK, were used as negative controls. NNK metabolites released from the hepatocytes into the medium were assayed as described above.

Sister chromatid exchanges (SCEs)

SCEs assay was performed on V79 cell line maintained in coculture with primary rat hepatocytes as an exogenous activating system. NNK-treated and control cells were incubated with 5-bromodeoxyuridine (5 µg/ml) for 28 hours, including 2 hours with colchicine (5 µg/ml). Cells were then harvested and slides prepared and scored for SCEs as previously described (15).

TABLE 1

<u>Inhibition of NNK mutagenicity in S. Thyphimurium (TA 1535)</u>
<u>by ellagic acid, curcumin and SKF-525A</u>

Inhibitor (nmol/dish)	Microsome (mg of protein)	His$^+$ revertants/ plates (Mean ± S.D.)*	% Inhibition (P)
None	1.8	480 ± 45	
Acide ellagique (800)	1.8	335 ± 42	30% (< 0.05)
Curcumin (160)	1.8	438 ± 46	N.S.**
None	1.4	346 ± 18	
SKF-525A (100)	1.4	234 ± 24	32% (< 0.005)

* n = 3: The numbers indicated do not include spontaneous revertants.

** N.S.: Not different from corresponding control.

RESULTS AND DISCUSSION

S. Thyphimurium was used to measure the capacity of some polyphenols to inhibit the activation of NNK to mutagenic intermediates. EA is a polyphenol present in soft fruits and vegetables such as grapes, strawberries, raspberries and some nuts regularly consumed by humans (16). As indicated in Table 1, EA was effective in inhibiting the activation of NNK. A 30% reduction in the number of revertants was achieved with 800 nmol EA/dish. In contrast, curcumin, a polyphenolic colorant isolated from *Curcuma*

TABLE 2

Effects of ellagic acid on the metabolism of NNK by
hamster lung explants

Groups	Metabolites (nnol/mg protein)		
	α-C hydroxylation	N-oxidation	NNA1
NNK (3.7 μM)	2.1 ± 0.7*	1.6 ± 0.3	1.0 ± 0.5
NNK (3.7 μM) +EA (100 μM)	1.7 ± 0.2	1.5 ± 0.1	1.0 ± 0.1

* Mean ± S.D. of 3 determinations.

** The difference between the means for the two treatments
is significant with $P < 0.05$.

longa, was ineffective. We observed that SKF-525A which
is a specific inhibitor of cytochrome P-450 monooxygenases
can reduce the mutagenicity of NNK. These enzymes, which
can activate various N-nitrosamines (17), are most likely
involved in the activation of NNK. Considering that mutagenicity and carcinogenicity of N-nitrosamines are well
correlated (18), these results are suggesting that EA could
be an effective inhibitor of NNK-induced carcinogenesis.

The modulation of NNK metabolism by EA has been studied with hamster lung explants. As shown in Table 2 and
Figure 1; lung tissues metabolize NNK by α-carbon hydroxylation, pyridine N-oxidation and carbonyl reduction.
α-Carbon hydroxylations are producing electrophilic intermediates which alkylate DNA and are consequently considered
activation pathways. The four metabolites 12, 13, 14, and
15, resulting from these oxidative pathways and released
in the culture medium. Pyridine N-oxidation yield the po-
lar metabolites 1 and 2. There is some indications that
the enzymes involved in these pathways are deactivating
NNK (10). Our results demonstrated that EA was inhibiting
the activation of NNK by α-carbon hydroxylation (Table 2).

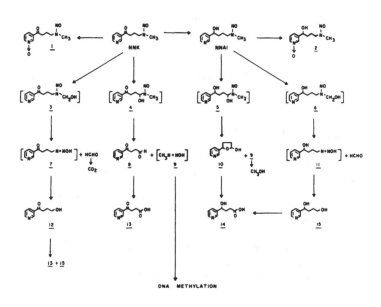

FIGURE 1:   Metabolic transformations of NNK.   Structures
in brackets are hypothetical intermediates.

TABLE 3

Effects of EA on methylation of lung explant DNA by NNK

Treatment	$\dfrac{O^6\text{-MeGua}}{\text{Gua}}$	$\dfrac{7\text{-MeGua}}{\text{Gua}}$	$\dfrac{O^6\text{-MeGua}}{7\text{-MeGua}}$
NNK (20.5 μM)	13.5 ± 1.5*	123 ± 17	0.11
NNK (20.6 μM) +EA (100 μM)	11.9 ± 1.9**	95 ± 10**	0.12

* Mean ± S.D. obtained from 10 determinations.

** The differences between the means for the two treatments are significant with $P < 0.05$ (O^6-MeGua/ Gua) and $P < 0.001$ (7-MeGua/Gua).

Methyldiazohydroxide 9 is an electrophilic intermediate generated during this activation (Figure 1) and can methylate DNA at the O^6-guanine and 7-guanine sites of DNA (19). The resulting O^6-methylguanine was miscoding during DNA replication and can activate oncogene (20,21). We observed that EA was protecting both O^6-guanine and 7-guanine sites of DNA (Table 3). Our results contrast with those of Dixit and Gold (22) who observed selective EA protection of the O^6-guanine site of salmon sperm DNA treated with N-methyl-N-nitrosourea. Results shown in table 3 are reflecting more an inhibition of NNK activation than a shielding of the DNA by EA as proposed by Dixit and Gold (22). Metabolism of NNK was studied in lung explants excised from hamsters who were fed a control diet or a diet supplemented with EA for two weeks. There was no difference in the levels of activation or deactivation of NNK, suggesting that chronic feeding with EA does not induce the enzymes involved in the metabolism of NNK (9).

The chemopreventive efficacy of EA, BHA, β-carotene + retinol and selenium was compared in A/J mice. NNK was administered in the drinking water during a 7 weeks period.

TABLE 4

Chemopreventive efficacies of ellagic acid, butylated
hydroxyanisole, β-carotene + all-trans-retinol

Chemopreventive agent (g/kg diet)	Total dose of NNK (mg/mouse)	Number of mice with tumors/ surviving mice	Number of tumors/ surviving mice ± S.E.
None (control -)	None	6/24	0.4 ± 0.1
None (control +)	9.2	28/28	15.7 ± 2.7
Ellagic acid (4)	9.4	24/25	7.5 ± 1.1*
2(3)-BHA (5)	9.1	13/19*	1.9 ± 0.4*
β-Carotene/ Retinol (2.14/0.009)	9.1	24/24	12.7 ± 3.1
Selenium (0.0022)	9.1	24/25	12.3 ± 2.5

* Different from control + ; $P < 0.01$.

This was the first time that this route was used to administer NNK to this species. It has the advantage of better
mimicking the almost continuous exposure of the smoker to
small quantities of this carcinogen. We have estimated
that the daily dose of NNK was 0.19 μg/day. We observed
that EA was inhibiting the multiplicity of lung adenomas
by 52% but not the number of tumor bearing animals (Table
4). Our results are similar to those of Lesca (23) who
treated A/J mice with benzo(a)pyrene (100 mg/Kg b.w) and
EA (100 mg/Kg b.w.). EA reduced the tumor multiplicity
by 53% but had no effect on the number of tumor-bearing
mice. Studies by Teel et al. (24) suggest that the chemo-

TABLE 5

Inhibition of NNK metabolism in rat hepatocytes by all-
trans-retinol*

Retinol Concentration (μM)	Metabolites (nM)		
	Keto acid	α-Carbon hydroxylation	Pyridine N-oxidation
0	135.6 ± 11.5**	156.8 ± 21.1	39.7 ± 25.2
0.18	115.2 ± 13.2	126.5 ± 13.8	21.8 ± 2.6
1.76	62.4 ± 28.5	77.2 ± 39.8	28.2 ± 22.3
3.52	59.1 ± 23.8	73.3 ± 33.8	24.6 ± 17.2
17.58	36.4 ± 16.1	50.3 ± 30.6	22.6 ± 20.0
35.16	28.6 ± 14.9	39.4 ± 26.3	14.2 ± 10.5

* Initial concentration of NNK was 2.27 μM.

** Mean ± S.D. (n = 3).

protective activity of EA is due to an inhibition of benzo
[a]pyrene activation to metabolites binding to DNA. Reduction of pulmonary cytochrome P-450 levels by chronic oral
feeding of EA as reported by Das et al. (25) further support our hypothesis that EA is protecting pulmonary tissues
by inhibiting P-450 mono-oxygenases involved in the activation of NNK. On-going investigations will determine if EA
has an anti-promoting activity.

BHA consumption in Canada is estimated to vary between
5.5 and 12.1 mg/person/day (26). In this study, we have

TABLE 6

Induction of SCEs in V79 cells cocultured with rat
hepatocytes and exposed to NNK

NNK (mM)	Retinol (mM)	SCEs frequency/chromosome
None (0.5% DMSO)		0.213 ± 0.012
None (0.5% DMSO)	0.070	0.220 ± 0.020
1	None	0.230 ± 0.035
1	0.070	0.225 ± 0.006
5	None	0.410 ± 0.027
5	0.070	0.340 ± 0.027
10	None	0.573 ± 0.129
10	0.070	0.458 ± 0.032
20	None	0.733 ± 0.106
20	0.070	0.570 ± 0.066
40	None	0.757 ± 0.215
40	0.070	0.635 ± 0.070

* Mean ± S.E. from 2 experiments and 30 metaphases per
experiment.

observed that the number of tumor bearing mice and the number of tumors per mouse was reduced significantly by BHA
treatment (Table 4). Previous studies have shown BHA was
inhibiting pulmonary carcinogenesis induced in A/J mice by
many chemical carcinogens including N-nitrosodimethylamine,
N-nitrosodiethylamine and benzo[a]pyrene (27,28,29). The
mechanism of chemoprotection by BHA has been studied extensively. BHA treatment increases phase II enzymes such as
glutathione-S-transferases but also increases hepatic metabolism of N-nitrosamines (29). Current understanding of
N-nitrosamine carcinogenesis suggest that glutathione con-

TABLE 7

Inhibition of NNK-induced SCEs in V79 cells cocultured
with rat hepatocytes by all-trans-retinol

NNK (mM)	Retinol (mM)	SCEs frequency/ chromosome
None	0.070	0.220 ± 0.020
20	0.017	0.638 ± 0.126
20	0.034	0.645 ± 0.024
20	0.070	0.443 ± 0.046
20	0.139	0.328 ± 0.024

* Mean ± S.E. from 2 experiments and 30 metaphases
  per experiment.

jugation does not play a role in the scavenging of reactive intermediates derived from N-nitrosamines (30).
Chronic feeding of mice with BHA supplemented diet increases hepatic P-450 enzymes but does not alter the levels
of P-450 reductases (31). Although BHA is also an inhibitor of mono-oxygenases, (32), our results and those of
Chung et al.(29) do not suggest that this inhibition is
responsible for the chemoprotection observed in this study.
Induction of hepatic metabolism by BHA treatment is likely
to reduce the exposure of pulmonary tissues to NNK. A similar mechanism was proposed by Morse et al. (33) who observed a chemoprotection of pulmonary carcinogenesis in
mice treated with NNK and indole-3-carbinol. Adding extra
selenium (2.2 mg sodium selenite/Kg diet) to AIN-76A diet
containing 0.35 mg selenium/Kg did not reduce the incidence or multiplicity of lung adenomas induced by NNK.

    Prospective and retrospective studies have suggested
that low intake of vegetables and fruits rich in carot-

enoids were associated to increased lung cancer risk (reviewed by Ziegler, 34). Chemoprotection by β-carotene would not require its conversion to retinol. The combination of β-carotene and retinol in chemoprevention interventions has been suggested by Goodman et al. (35). Mehta et al. (36) reported that retinol or β-carotene administered singly in the diet were not preventing N-nitrosodiethylamine-induced carcinogenesis in Syrian golden hamster. In contrast, a combination of β-carotene and retinol significantly reduced the number of lung adenosquamous carcinoma induced by this N-nitrosamine. We observed that this regimen was not protecting lung tissues from NNK induced carcinogenesis in A/J mice (Table 4).

The effects of retinol on the metabolism of NNK was studied in freshly isolated hepatocytes. Retinol inhibited the formation of the keto acid 13 which is the major metabolite generated by α-carbon hydroxylation of NNK (Table 5). We used the sum of the metabolites 12, 13, 14, and 15, as an index of total α-carbon hydroxylation of NNK. This index was reduced by 50% when hepatocytes were cultured with 1.76 μM retinol. In contrast, total pyridine-N-oxidation as measured by the sum of the metabolites 1 and 2 was reduced by only 29%. These results suggest that retinol could inhibit the initiation of carcinogenesis by NNK. Previous studies have demonstrated that retinol inhibits the mutagenicity (37, 38) and SCEs (39,40) induced by several procarcinogens including N-nitrosodimethylamine and N-nitrosodiethylamine. Huang et al. (30) have proposed that retinol inhibits selectively some forms of cytochrome P-450. Previous results from this laboratory suggested that cytochrome P-450 are involved, not only in the α-carbon hydroxylation, but also in the pyridine-N-oxidation of NNK (40). Thus, retinol would inhibit preferentially the isozymes involved in the α-carbon hydroxylation of NNK. We have observed that inhibition of NNK activation resulted in a reduction of SCEs induced in V79 cells. (Tables 6 and 7).

CONCLUSIONS

Results from this study and those of Lesca (23) strongly suggest that EA could be effective in preventing the development of cancer induced by tobacco carcinogens. Our results extend previous observations that EA is a versatile and non-toxic anticarcinogen effective against a wide range

of chemical carcinogens. Future experimental studies
should focus on the efficacy of EA as antipromoter. Considering that EA is well tolerated by humans (41) its application in chemoprevention interventions should be considered. The food antioxidant BHA is a good inhibitor of pulmonary carcinogenesis induced by NNK. Future studies
should determine if this inhibition results from an induction of hepatic metabolism. Retinol inhibits more effectively the activation that the deactivation pathways of
NNK. This inhibition results in a dose-dependent reduction
of the genotoxicity of NNK. These data are contributing to
a better understanding of the role nutrients in preventing
carcinogenesis assosiated with tobacco smoking.

ACKNOWLEDGMENTS

The technical assistances of Carole Bergeron, Francine
Giguère and Lili Liu are appreciated. This study was sup-
ported by grants from NCI (Canada) and the Cancer Research
Society Inc.

REFERENCES

1. United States Department of Health and Human Services.
The Health Consequences of Smoking. Cancer. USPHS Publication No 82-50179, p. 322 Washington, DC: Government Printing Office, 1982.

2- Hoffmann, D., Schmeltz, I., Hecht, S.S. and Wynder,
E.L.: Tobacco carcinogenesis. In: H.V. Gelboin and
P.O. Ts'o (eds). Polycyclic Hydrocarbons and Cancer
Vol. 1 pp. 85-117, New York: Academic Press Inc. 1978.

3. Hecht, S.S. and Hoffmann,D. Tobacco-specific nitrosamines, an important group of carcinogens in tobacco
and tobacco smoke. Carcinogenesis, 9: 875-884, 1988.

4. Byers, T.E., Graham, S. Haughey, B.P. Marsshall, J.R.
and Swanson, M.K. Diet and lung cancer risk: finding
from the western New York diet study. Am. J. Epidemio.
125: 351-363, 1987.

5. Hecht, S.S., Chen, C.B., Dong, M., Ornaf, R.M., Hoffmann, D. and Tso, T.C. Studies on non-volatile nitrosamines in tobacco. Beitr. Tabakforsch., 9: 1-6, 1977.

6. Maron, D.M., and Ames, B. N. Revised methods for the Salmonella mutagenicity test. Mutat. Res., 113: 173-215, 1983.

7. Guttenplan, J.B. Enhanced mutagenic activities of N-nitroso compounds in weakly acidic media. Carcinogenesis,. 1: 439-444, 1980.

8. Mossman, B.T. and Craighead, J.E.. Use of hamster tracheal organ cultures for assessing the cocarcinogenic effects of inorganic particulates on the respiratory epithelium. Prog. Exp. Tumor Res. 24: 37-47, 1979.

9. Castonguay, A., Allaire, L., Charest, M., Rossignol, G. and Boutet, M. Metabolism of 4-(methylnitrosamino)-1-(3-pyridyl)-1-butanone by hamster respiratory tissues cultured with ellagic acid. Cancer Lett. (In press).

10. Castonguay, A., Lin, D., Stoner, G.D., Radok, P., Furuya, K., Hecht, S.S., Schut, H.A.G. and Klaunig, J.E. Comparative carcinogenecicity in A/J mice and metabolism by cultured mouse peripheral lung of N'-nitrosonornicotine, 4-(methylnitrosamino)-1-(3-pyridyl)-1-butanone and their analogues. Cancer Res. 43: 1223-1229, 1983.

11. Lowry, O.H., Rosebrough, N.J., Farr, L., and Randall, R.J. Protein measurement with the folin phenol reagent. J. Biol. Chem., 193: 265-275, 1951.

12. Daoud, A.H., and Irving, C.C. Methylation of DNA in rat liver and intestine by dimethylnitrosamine and N-methylnitrosourea. Chem.-Biol. Interact., 16: 135-143, 1977.

13. Milligan, J.R., Hirani-Hojatti, S., Catz-Biro, L., and Archer, M.C. Methylation of DNA by three N-nitrosocompounds. Evidence for a common methylating intermediate. Chem-Biol. Interact., (In Press).

14. Bradley, M.O. and Sina, J.S. Methods for detecting
     carcinogens and mutagens with the alkaline elution/
     rat hepatocyte assay. In "Handbook of mutagenicity
     test procedures". Second edition B.J. Kilbey, M.
     Legator, W. Nichols and C. Ramel (eds) Elsevier
     Science Publishers BV1984, pp 71-82, 1984.

15. Alaoui-Jamali, M.A., Lasne, C., Antonakis, K. and
     Chouroulinkov, I. Absence of genotoxic effects in
     cells exposed to four ketonucleoside derivatives. Mu-
     tagenesis, 6: 411-417, 1986.

16. Bate-Smith, E.C. Detection and determination of el-
     lagitannins. Phytochemistry, 11: 1153-1156, 1972.

17. Yang, C.S. Tu, Y.Y. Koop, D.R. and Coon, M.J. Meta-
     bolism of nitrosamines by purified rabbit liver cyto-
     chrome P-450 isozymes. Cancer Res., 45: 1140-1145,
     1985.

18. Guttenplan, J.B. N.-Nitrosamines: bacterial mutagene-
     sis and *in vitro* metabolism. Mutat. Res., 186: 81-
     134, 1987.

19. Hecht, S.S. and Hoffmann, D. Tobacco-specific nitro-
     samines, an important group of carcinogens in tobacco
     and tobacco smoke. Carcinogenesis, 9: 875-884, 1988.

20. Loechler, E.L., Green, C.L. and Essigman, J.M. *In vivo*
     mutagenesis by O^6-methylguanine built into a unique
     site in a viral genome. Proc. Ntl. Acad. Sci. USA, 81,
     6271-6275, 1984.

21. Barbacid, M. Oncogenes and human cancer: cause or
     consequence? Carcinogenesis, 7: 1037-1042, 1986.

22- Dixit, R. and Gold, B. Inhibition of N-Methyl-N-nitro-
     sourea-induced mutagenicity and DNA methylation by el-
     lagic acid. Proc. Ntl. Acad. Sci. USA 83: 8039-8043,
     1986.

23. Lesca, P. Protective effects of ellagic acid and other
     plant phenols on benzo[a]pyrene-induced neoplasia in
     mice. Carcinogenesis, 4: 1651-1653, 1983.

24. Teel, R.W., Dixit, R. and Stoner, G.D. The effect of ellagic acid on the uptake, persistence, metabolism and DNA-binding of benzo[a]pyrene in cultured explants of strain A/J mouse lung. Carcinogenesis, 6: 391-395, 1985.

25. Das, M. Bickers, D.R., and Mukhtar, H. Effect of ellagic acid on hepatic and pulmonary xenobiotic metabolism in mice: studies on the mechanism of its anticarcinogenic action. Carcinogenesis, 6: 1409-1413, 1985.

26. Kirkpatrick, D.C. and Lauer, B.H. Intake of phenolic antioxidants from foods in Canada. Fd Chem. Toxic., 24: 1036-1037, 1986.

27. Wattenberg, L.W. Inhibition of carcinogenic effects of diethylnitrosamine (DEN) and 4-nitroquinoline-N-oxide (NQO) by antioxidants. Fed. Proc., 31: 633, 1972.

28. Speier, J.L., Lam, L.K.T., and Wattenberg, L. W. Effects of administration to mice of butylated hydroxyanisole by oral intubation of benzo[a]pyrene-induced pulmonary adenoma formation and metabolism of benzo[a] pyrene. J. Ntl. Cancer Inst., 60: 605-609, 1978.

29. Chung F.-L, Wang, M., Carmella, S.G. and Hecht, S.S.. Effects of butylated hydroxyanisole on the tumorigenicity and metabolism of N-nitrosodimethylamine and N-nitrosopyrrolidine in A/J mice, Cancer Res., 46: 165-168, 1986.

30. Tacchi, A.M., Jensen, D.E. and Magee, P.N.. Effect of glutathione modulation using buthionine sulfoximine on DNA methylation by dimethylnitrosamine in the rat. Biochem. Pharm. 36: 881-885, 1987.

31. Speier, J.L., Wattenberg, L.W. Alterations in microsomal metabolism of benzo[a]pyrene in mice fed butylated hydroxyanisole. J. Natl. Cancer Inst. 55: 469-472, 1975.

32. Yang, C.S. Strickhart, F.S. and Woo, G.K. Inhibition of the mono-oxygenase system by butylated hydroxyanisole and butylated hydroxytoluene. Life Sci. 15: 1497-1505, 1974.

33. Morse, M.A., LaGreca, S.D. and Chung, F.-L. Inhibitory effects of indole-3-carbinol on NNK-induced tumorigenecity and O^6-methylguanine formation in A/J mouse lung. Proc. Am. Assoc. Cancer Res. 30: 178, 1989.

34. Ziegler, R.G. A review of epidemiologic evidence that carotenoids reduce the risk of cancer. J. Nutr., 119: 116-122, 1988.

35. Goodman, G.E., Omenn, G.S., Feigl, P., Kleinman, G.D., Lund, B., Thomas, D.D., Henderson, M.M., and Prentice, R. Chemoprevention of lung cancer with retinol/beta-carotene. In: F.L. Meyskens and K.n. Prasad (eds). Vitamin and cancer. pp. 341-350, Clifton, N.J. Humana Press, 1986.

36. Mehta, R.G., Rao, K.V.N., Detrisac, C.J., Kelloff, G.J. and Moon, R.C. Inhibition of diethylnitrosamine-induced lung carcinogenesis by retinoids Proc. Am. Assoc. Cancer Res., 29: 129, 1988.

37. Busk, L., and Ahlborg, U.G. Retinol (vitamin A) as a modifier of 2-aminofluorene and 2-acetyl-aminofluorene mutagenesis in Salmonella/microsome assay. Arch. Toxicol, 49, 169-174, 1982.

38. Huang, C.C. Retinol (vitamin A) inhibition of dimethylnitrosamine (DMN) and diethylnitrosamine (DEN) induced sister-chromatid exchanges in V79 cells and mutations in Salmonella-microsome assay. Mutat. Res. 187: 133-140, 1987.

39. Huang, C.C., Hsueh, J.L. Chen, H.H. and Batt, T.R. Retinol (Vitamin A) inhibits sister chromatid exchanges and cell cycle delay enduced by cyclophosphamide and aflatoxin B1., in Chinese hamster V79 cells, Carcinogenesis, 3, 1-5, 1982.

40. Charest, M., Rossignol, G. and Castonguay, A. *In vitro* and *in vivo* modulation of the bioactivation of 4-(methylnitrosamino)-1-(3-pyridyl)-1-butanone in hamsters lung tissues. Chem. Biol. Intereact. (In Press).

41. Girolami, A. and Cliffton, E.E. Hypercoagulable state induced in humans by the intravenous administration of purified ellagic acid. Thromb. Diath. Haemorrh. 17: 165-175, 1967.

Nutrients and Cancer Prevention K. N. Prasad and F. L. Meyskens, Jr., eds. © 1990 The Humana Press

MECHANISMS OF SPECIFIC NUTRIENTS IN THE PREVENTION

OF CANCER

Michael J. Hill   DSc FRCPath

PHLS-CAMR, Salisbury, Wiltshire SP4 0 J G, United Kingdom

INTRODUCTION

Many dietary intervention protocols for cancer prevention have been proposed, often with little justification. However, in recent years our understanding of the mechanisms of carcinogenesis, particularly in the gastrointestinal tract, has increased enormously and we are now in a position to propose dietary interventions with a solidly rational basis, and to devise rational procedures for their rapid evaluation. In this presentation I will discuss the mechanism of action of three specific nutrients in the prevention of cancer of the gastrointestinal tract, namely ascorbic acid in the primary prevention of gastric cancer and calcium supplements or caecal acidification in the primary prevention of colorectal cancer. In both cancers it will first be necessary to review the state of our current knowledge of the mechanism of carcinogenesis, in order to be able to put the role of the specific nutrient into context.

GASTRIC CARCINOGENESIS

Causation

In 1975 Correa et al[7] postulated a
histopathological sequence in gastric
carcinogenesis of the intestinal type (Fig 1),
the initial lesion of which was gastric atrophy
(GA) leading to chronic atrophic gastritis
(CAG). In a proportion of CAG patients the
lesion progresses to intestinal metaplasia (IM).
in some cases of which increasingly severe
epithelial dysplasis (ED) develops leading,
ultimately, to gastric cancer. Correa et al
proposed a mechanism for this sequence: at the
initial stage gastric acid secretion is
decreased to the point where the gastric milieu
can no longer be acidified to below pH 4 and so
is no longer a selfsterilising environment. In
consequence a resident bacterial flora can
establish itself in the stomach and can reduce
nitrate to nitrite and catalyse the formation of
N-nitroso compounds in the luminal contents.
These latter carcinogens were postualted to be
responsible for the progression of the gastric
lesion through IM and ED to gastric cancer. This
model only applies to gastric cancers of the
intestinal type (on the classification of
Lauren, ref 20); although such cancers account
for the majority of gastric cancers in almost
all countries, we have no hypotheses for the
causation of gastric cancers of the other major
histological type, the so-called diffuse type.

Multistage models such as that proposed by
Correa et al are often interpreted in the
context ofthe classical two-stage
inititation-promotion model of carcinogenesis.
It is important to note that, to date, oncogenes
have only been reported at the final stages
(severe epithelial dysplasia and gastric
carcinoma) and so the early stages should be
considered as either increasing the sensitivity

of the mucosa to the action of local carcinogens
or as permitting an increased rate of production
of locally acting carcinogens.
The Correa hypothesis is a very good one because
it is so readily testable at all stages. The
consequences of

Fig 1

The histopathological sequence in gastric
carcinogenesis (based on Correa *et al* 1975).

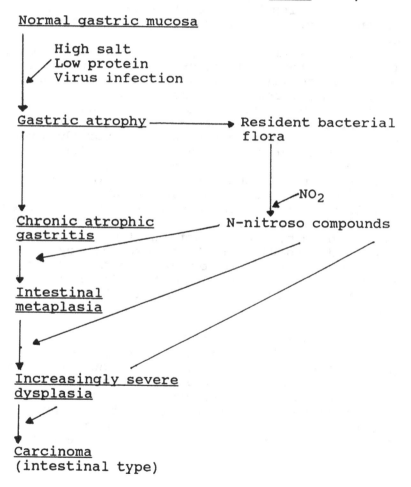

Normal gastric mucosa

High salt
Low protein
Virus infection

Gastric atrophy ──────→ Resident bacterial
flora

NO_2

Chronic atrophic
gastritis ── N-nitroso compounds

Intestinal
metaplasia

Increasingly severe
dysplasia

Carcinoma
(intestinal type)

the hypothesis are clear; if the proposed mechanism is correct then it implies that;
(i) loss of gastric acidity should carry an excess risk of malignancy regardless of the cause (ie whether due to natural ageing, poor diet, gastric surgery, pernicious anemia, immune deficiency etc):
(ii) the disease states associated with gastric hypochlorhydria or achlorhydria should be accompanied by gastric juice analyses rich in bacteria, nitrite and N-nitroso compounds;
(iii) the gastric juice analyses should be correlated with the rate of progression from IM through increasingly severe dysplasia to carcinoma;
(iv) it is unlikely that, under conditions that favour the formation of N-nitroso compounds, only the locally acting N-nitroso compounds will be formed and some of those that are target-organ-specific will also be produced. Consequently, if sufficient locally-acting carcinogen is produced to account for the excess risk of gastric cancer there should also be an excess risk of tumours at other sites corresponding to the target organs of the other principal N-nitroso compounds produced;
(v) if the postulated mechanism is correct then chronic bacterial infection at other sites, if accompanied by the production of N-nitroso compounds. should also be accompanied by local carcinogenesis. Examples would be the urinary bladder, the sigmoid colon of patients with ureterosigmoidostomy, the infected uterine cervix etc.

This hypothesis has been discussed in detail elsewhere [13] [14] [15] and all of the above predictions have been confirmed. Thus there is now a large body of evidence, summarised in Table 1, supporting the hypothesis mechanism. Two important factors need to be taken into account in interpreting the literature: the first is the confusion caused by problems with

the assay of N-nitroso compounds and the second
is the wide variation in the ability of
bacterial strains to N-nitrosate. In early
studies only the volatile N-nitroso compounds
were assayed because these were the only ones
for which there were reliable assay procedures.
In 1980 Walters et al[43] described the first
techniques for the assay of total N-nitroso
compounds (TNNC) and demonstrated that the
volatile fraction was an

Table 1

Evidence supporting the proposed histopathological
sezuence. (For details and reference see ref 14).

Prediction	Observation
1. Relation between loss of gastric acid and increased risk of gastric cancer.	Increased risk of gastric cancer seen in a range of diseases involving hypoacidity.
2. Gastric juice analyses related to gastric pH.	In 23 studies reported between 1980 and 1985, the gastric flora and gastric juice nitrite concentration increased with increaseing pH. Total N-nitroso compounds also increased with gastric pH.
3. Gastric juice analyses should correlate with disease progression.	Severity of dysplasia correlate with gastric bacteria and nitrite.
4. Cancer at other sites associated with gastric atrophy.	Many reports of epigastric cancers, eg the colon, biliary tract and pancreas.
5. Local cancers at other sites with similar conditions.	Similar sets of conditions associated with cancer of the bladder, cervix and colon in urine diversion.

insignificant contributer to the total. Using
their technique numerous groups have reported a
good correlation between gastric juice pH, TNNC
concentration and risk of gastric cancer in
groups of patients with various gastric
lesions[38 40]. This was in agreement with the
hypothesis of Correa al et al[7]. However, in all
such studies the samples were stored. often for
prolonged periods subsequently shown to be
unacceptable. In order to speed up the assay
Bavin et al[1] streamlined the technique and used
a different sample stabilisation procedure.
Using this method they obtained results showing
no relation between gastric juice pH and TNNC
concentration, in contradiction to the
hypothesis of Correa et al. In an attempt to
resolve thls conflict Pignatelli et al[36]
examined both methods critically and in detail:
from these experiments they devised a new
technique which is an improvement on both of the
previous ones. Provided that samples are assayed
within 4 weeks the method gives reproducible and
reliable results: using this new improved assay
method Pignatelli et al found a good correlation
between pH and TNNC concentration in support of
the hypothesised mechanism of gastric
carcinogenesis.

The stomach is supplied with a regular inoculum
of bacteria in swallowed saliva and food. In the
acid stomach these organisms are rapidly killed:
those still alive are unable to metabolise at
such an unfavourable pH and so no nitrite or
N-nitroso compound is formed by bacterial action
in the acid stomach. When acid secretion is
decreased until the luminal pH fails to fall
below 4 at any time during the day, the gastric
contents are no longer self-sterilising and a
resident bacterial flora establishes from those
swallowed organisms best suited to the gastric
milieu. Those members of this new resident flora
that utilise nitrate are usually
nitrate-assimilators: such organisms have been
shown by Calmels et al[5] and by Leach et al [21] to

catalyse the N-nitrosation reaction, but only at a low rate. In a proportion of cases the resident flora will include nitrate dissimulators; such organisms have been shown by Leach et al[22] to produce N-nitroso compounds at rates that are 100-1000 times those achieved by the more common assimilators. Thus it is not enough simply to know that the stomach is colonised. but it is also necessary to know the composition of that flora and whether it contains nitrate dissimulating organisms. Techniques for the rapid detection and assay of these latter organisms are currently being developed in this laboratory.

Mechanism of Prevention

On the Correa model gastric cancer can be prevented at any of the stages. There are no hypotheses on the causation or the means of prevention of gastric atrophy and the consequent loss of gastric acidity. However. specific nutrients have been suggested for the prevention of the later stages, the progression from IM through increasingly severe ED to gastric cancer.

If N-nitroso compounds are responsible for this progression then gastric cancer should be preventable by inhibiting N-nitroso compound formation. either by scavenging the precurser nitrite[28] or by inhibiting the N-nitrosation reaction itself. It has been clearly established that ascorbic acid is a potent scavenger of nitrite[27] . Ascorbic acid is a powerful reducing agent which readily reduces nitrite to nitric oxide. Since the ascorbate ion reacts with nitrite 230 times faster than does the free acid and since the acid dissociation constant of ascorbic acid is 4.3 the scavenging action is most potent below pH 5: this range includes the pH of the normal acid stomach even after a meal 26, 41 and the resting gastric pH of persons with moderate hypochlorhydria. Although the optimal pH is below 5 ascorbate has some activity even at neutral pH values. It has been shown to be an effective scavenger of nitrite *in vivo* in the stomach of the rat 6 . the mouse[29] and the human[39] . In both of the rodents studies cited the scavenging of the nitrite prevented the formation of N-nitroso compounds with co-administered amines: this was confirmed by the absence of tumour formation at the target site of the putative nitrosamine, in contrast to the observations in animals fed nitrite and amine but no ascorbate .

It had been assumed that the inhibition by ascorbic acid of nitrosation of for example, morpholine in the rodent stomach was simply due to the removal of the precurser nitrite. However, recent studies by Mackerness *et al*[24] have shown that ascorbate is also able to inhibit the bacterial N-nitrosation reaction at neutral pH, possibly by competetive attachment to the enzyme binding site. This affect on bacterial nitrosation is of importance because Leach *et al*[21] have demonstrated that in the neutral stomach the bacterial formation of N-nitroso compounds is more important than the acid-catalysed reaction by several orders of magnitude.

Several groups are currently planning dietary interventions with ascorbic acid in the prevention of gastric cancer. A problem with such studies is the lack of detailed knowledge of the rate of progression through the various stages of the histopathological sequence. However, the studies are being undertaken with considerable optimism because of the well documented protective effect against gastric carcinogenesis of either ascorbic acid[2] or of foods rich in ascorbic such as fresh fruits and salad vegetables[19]

COLORECTAL CANCER

Causation

As with gastric cancer, in colorectal cancer there is a clearly identified precancerous lesion and a widely recognised and accepted histopathological sequence. Morson[30] [31] summarised the data showing that almost all colorectal cancers arise in preformed benign adenomas. He has identified the factors determining the risk of malignancy in an adenoma [31] [32] [33], the principal of which are size, severity of epithelial dysplasia and villousness (Table 2). Epidemiological studies (summarised by Morson *et al*[33]) show that, while many aspects of the geographical distribution of the two lesions is similar, there are clear examples of groups of centres where the prevalence of adenomas is similar but the incidence of carcinomas is different (eg Tromso, Oslo and Liverpool) and *vice versa* (eg Colombia, Iran and Johannesburg blacks). Similarly the distribution of

Table 2

Factors determining the malignant potential of an adenoma (for details see reference 33)

Factors	Percentage containing malignancy
Size 0-3 mm	0.1%
3-10 mm	1.3%
10-20 mm	9.5%
more than 20 mm	46.0%
Villousness tubular	4.9%
villous	40.7%
tubulovillous	22.5%
Dysplasia mild	5.7%
moderate	18.0%
severe	34.5%

the two lesions along the colorectum differs
markedly, suggesting that the precursor adenoma
has a causation that differs from that of the
progression to carcinoma. In 1978 Hill et al[16]
proposed a mechanism of the adenoma-carcinoma
sequence in the large bowel, the first stage of
which was the formatlon of a small adenoma by
the action of environmental factors, termed E1
(Fig 2). There is a familial/genetic component
in the causation of adenomas[4]; it was proposed
that this takes the form of an increased
sensitivity to the adenogenic effects of E1.
with those carrying the gene being termed
`adenomaprone'. Most adenomas remain small and
such adenomas have a low risk of malignancy. A
small proportion grow to a large size: this
proportion varies between populations and
between subsites in the colon and is determined
by environmental factors E2 that differ from
those causing adenoma formation (E1). Whereas
many large adenomas become severely dysplastic
and progress to malignancy many do not. and so
the increase in severity of dysplasia is not
inevitable and must be caused. The factor
responsible for this is termed factor C, which
is much more active on large than on small
adenomas.

It is common for the adenoma-carcinoma sequence
in the colon to be discussed in terms of the
classical two-stage initiation/promotion model
of chemical carcinogenesis. However, the usual
markers of carcinogenesis (eg oncogene
expression, chromosonmal abnormality etc) have
only been reported in the later stages of severe
dysplasia and carcinoma. As with the situation
in the stomach, therefore, the relevant model is
one of pre-cancer progressing to cancer and the
terms `initiation' and `promotion' cannot, as
yet, be applied to any of the identified stages
of the hypothetical sequence. In particular. the
use of the term `promotion' to describe
theprogression from the adenoma to carcinoma is
inappropriate.

We have studied the role of bile acid metabolites in colorectal carcinogenesis [12] [13] [35]; Table 3 summarises the information on the tumour promoting action of bile acids, particularly the two principal bacterial metabolites found in faeces (deoxycholic and lithocholic acids), whilst Table 4 summarises the evidence of a role for bile acids in human colorectal carcinogenesis. Of particular interest in the context of the present

Fig 2

Mechanism of the adenoma-carcinoma sequence in the colorectum.

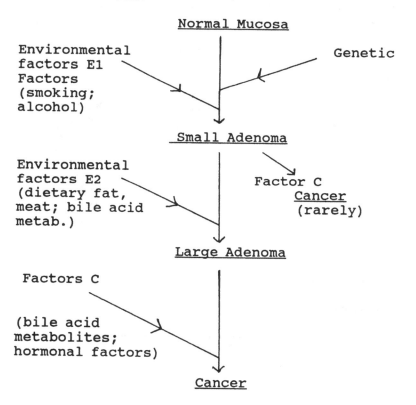

Normal Mucosa

Environmental factors E1 Factors (smoking; alcohol)

Genetic

Small Adenoma

Environmental factors E2 (dietary fat, meat; bile acid metab.)

Factor C
Cancer
(rarely)

Large Adenoma

Factors C

(bile acid metabolites; hormonal factors)

Cancer

Table 3

Evidence from experimental models that bile acids are
tumour promoters, mutagens or co-mutagens (for details
see ref 13).

Test Systems	Bile Acid Used	Observation
1. Rats treated with colon carcinogens	Deoxycholic acid Lithocholic acid	Colon tumour promotion
2. Skin painting on rats	Deoxycholic acid	Skin co-carcinogens
3. Subcutaneous injection in rats	Range of bile acids	Co-carcinogens
4. Bacterial mutagenesis	Range of bile acids	Mutagenicity promotion increased by less of 7-hydroxyl; decreased by hydroxyl oxidation; increase by inversion at C-5
5. Hamster embryo cell transformation	Lithocholic acid	Mutagenicity

Table 4

Evidence that bile acids are implicated in the causation of colorectal cancer (for further details and references see references 12 and 13).

Type of Study	Observation
Comparision of populations	Faecal bile acid (FBA) concentration correlated with incidence of colorectal cancer (CRC) in many studies from many laboratories.
High risk patient groups	The risk of CRC correlates with the FBA concentration in ulcerative colitics and in adenoma patients.
Animal and _in vivo_ studies	1. Bile acids are promoters of colorectal carcinogenesis and of mutagenesis. 2. Changes in the FBA concentration due to dietary or surgical manipulations produce parallel changes in the CRC prevalence.
Bile acid binding sites	Deoxycholic acid binding sites detected in a high proportion of colorectal cancers, but only a low percentage of controls.
Bile acid kinetics	Deoxycholic acid turnover and colonic absorption is faster in adenoma patients than in controls.

discussion is their role in the various stages
of the adenoma-carcinoma sequence. The rate of
formation of new adenomas in patients who have
had an adenoma resected is unrelated to the
faecal bile acid (FBA) concentration or to the
FBA profile, indicating that bile acid
metabolites are not related to factor E1.
However, adenoma size is strongly correlated
with the FBA concentration[13 17] and with the
bile acid profile[35], particularly the ratio of
the two principal faecal bile acids lithocholate
to deoxycholate (LA/DC). Further, the severity
of epithelial dysplasia has been related to the
FBA concentration confirming the toxic effects
of bile acids on the colorectal mucosa observed
in rodents[44].

This is evidence that bile acid metabolites are
related to factors E2 and C; the role of bile
acids in the various stages is summarised in
Table 5. Table 6 summarises the current state of
knowledge of the identity of E1, E2 and C.
Colorectal carcinogenesis can potentially be
inhibited by interfering with any or all of the
stages of adenoma-carcinoma sequence.

Mechanism of Prevention

Dietary interventions have been proposed with
the aim of decreasing the FBA concentration in
free solution and the degree of degradation of
the bile acids by bacterial action in the colon.

Newmark et al[34] have proposed that the FBA
concentration in solution can be decreasd by
precipitation as calcium soaps: since the free
bile acids in the colon cause mucosal damage,
such damage could potentially be decreased by
increasing the colonic concentration of calcium.
A high proportion of the normal dietary intake
of calcium is absorbed from the small bowel. but
the capacity for absorption of calcium is

limited. Higher than normal intakes of calcium should, therefore. result in increased faecal concentrations of the cation being available for binding bile acids. There is some epidemiological evidence (eg reference 10), and a large body of data from animal experiments has been

Table 5

The role of bile acids in the individual stages of the adenoma-carcinoma sequence.

Patient Group	Stage	Involvement
Adenoma patients	Adenoma formation	No role
	Adenoma growth	Correlated with size of the largest adenoma
	Dysplasia	Correlated with severity of dysplasia
Ulcerative colitics	Adenoma formation	No relation
	Adenoma growth	No information
	Dysplasia	Correlated with severity of dysplasia

Table 6

Information on the identity of the factors
causing the various stages in the adenoma-
carcinoma sequence.

Stage   Possible Causal Factor

Adenoma   Genetic predisposition/
formation   familial factors; alcohol
                             consumption? Smoking?

Adenoma   Fat/meat (fibre protective?);
growth   Bile acid metabolites

Dysplasia   Bile acid metabolites;
                             Mucosal damage?
                             Inflammatory bowel disease?
                             Hormonal factors

---

accumulated in support of the hypothesis. Wargovlch et al[44] reported the toxic damage caused in the colonic mucosa by bile acids: Newmark et al[34] suggested that this damage was caused by the abstraction of calcium ions from the mucosal cells causing a loss of membrane integrity and function. Saturation of the faecal bile acids with calcium ions prevents this ion abstraction and so prevents the toxic damage. When deoxycholic acid is administered per rectum to rats mucosal damage ensues: when the bile acid was administered as the calcium salt no damage to the mucosa was seen. Further, when the deoxycholate was administered per rectum and high doses of calcium were given per os no mucosal damage was seen and the faecal bile acids were in the form of calcium soaps. In a small trial Lipkin and Newmark[23] observed that in patients with a hereditary predisposition to colorectal cancer administration of dietary supplements of calcium led to a more healthy pattern of tritiated thymidine incorporation in the colonic mucosa. Numerous trials are in progress in which the effect of dietary supplements of calcium on the rate of formation of new adenomas is being monitored. It is important to note that, as yet, we have no good hypotheses on the causation of adenoma formation and so have no good reason for thinking that calcium supplements will have any beneficial effect at that stage of the adenoma-carcinoma sequence. In contrast, we have good evidence that bile acids are important in the causation of adenoma growth and that, therefore, calcium might be expected to have a beneficial effect in inhibiting that stage of the sequence. The European group for Cancer Prevention (ECP) is currently conducting such a study.

It is well established that the bacterial enzymes responsible for the production of the major faecal bile acid metabolites, the 7-dehydroxylase, has a pH-optimum of between 7 and 8; further, as well as having a low activity at acidic pH values, the enzyme is not produced at pH values below 6 (reference 25). In consequence, since it is the products of the action of this enzyme that are responsible for the mucosal toxicity, it has been proposed [11],[42] that acidification of the colonic contents by dietary supplements of lactulose or other non-absorbed sugars or sugar alcohols should decrease the risk of colorectal carcinogenesis. Bown et al[3] showed that lactulose administration caused a fall. ln caecal pH from 6-7 to below 4.5, whilst Fadden et al[8] showed that when lactulose was fed to pigs it caused a decrease in the rate of dehydroxylation of the caecal bile acids. Further, Felix[9] showed that in minipigs fed lactitol the rate of formation of both lithocholate and deoxycholate was greatly decreased at all subsites in the colon. In a recent report by Rafter et al[37] it was demonstrated that an acidification of the caecal contents also caused precipitation of the colonic bile acids. Thus the bile acids in solutlon (and therefore available to cause mucosal damage) were at a lower concentration (due to precipitation) as well as less extensively bacterially degraded. Since lithocholate is more hydrophobic than is deoxycholate it is more readily precipitated both by calcium and by acidification: in consequence both interventions are likely not only to yield a lower FBA concentration but also to give a more favourable FBA profile with a lower ratio LA/DC. This has been confirmed in this laboratory (Fernandez, in prepartion) with calcium supplements.

CONCLUSION

In parts of Europe (eg Portugal, Northern Italy, Hungary) gastric cancer is still a major cause of cancer death, whilst in others (eg Germany, UK, Denmark, Sweden) colorectal cancer is very prevalent. It is important, therefore, that dietary advice designed to decrease the risk of, or example, colorectal cancer in one part of Europe should not inadvertently increase the risk of gastric cancer elsewhere. In this context, the proposed interventions are ideal. If calcium is recommended to prevent colorectal cancer, it will presumably be from dairy products which are known to protect against gastric cancer[13]. Similarly, ascorbic acid (and fresh fruits, salads etc), as well as protecting against gastric cancer, is also known to be protective against colorectal cancer (see, for example, the paper by Kuhn in this volume). Such dietary advice can therefore be given in the knowledge that it is unlikely to lead to unwanted malignancies elsewhere.

REFERENCES

1. Bavin M, Darkin DW, Viney NJ. Total N-nitroso groups in gastric juice. IARC Scientific Publication No 41, Lyon, 337-344 (1982).

2. Bjelke E. Epidemiological studies of cancer of the stomach, colon and rectum. Scand. J. Gastro. 9: Supplement 31 (1984).

3. Bown RL, Gibson JA, Sladen GE, Hicks B, Dawson AM. Effects of lactulose and other laxatives on ideal and colonic pH as measured by a radiotelemetry device. Gut 15: 999-1004 (1974).

4. Burt RW, Bishop T, Cannon LA, Dowdle DA. Lee RG, Skolnich LH. Dominant inheritance of adenomatous colonic polyps and colorectal cancer. New Eng. J. Med. 312: 1540-1544 (1985).

5. Calmels S, Ohshima H. Vincent P et al. Screening microorganisms for nitrosation catalysis at pH7 and kinetic studies on nitrosamine formation from secondary amines by E.coli strains. Carcinogenesis 6: 911-915 (1985).

6. Cardesa A. Mirvish SS, Haven GT, Shubik P. Inhibitory effect of ascorbic acid on the acute toxicity of dimethylamine plus nitrite in the rat. Proc. Soc. Exp. Biol. Med. 145: 124-128 (1974).

7. Correa P. Haenszel W, Cuello C, Tannenbaum S. Archer M. A model of gastric cancer epidemiology. Lancet ii 5 8 - 6 0 (1 9 7 5) .

8.   Fadden K, Owen R, Hill MJ <u>et al</u>. Steroid degradation along gastrointestinal tract: the use of the cannulated pig as a model system. <u>Trans. Biochem. Soc</u>. 12: 1105-6 (1984).

9.   Felix YF. Thesis for Fellowship of the Institute of Med. Lab. Sciences (London) 1987.

10. Garland C, Shekelle RB, Barrett-Conner E, Criqui MH, Rossof AH, Paul D. Dietary vitamin D and calcium and risk of colorectal cancer. <u>Lancet</u> i: 307-309 (1985).

11. Hill MJ. Steroid nuclear dehydrogenation and colon cancer. <u>Amer. J. Clin. Nutr.</u> 27: 1475-1480 (1974).

12. Hill MJ. Mechanisms of colorectal carcinogenesis. In (eds J. Joossens, J Geboers, MJ Hill) <u>Diet and Human Carcinogenesis</u> Excerpta Medica, Amsterdam. 149-164 (1985).

13. Hill MJ. Microbes and Human Carcinogenesis, Edward Arnold, London (1986).

14. Hill MJ. Gastric carcinogenesis: luminal factors. In (eds PI Reed, MJ Hill) <u>Gastric Carcinogenesis</u> Excerpta Medica. Amsterdam. 187-200 (1988).

15. Hill MJ. N-nitroso compounds and lung cancer. In (ed MJ Hill) N-nitroso <u>Compounds: toxicology and bacteriology</u> Ellis Horwood, Chichester. 142-162 (1989)

16. Hill MJ, Morson BC. Bussey HJR. Aetiology of adenomacarcinoma sequence. <u>Lancet</u> i: 245-247 (1978).

17.   Hill MJ, Morson BC, Thompson MH. The role
       of faecal bile acids in large bowel
       carcinogenesis. Br. J. Cancer 48: 143
       (1983).

18.   Hll MJ. Melville D, Lennard-Jones J. Neale
       K, Ritchie JK. Faecal bile acids dysplasia
       and carcinoma in ulcerative colitis.
       Lancet ii: 183-186 (1987).

19.   Judd P. Dietary factors in the aetiology
       of gastric cancer. In (eds PI Reed, MJ
       Hill) Gastric Carcinogenesis. Excerpta
       Medica, Amsterdam. 87-98 (1988).

20.   Lauren P. The two histological main types
       in gastric carcinoma: diffuse and
       so-called intestinal type. Acta Path. Mic.
       Scand 64: 31-49 (1965).

21.   Leach S. Challis B, Cook AR. Hill MJ,
       Thompson MH. Bacterial catalysis of the
       N-nitrosation of secondary amines. Trans.
       Biochem. Soc. 13: 380-381 (1985).

22.   Leach S. Mechanisms of endogenous
       N-nitrosation. In (ed MJ   Hill)
       Nitrosamines: Toxicology and Microbiology
       Ellis Horwood, Chichester. 69-87 (1987).

23.   Lipkin M. Newmark H. Effect of added
       dietary calcium on colonic epithelial cell
       proliferation in subjects at high risk for
       familial colonic cancer. N. Eng. J. Med.
       313: 1381-1384 (1985).

24.   Mackerness C, Leach S, Thompson MH, Hill
       MJ. The inhibition of bacterially mediated
       N-nitrosation by vitamin C: Relevance of
       the inhibition of endogenous nitrosation
       in the achlorhydric stomach. Carcingenesis
       10: 397-399 (1989).

25.   Midvedt T, Norman A. Breakdown of bile
       salts by intestinal bacteria. Acta Path.
       Mic. Scand. 71: 629-638 (1967).

26. Milton-Thompson G, Lightfoot N. Ahmet Z. Intragastric acidity, bacteria, nitrite and N-nitroso compounds before, during and after cimetidine treatment. Lancet i: 1091-1094 (1982).

27. Mirvish SS. Effects of vitamins C and E on N-nitroso compound formation. carcinogenesis and cancer. Cancer 58: 1842-1850 (1986).

28. Mirvish SS, Wallcave L. Eagen M, Shubik P. Ascorbate-nitrite reaction: possible means of blocking the formation of carcinogenic N-nitroso compounds. Science 177: 65-68 (1972).

29. Mirvish SS, Cardesa A, Wallcave L. Shubik P. Induction of mouse lung adenomas by amines or ureas plus nitrite and by N-nitroso compounds: effect of ascorbate, gallic acid, thiocyanate and caffeine. J. Nat. Cancer Nut. 55: 633-636 (1975).

30. Morson BC. Factors influencing the prognosis of early cancer of the rectum. Proc. Roy. Soc. Med. 59: 607-608 (1966).

31. Morson BC. The polyp-cancer sequence of the large bowel. Proc. Roy. soc. Med. 67: 451-457 (1974).

32. Morson BC, Konishi F. Dysplasia of the colon and rectum. In (ed R Wright) Recent Advances in Gastrointestinal Pathology. R Saunders, London. 331-343 (1980).

33. Morson BC, Bussey HJR. Day D, Hill MJ. Adenomas of the large bowel. Cancer Surveys 2: 457-477 (1983).

34. Newmark H, Wargovich MJ, Bruce WR. Colon cancer and dietary fat, phosphate and calcium: A hypothesis. J. Nat Cancer Inst. 74: 1323-1325 (1984).

35. Owen RW, Thompson MH, Hill MJ, Wilpart M. Mainguet P, Roberfroid M. The importance of the ratio of lithocholic to deoxycholic acid in large bowel carcinogenesis. <u>Nutr. Cancer</u> 9: 67-71 (1987).

36. Pignatelli B, Richard I, Bourgade M. Bartsch H. An improved method for analysis of total N-nitroso compounds in gastric juice. <u>Analyst</u> 112: 945-949 (1987).

37. Rafter J, Eng WS, Furrer R, Medline A, Bruce WR. Effects of calcium and pH on the mucosal damage produced by deoxycholic acid in the rat colon. <u>Gut</u> 27: 1320-1329 (1986).

38. Reed PI, Smith PL, Hines K. Gastric juice N-nitrosamines in health and gastroduodenal disease. <u>Lancet</u> ii: 550-552 (1981).

39. Reed PI, Summers K, Smith P. Walters CL, Bartholomew B, Hill MJ. Vennitt S, Hornig D, Boneour, J-P. Effect of ascorbic acid treatment on gastric juice nitrite and N-nitroso compounds concentrations in achlorhydric subjects. <u>Gut</u> 24: 492-493 (1983).

40. Sharma BK. Santana IA, Wood EC, Walt R, Pereira M, Noone P. Pounder R. Smith P, Walters CL. Intragastric bacterial activity and nitrosation before, during and after treatment with omeprazole. <u>Brit. Med. J.</u> 289: 717-719 (1984).

41. Thomas JM, Misiewicz J, Cook A. Hill MJ, Smith P. Walters CL, Forster J, Martin L, Woodings D. Effects of one years treatment with ranitidine and of truncal vagotomy on gastric contents. <u>Gut</u> 28: 726-738 (1987).

42. Thornton JR. High colonic pH promoter colorectal cancer. <u>Lancet</u> i: 1081-1083 (1981).

43.   Walters CL, Hart RJ, Keefer L. Newberne P. The sequential determination of nitrite. N-nitroso compounds and nitrate and its application. IARC Scientific Publication No 31 Lyon 389- 393 (1980).

44.   Wargovich MJ, Eng V, Newmark HL, Bruce WR. Calcium ameliorates the toxic effect of deoxychoic acid on colonic epithelium. Carcinogenesis 4: 1205-1207 (1983).

Preclinical Studies
in Cancer Prevention and Treatment

Nutrients and Cancer Prevention K. N. Prasad and F. L. Meyskens, Jr., eds. © 1990 The Humana Press

REDUCTION OF ULTRAVIOLET-INDUCED IMMUNOSUPPRESSION AND
ENHANCED RESISTANCE TO ULTRAVIOLET-INDUCED TUMORS BY
RETINYL PALMITATE AND CANTHAXANTHIN

Helen L. Gensler

Department of Radiation Oncology and Cancer Center
University of Arizona College of Medicine
Tucson, AZ 85724

INTRODUCTION

There is strong evidence that UV irradiation is a
causal factor in human nonmelanoma skin cancer (1-3), and
that immunosuppression is a high risk factor for skin
cancer in humans (4,5). The use of animal model systems to
investigate the sequence of events which lead to the
induction and progression of skin tumors following chronic
ultraviolet irradiation has clearly shown that the
genotoxic effect of UV irradiation is only one of the
components involved in this process. Immunological factors
are also critically important in the pathogenesis of UV
induced skin cancers (6,7). Most tumors induced by UV
irradiation are highly antigenic and cannot grow in normal
syngeneic mice. However, they can grow in immunodepressed
or UV irradiated mice. The inability to reject antigenic,
syngeneic UV-induced tumors can be transferred from UV
irradiated mice to naive recipients with splenocytes
bearing an Lyt-1$^+$, Lyt-2$^-$, L3T4$^+$, Ia$^-$ phenotype(8). This
anergy has been found to be critical in photocarcinogenesis
(9). Significantly, the suppression induced by UV
irradiation appears to be restricted to contact
hypersensitivity reactions and rejection of tumors induced
by UV radiation or some chemicals (10,11). Antibody
formation, mitogen reactivity, and allograft rejection are
reported to be normal in UV irradiated mice (12-14).

That immunologic factors, and especially

immunosuppression, are related to human skin cancer
induction is evident from the high incidence of cutaneous
malignancies in immunosuppressed organ transplant
recipients. In Australia and New Zealand, renal transplant
recipients were treated with azathioprine, prednisone, and
some with antilymphocyte globulin (4). Of those patients
surviving 15 years of immunosuppression, 44% developed
cutaneous cancer. The increase in transplant recipients was
primarily of invasive squamous cell carcinoma, which
occurred at approximately 40 times the rate found in a
control population (4).

Retinoids have been found to prevent murine
photocarcinogenesis (15,16) as well as chemically induced
cutaneous tumor promotion (17-19). An additional activity
of retinoids is prevention of immunosuppression, e.g.
neonatal tolerance (20), post-operative immunosuppression
(21) and postburn immunosuppression (22). Canthaxanthin, a
carotenoid which is not a provitamin A, has been shown to
delay or prevent photocarcinogenesis in the albino,
hairless SKH/hr-1 mouse, at concentrations of 0.7% or 2% in
the diet, respectively (23). Canthaxanthin has also been
reported to be an immunostimulant (24).

The experiments presented here were designed to address
the hypothesis that retinyl palmitate and/or canthaxanthin
prevents the suppression of immune functions in pigmented
UVB irradiated mice, thereby enhancing host resistance to
antigenic UV-induced tumors and reducing
photocarcinogenesis.

MATERIALS AND METHODS

Specific-pathogen-free C3H/HeN mice were used in this
study because this strain has been previously used to
delineate the immunosuppression induced by UV irradiation.
The diets consisted of the basal diet (AIN76A) supplemented
with 1% canthaxanthin, 120 IU retinyl palmitate per g diet,
or the combination of both. The retinyl palmitate and
canthaxanthin were supplied by Dr. H. Bhagavan of Hoffmann-
La Roche. All diets not containing canthaxanthin beadlets
contained placebo beadlets. The designated diets were
administered for 18 weeks before UV irradiation, and
throughout the experiment. This time allowed for
immunomodulatory effects and local accumulation of retinyl
palmitate and canthaxanthin (23,25). UV irradiation

consisted of five 30 min treatments per week for 12 or 24 weeks for the immunomodulatory or photocarcinogenesis experiments, respectively. The UV source was a bank of 6 Westinghouse FS40 lamps which delivered to the mice a total of 4.95×10^5 or 9.9×10^5 Jm^{-2}, respectively. Eighty percent of the energy output of these lamps was in the UVB range (280-320nm). In the photocarcinogenesis study, UV irradiation was terminated when 25% of the control irradiated mice had tumors. In the direct tumor challenge assay, 12 mice per group received bilateral subcutaneous injections of 2×10^6 UV20 tumor cells in unirradiated skin, and challenge growth was recorded at 3 day intervals. In the passive transfer assay, 10^8 splenocytes from UVB irradiated donors were injected into the lateral tail vein of each naive recipient. On the following day, challenges of 10^6 UV20 tumor cells were injected subcutaneously into the flanks of recipient mice. Growth of these challenges were recorded at 3 day intervals.

RESULTS

The ability of dietary retinyl palmitate, canthaxanthin, or the combination of both, to prevent induction of immunosuppression by UVB irradiation was assessed by passive transfer of splenocytes (26). Growth of UV20 tumor challenges in recipients of splenocytes from UV irradiated mice fed the basal diet, or the basal diet supplemented with retinyl palmitate, canthaxanthin, or both, are presented in Figure 1. Recipients of splenocytes from UV irradiated mice fed the basal diet had little ability to reject a UV20 tumor challenge, with growth of 95% of challenges. However, if the UV irradiated splenocyte donors had been fed with the combination of retinyl palmitate and canthaxanthin, the recipients rejected the UV20 tumor challenges as effectively as did the mice which received splenocytes from unirradiated mice. The combination was more active at reduction of UV-induced immunosuppression than was either retinyl palmitate or canthaxanthin administered as single agents.

The influence of dietary retinyl palmitate and/or canthaxanthin on resistance of UV irradiated mice to a syngeneic, antigenic, UV-induced tumor was also measured. The growth of UV20 tumor challenges implanted in UV irradiated and unirradiated mice is shown in Figure 2. The

DONORS

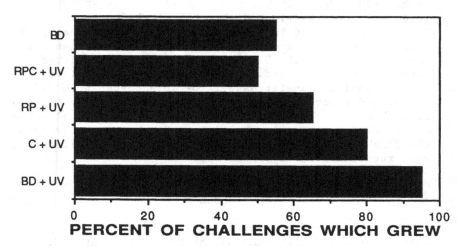

Figure 1. Passive transfer of immunosuppression with splenocytes from UV irradiated donors treated with retinyl palmitate and/or canthaxanthin. Mice were fed the basal diet supplemented with 1% canthaxanthin, 120 IU retinyl palmitate per g diet, or the combination of both, for 18 weeks before UV irradiation was started. After 12 weeks of UV radiation treatments, yielding a cumulative dose of 4.5 X 10^5 Jm^{-2}, spleens were removed and used as the source of splenocytes for the passive transfer assay. 10^8 splenocytes were injected intravenously into each naive syngeneic recipient. Within 24 h, 10^6 UV20 tumor cells were injected intradermally into the flank of each splenocyte recipient. Tumor growth or rejection of 20 challenges per group was assessed at 3 weeks post challenge. BD, basal diet; RP, retinyl palmitate; C, canthaxanthin; RPC, retinyl palmitate plus canthaxanthin.

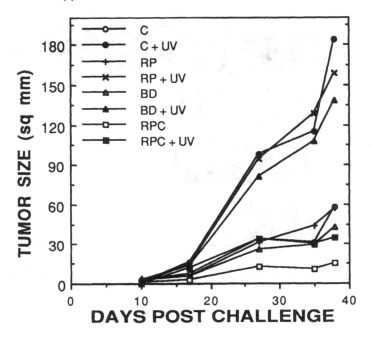

Figure 2. Growth of UV20 tumor implants in UV irradiated mice which had been fed the basal diet supplemented with retinyl palmitate and/or canthaxanthin. Mice were treated as described in the legend of Figure 1. After 12 weeks of UV radiation treatments, 2 X 10^6 UV20 tumor cells were injected in the unirradiated ventral skin of dorsally irradiated mice. Values represent the means of 24 challenges per group of mice. Symbols are presented in the legend of Figure 1.

enhanced tumor growth found in UV irradiated mice as compared with unirradiated mice was not found in UV irradiated mice fed the combination of retinyl palmitate plus canthaxanthin. Neither agent alone overcame the increased susceptibility of UV irradiated mice to an antigenic, UV-induced tumor.

The mean primary tumor burden per mouse, i.e. total tumor area per mouse, at 27.5 weeks after the first UV exposure is presented in Figure 3. Dietary canthaxanthin

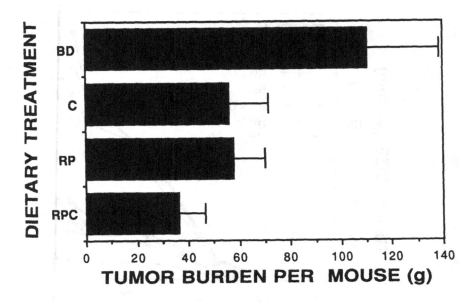

Figure 3.   Primary UV-induced tumor burden per mouse in
mice treated with retinyl palmitate and/or canthaxanthin.
Mice were treated as described in the legend of Figure 1
except that these mice underwent 24 weeks of UVB
irradiation. The tumor area per mouse was calculated as the
total tumor area (length x width of each tumor) per mouse
at 27.5 weeks after the first UV exposure. Values represent
the means of 25-30 mice per group ± SEM. Symbols are
presented in the legend of Figure 1.

(P=0.0081, analysis of variance), or retinyl palmitate
(P=0.0135) yielded significantly lower tumor burdens per
mouse than was found in mice fed the basal diet. The
combination resulted in a lower tumor burden than was found
in mice fed either agent individually.
    The body weights of the UV irradiated mice are
presented in Figure 4. Using analysis of covariance, the
overall difference of the means was significant, and this
significance was due to a lower body weight of mice fed the
basal diet supplemented with the combination of retinyl

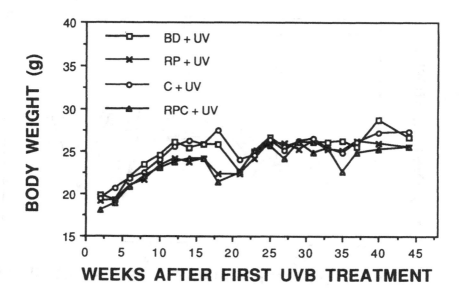

WEEKS AFTER FIRST UVB TREATMENT

Figure 4. Body weights of UV irradiated mice fed the basal diet supplemented with retinyl palmitate and/or canthaxanthin. The duration of the UV radiation treatment period was 24 weeks. Values are the means of 20 mice per group. Symbols are presented in the legend of Figure 1.

palmitate plus canthaxanthin. Based on the least square means, this group weighed 1.5g less than the other groups of mice. The average food consumption per week was similar in all UV irradiated mice, regardless of dietary treatment, as indicated by the Student t test. The daily food consumption per mouse is presented in Figure 5.

DISCUSSION

The combination of dietary retinyl palmitate and canthaxanthin was more effective than either agent alone at preventing UV-induced immunosuppression, at enhancing resistance to an antigenic UV-induced tumor, and at limiting growth of primary UV-induced tumors. Thus, by

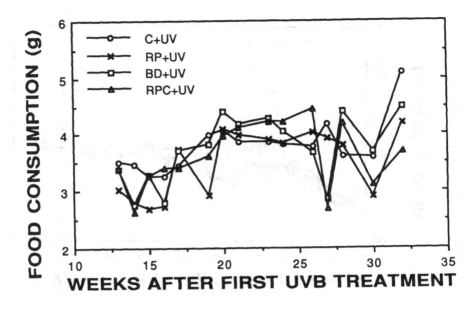

Figure 5. Daily food consumption per UV irradiated mouse
fed the basal diet supplemented with retinyl palmitate
and/or canthaxanthin. The duration of the UV radiation
treatment period was 24 weeks. Values are the means of 20
mice per group. Symbols are presented in the legend of
Figure 1.

three different parameters, the combination of these
compounds achieved a greater effect than did individual
agents. The correlation of these three parameters suggests
that prevention of immunosuppression is a mechanism which
could account for the ability of dietary retinyl palmitate
and canthaxanthin to limit growth of UV-induced tumors.

     The mechanisms by which retinyl palmitate and/or
canthaxanthin prevent UV-induced immunosuppression have not
yet been defined. Retinoids have a number of
immunomodulating activities: 1) stimulation of cytotoxic T
cells (27), 2) stimulation of interleukin-2 production
(28,29), and 3) stimulation of macrophages (30). A
potential mechanism for canthaxanthin immunomodulation is
by quenching high energy oxygen species induced by UV

irradiation (31), thereby reducing oxidation of sterols. The oxidized sterols, e.g. 25-hydroxycholesterol or activated vitamin D_3, are strong immunosuppressants (32,33).

Specific or restricted immunosuppression appears to be a general mechanism by which immunogenic tumors are able to grow in an otherwise immunocompetent host. The immunogenicity in syngeneic hosts of many tumors induced by chemicals or ultraviolet irradiation is well established (34-36). Immunization can be demonstrated by removing established tumor implants surgically or with ligation, or by injection of heavily x-irradiated tumor cells. Subsequent implants of the same tumor cell line are rejected, and this capacity for specific rejection can be transferred to naive mice with lymphoid cells. The Meth A fibrosarcoma, which was originally induced by methylcholanthrene, a mastocytoma (P815), and the P388 lymphoma are examples of immunogenic tumors which grow progressively in a host by inducing a specific immunosuppression (37-39). In mice which had not been previously immunized, immunity developed early after implantation. This immunity, or ability to reject tumor cells, could be passively transferred to a recipient with Ly-2$^+$ lymphocytes from a tumor bearing animal. Continued growth of the immunogenic tumor was found to result in the loss of established host immunity to the tumor, measured by loss of the ability to reject a challenge implant. This decay of immunity resulted from the generation of suppressor lymphocytes, as demonstrated by the ability of L3T4$^+$ splenocytes from mice with a large tumor to prevent the expression of passively transferred immunity to the same tumor (40). This suppression was specific for the tumor which induced it. Significantly, the induction of an immunosuppression which down-regulates the tumoricidal capacity of the host masks the apparent immunogenicity of the tumor, which is detectable by transplantation techniques only before the immunosuppression. In contrast to tumor-induced suppression, UV-induced immunosuppression has not been found to regulate an established immunity (41).

The finding that dietary retinyl palmitate and canthaxanthin prevented ultraviolet-induced immunosuppression and enhanced host resistance to

autochthonous as well as implanted UV-induced tumor
implants suggests that modulation of immunosuppression may
be an important mechanism for chemoprevention of
immunogenic tumors.

ACKNOWLEDGMENTS

I thank Karen Holladay for expert technical assistance
in the studies reported here and Dr. Hemmige Bhagavan,
Hoffmann-La Roche, for kindly providing retinyl palmitate
and canthaxanthin. This research was supported by NIH Grant
CA-27502.

REFERENCES

1.   Engel, A., Johnson, M.L. and Haynes, S.G. Health
      effects of sunlight exposure in the United States.
      Arch. Dermatol. 124:72-79, 1988.
2.   Forbes, P.D. and Davies, R.E. Photobiology of
      experimental ultraviolet photocarcinogenesis. In: R.W.
      Daynes and J.D. Spikes, (eds.), Experimental and
      Clinical Photoimmunology, Vol. 1, pp. 43-60. Boca
      Raton, Florida: CRC Press, 1986.
3.   Kraemer, K.H., Lee, M.M. and Scotto, J. Xeroderma
      pigmentosum, cutaneous, ocular, and neurologic
      abnormalities in 830 published cases. Arch. Dermatol.,
      123:241-250, 1987.
4.   Sheil, A.G. Cancer after transplantation. World J.
      Surg. 10:389-396, 1986.
5.   Penn, I. Cancer is a complication of severe
      immunosuppression. Surg. Gynecol. Obst., 162:603-610,
      1986.
6.   Kripke, M.L. Immunological unresponsiveness induced by
      ultraviolet radiation. Immunol. Rev. 80:87-102, 1984.
7.   Daynes, R.A., Bernhard, E.J., Gurish, M.F. and Lynch,
      D.H.
      Experimental photoimmunology: Immunologic
      ramifications of UV-induced carcinogenesis. J. Invest.
      Dermatol., 77:77-85,1981.
8.   Ullrich, S.E. and Kripke, M.L. Mechanisms in the
      suppression of tumor rejection produced in mice by
      repeated UV irradiation. J.immunol., 133:2786-2790,
      1984.

9.   Fisher, M.S. and Kripke, M.L. Suppressor T lymphocytes control the development of primary skin cancers in ultraviolet-irradiated mice. Science, 216:1133-1134, 1982.

10. Noonan, F.P., Kripke, M.L., Pedersen, G.M., and Greene, M.I. Suppression of contact hypersensitivity in mice by ultraviolet irradiation is associated with defective antigen presentation. Immunology, 43:527-533, 1981.

11. Roberts, L.K., and Daynes, R.A. Modification of the immunogenic properties of chemically induced tumors arising in hosts treated concomitantly with ultraviolet light. J. Immunol. 125:438-447, 1980.

12. Spellman, C.W., Woodward, J.G., and Daynes, R.A. Modification of immunolgical potential by ultraviolet radiation. I. Immune status of short term UV-irradiated mice. Transplantation 24:112-119, 1977.

13. Kripke,M.L., Lofgreen, J.S., Beard, J., Jessup, JM., and Fisher, M.S. In vivo immune response of mice during carcinogenesis by ultraviolet irradiation. J. Natl. Cancer Inst., 59:1227-1230, 1977.

14. Norbury, K.C., Kripke, M.L., and Budman, M.B. In vitro reactivity of macrophages and lymphocytes from ultraviolet-irradiated mice. J. Natl. Cancer Inst., 59:1231-1235, 1977.

15. Connor, M.J., Lowe, N.J., Breeding, J.H. and Chalet, M. Inhibition of ultraviolet-B skin carcinogenesis by all-trans-retinoic acid regimens that inhibit ornithine decarboxylase induction. Cancer Res., 43:171-174, 1983.

16. Epstein, J.H. and Grekin, D.A. Inhibition of ultraviolet induced carcinogenesis by all-trans-retinoic acid. J. Invest. Dermatol., 76:178-180, 1981.

17. Boutwell, R.K., Verma, A.K., Takigawa, M., Loprinzi, C.L. and Carbone, P.P. Retinoids as inhibitors of tumor promotion. In: J.H. Saurat, (ed.) Retinoids: New Trends in Research and Therapy, pp. 83-96. Basel, Karger, 1985.

18. Gensler, H.L., Watson, R.R., Moriguchi, S. and Bowden, G.T. Effects of dietary retinyl palmitate or 13-cis-retinoic acid on the promotion of tumors in mouse skin. Cancer Res., 47:967-970, 1987.

19. Gensler, H.L., Sim, D.A. and Bowden, G.T. (1986) Influence of the duration of topical 13-cis-retinoi acid treatment on inhibition of mouse skin tumor promotion. Cancer Res., 46:2767-2770, 1986.

20. Malkovsky, M., Hunt,R., Palmer, L., Dore, C. and
    Medawar, P.B. Retinyl acetate-mediated augmentation of
    resistance to a transplantable 3-methylcholanthrene-
    induced fibrosarcoma. Transplantation, 38:158-161,
    1984.

21. Cohen, B.E., Gill, G., Cullen, P.R., and Morris, P.J.
    Reversal of postoperative immunosuppression in man by
    vitamin A. Surg. Gynecol. Obstet., 149:658-662, 1979.

22. Fusi, S., Kupper, T.S., Green, JD.R., and Ariyan, S.
    Reversal of postburn immunosuppression by the
    administration of vitamin A. Surgery, 96:330-334,
    1984.

23. Mathews-Roth, M.M. and Krinsky, N.I. Carotenoid dose
    level and protection against UV-B induced skin tumors.
    Photochem. Photobiol. 42:35-38, 1985.

24. Bendich, A. and Shapiro, S.S. Effect of β-carotene and
    canthaxanthin on the immune responses of the rat. J.
    Nutr. 116:2254-2262, 1986.

25. Peng, Y.M., Alberts, D.S., Xu, M.J., Watson, R.R.,
    Gensler, H.L. and Bowden, G.T. Effects of high dietary
    retinyl palmitate and selenium on tissue distribution
    of retinoids in mice exposed to tumor initiation and
    promotion. J. Nutr. Growth Cancer, 3:38-45, 1986.

26. Gensler, H.L. Reduction of immunosuppression in UV-
    irradiated mice by dietary retinyl palmitate plus
    canthaxanthin. Carcinogenesis, 10:203-207, 1989.

27. Dennert, G., Crowley, C., Kouba, J. and Lotan, R.
    Retinoic acid stimulation of the induction of mouse
    killer T-cells in allogeneic and syngeneic systems. J.
    Natl. Cancer Inst., 62:89-94, 1979.

28. Colizzi, V. and Malkovsky, M. Augmentation of
    interleukin-2 production and delayed hypersensitivity
    in mice infected with Mycobacterium bovis and fed a
    diet suppplemented with vitamin A acetate. Infect.
    Immun., 48:581-583, 1985.

29. Dennert, G. Immunostimulation by retinoic acid. In: J.
    Nugent, and S. Clark, S. (eds), Retinoids,
    Differentiation and Disease, Ciba Foundation Symposium
    113, pp. 117-131. London: Pitman, 1985.

30. Watson, R.R., Moriguchi, S. and Gensler, H.L. Effects
    of dietary retinyl palmitate and selenium on
    tumoricidal capacity of macrophages in mice undergoing
    tumor promotion. Cancer Lett., 36:181-187, 1987.

31. Krinsky, N.I. and Deneke, S.M. Interaction of oxygen
    and oxyradicals with carotenoids. J. Natl. Cancer
    Inst., 69:205-210, 1982.

32. Sprangrude, G.J. and Daynes, R.A. Oxygenated sterols as immunosuppressive agents. In: R.A. Daynes and G. Krueger (eds), <u>Experimental and Clinical Photoimmunology</u>, Vol.II, pp. 89-102. Boca Raton, Florida, CRC Press, 1986.

33. Rigby, W.F. The immunobiology of vitamin D. Immunol. Today, 9:54-62, 1988.

34. Klein, G. Tumor antigens. Annu. Rev. Microbiol. 20:223-252, 1966.

35. Hellstrom, D.E. and Hellstrom, I. Cellular immunity against tumor antigens. Adv. Cancer Res. 12:167-223, 1969.

36. Hostetler, L.W., Romerdahl, C.A. and Kripke, M.L. Specificity of antigens on UV radiation-induced antigenic tumor cell variants measured <u>in vitro</u> and <u>in vivo</u>. Cancer Res., 49:1207-1213, 1989.

37. North, R.J. and Dye, E.S. Ly-1+2- suppressor T cells down-regulate the generation of Ly-1-2+ effector T cells. Immunology, 53:47-56, 1985.

38. North, R.J. and Bursuker, I. The generation and decay of the immune response to a progressive fibrosarcoma: Ly-1+2- suppressor T cells down-regulate the generation of Ly-1-2+ effector T cells. J. Exp. Med., 159:1295-1311, 1984.

39. Dye, E.S. and North, R.J. Specificity of the T cells that mediate and suppress adoptive immunotherapy of established tumors. J. Leukocyte Biol., 36:27-38, 1984.

40. DiGiacomo, A. and North, R.J. T cell suppressors of antitumor immunity. The production of Ly-1-2+ suppressors of delayed sensitivity precedes the production of suppressors of protective immunity. J. Exp. Med., 164:1179-1192, 1986.

41. Kripke, M.L., and Fisher, M.S. Immunologic parameters of ultraviolet carcinogenesis. J. Natl. Cancer Inst., 57:211-215, 1976.

Nutrients and Cancer Prevention K. N. Prasad and F. L. Meyskens, Jr., eds. © 1990 The Humana Press

RETINOIDS AND PREVENTION OF EXPERIMENTAL CANCER

Richard C. Moon

IIT Research Institute

10 West 35th Street, Chicago, IL   60616

A dietary vitamin A deficiency results in clinical symptoms manifested by growth retardation, degeneration of reproductive organs, metaplasia and hyperkeratinization of epithelial tissues (1). Moreover, animals deficient in vitamin A are more susceptible to chemical carcinogens than are non-deficient animals (2,3). It has also been well documented that, the exogenous administration of retinoids to experimental animals suppress epithelial carcinogenesis in several organs (4,5). Similarly, in vitro studies have shown that the expression of malignant phenotype is also suppressed by certain retinoids (6).

During the last decade, several retinoids have been evaluated in our laboratory for their efficacy against urinary bladder, tracheal, esophageal, and mammary carcinogenesis induced by chemical carcinogens. Although several examples may be cited relative to the efficacy of retinoids against epithelial carcinogenesis, we shall limit our discussion to a brief review of the effect of these agents on cancer of the mammary gland, urinary bladder and respiratory tract.

MAMMARY CANCER: RETINOIDS AS SINGLE AGENTS

The initial study demonstrating the effectiveness of retinoids as chemopreventive agents in chemically-induced mammary carcinogenesis was conducted in our laboratory using 7,12-dimethylbenz(a)anthracene (DMBA)-treated

197

Sprague-Dawley female rats and retinyl acetate (7); DMBA-treated animals receiving a diet supplemented with the retinoid exhibited a significant reduction in mammary cancer incidence and multiplicity from that of control rats fed a placebo diet. Since then a number of retinoids have been evaluated for chemopreventive activity against both DMBA and N-methyl-N-nitrosourea (MNU)-induced mammary carcinogenesis as well as against mammary cancer development in both mammary tumor virus positive and mammary tumor virus negative mice (5). All active compounds are effective in decreasing tumor multiplicity and increasing latency at retinoid concentrations which are non-toxic. Since N-(4-hydroxyphenyl)retinamide (4-HPR) has been found to be the most effective retinoid against mammary carcinogenesis, when both toxicity and efficacy are taken into consideration, it has been used as the retinoid of choice in a majority of such experiments.

The exact time of carcinogen exposure in the human population is unknown; thus, it is of clinical importance to determine how long after the carcinogenic insult retinoid administration can be delayed and still maintain chemopreventive efficacy. Generally, retinoids are most effective in inhibiting mammary carcinogenesis when administered shortly after carcinogen treatment. However, McCormick and Moon (8) showed that retinoid treatment can be delayed in the rat mammary tumor model for as long as 16 weeks after carcinogen administration and still retain its chemopreventive effectiveness, although in groups of animals in which retinoid treatment was initiated 20 weeks after carcinogen administration, the ability of retinoids to inhibit carcinogenesis was lost. These findings indicate that retinoid administration can be delayed for as long as 4 months but not for 5 months. It was apparent, therefore, that a "critical" point exists in tumor development beyond which retinoids may be ineffective. Such a delay corresponds to approximately ten years in the human being.

Toxicity which may accompany administration of a retinoid is also of concern in long term chemoprevention studies. For example, retinyl acetate and 4-HPR are both effective inhibitors of chemical carcinogenesis of the rat mammary gland, but the patterns of metabolism and organ distribution of the two compounds are quite different. Chronic dietary treatment with high doses of retinyl acetate results in an accumulation of retinyl esters in the liver, a process frequently accompanied by significant hepatic toxicity. On the other hand, dietary administration of 4-HPR results in a much higher concentration of retinoid in the mammary gland, but with relatively little liver accumulation (9). In addition, 4-HPR is active both in mice and rats. Therefore, as a result of its organ distribution, it would appear that 4-HPR is preferable to retinyl acetate for use in the prevention of experimental breast cancer.

In an effort to more closely simulate the clinical situation, we conducted two experiments in which retinoid treatment was not initiated until after the surgical removal of the first palpable tumor (10). Very little quantitative inhibition of mammary tumorigenesis was evident until approximately 50 days following tumor excision, after which a significantly reduced rate of tumor appearance was noted in the retinoid-treated group in comparison to control animals. These studies suggest that retinoids inhibit cancer by suppressing the progression of early lesions. If the retinoid offered any protection against the proliferation of fully established cancers, the effect would not have been delayed for 50 days after tumor excision. Thus, as noted earlier, there must be a crucial step(s) by which retinoid-responsive preneoplastic or early neoplastic lesions become retinoid resistant.

Although the evidence supporting the inhibitory activity of retinoids on mammary cancer in rats is substantial, only a few studies describing the use of retinoid in mammary tumorigenesis in mice have been reported. In the initial study by Maiorana and Gullino (11), it was found that retinyl acetate did not influence (neither inhibited nor enhanced) tumor incidence, latency, or tumor number in C_3H-A^{vy} female mice positive for the mammary tumor virus (MTV). However, using C_3H mice negative for the MTV it was found that the number of hyperplastic alveolar nodules (putative precancerous lesions) developing in animals receiving dietary 4-HPR, was significantly less than that of control mice receiving the placebo diet, while retinyl acetate did not affect noduligenesis in these experiments (5). Welsch et al. (12) on the other hand, have reported an enhancement of tumor development in nulliparous and multiparous mice of the GR strain fed a diet supplemented with retinyl acetate, but inhibition with 4-HPR in C_3H mice (13).

MAMMARY CANCER: RETINOIDS AND OTHER AGENT COMBINATIONS

Even though retinoids can significantly inhibit experimental carcinogenesis of various organs, a totally effective retinoid that can reduce the cancer incidence to zero is yet to be developed. It is, however, possible to enhance the inhibition achieved by retinoids if a combination of retinoid with other growth modifiers is employed.

Recent studies by several investigators have demonstrated such interaction between retinoids and other modifiers of mammary carcinogenesis. In most cases, combined treatment affords greater protection against mammary carcinogenesis than either treatment alone. Carcinogen-induced rat mammary cancer models are subject to inhibition by both retinoids and modification of host hormonal status. It is well known that ovarian hormone-dependent tumors regress following ovariectomy of the tumor-bearing animal. Similarly, if animals are ovariectomized shortly after carcinogen administration, only the ovarian hormone-independent tumors appear, and cancer incidence is low. The combination of ovariectomy (2 weeks postcarcinogen administration) and retinyl acetate result in a synergistic inhibition of tumor incidence and multiplicity (10). Similar results were obtained with 4-HPR. In a more recent study, it was demonstrated that tamoxifen and 4-HPR, when used in combination, were much more effective in inhibiting mammary carcinogenesis than either agent alone (14). A similar synergistic inhibition has been demonstrated in the MNU-induced mammary carcinogenesis model by concomitant administration of retinyl acetate and 2-bromo-α-ergocryptine, an inhibitor of pituitary prolactin secretion (15). Since the blood prolactin levels of the retinyl acetate-treated rats were similar to those of control animals, the enhanced combination effect was probably not due to a further suppression of prolactin secretion but to an effect at the level of the mammary parenchymal cell. Although hormonal modification of experimental mammary tumorigenesis is well established, the evidence cited above indicates that the retinoids also effectively alter mammary tumorigenesis. These data suggest the existence of populations of preneoplastic and/or neoplastic cells displaying differential sensitivity to the retinoids and hormones. Whether retinoids preferentially suppress the growth of hormone-dependent cell populations, reverse the neoplastic potential of these cells, or induce terminal differentiation of preneoplastic cells, as has been demonstrated in C3H 10T1/2 cells (16), is presently unknown.

Combination chemoprevention has also been demonstrated with retinoids and other agents that inhibit development of mammary cancer. Thompson et al. (17) were the first to show an enhanced inhibition of MNU-induced rat mammary carcinogenesis with retinyl acetate and selenium. The effect was confirmed by Ip and Ip (18) using the DMBA-induced mammary tumor model. Although both groups of workers found that the combined effect of retinyl acetate and selenium was substantially greater than the effect of either treatment alone, both studies were complicated by the significant reduction in food intake and body weight gain in animals receiving these chemopreventive agents. Attempts to combine modalities for prevention of mammary cancer are not always successful. For example, 4-HPR and MVE-2 (a maleic anhydride-divinyl ether copolymer), immunostimulatory agents, are both effective inhibitors of MNU-induced mammary carcinogenesis in rats. However, the combination of 4-HPR and MVE-2 was no more effective in inhibiting cancer than either agent alone (19).

URINARY BLADDER CANCER

The induction of urinary bladder cancer by MNU or N-butyl-N-(4-hydroxybutyl)nitrosamine (OH-BBN) is sensitive to modulation by retinoids. Sporn et al. (20) were the first to demonstrate the efficacy of 13-cis-retinoic acid in inhibiting the incidence as well as reducing the severity of bladder neoplasms induced by the intravesical administration of MNU to female Wistar-Lewis rats.

In the attempt to improve upon the therapeutic index attained with 13-cis-retinoic acid, extensive studies were undertaken in our laboratory to identify retinoids with increased chemopreventive activity when administered at nontoxic levels in the diet. Using an experimental model in which C57BL/6 x DBA/2 F_1 mice are treated with OH-BBN, a large number of synthetic n-alkyl amide derivatives of retinoic acid have been identified which possess a greater activity:toxicity ratio than that seen with 13-cis-retinoic acid (21).

These studies showed once again that modifications of the basic retinoid structure can have a significant effect on anticancer activity. For example, the addition of an ethylamide or a hydroxyethylamide group to all-trans-retinoic acid results in compounds which are highly effective chemopreventive agents for bladder cancer, but much less toxic than is all-trans-retinoic acid. Similarly, addition of the ethylamide or hydroxyethylamide group to 13-cis-retinoic acid results in the formation of a less toxic retinoid, with equal or greater cancer-inhibitory activity. Conversely, however, changing the aromatic ring of the highly active ethyl retinamide to a trimethylmethoxyphenyl group produces a compound with little or no cancer-inhibitory activity in the bladder.

Consistent with the findings reported for retinoid action in the mammary gland, the onset of retinoid administration can be delayed for some time with retention of chemopreventive activity against urinary bladder carcinogenesis (22). Delaying the administration of a dietary supplement of 13-cis-retinoic acid for 5 or 9 weeks after the final administration of OH-BBN to F344 rats, resulted in no loss of chemopreventive effect when compared to a group for which retinoid supplement was begun 1 week after the cessation of OH-BBN treatment; all retinoid groups showed a statistically significant inhibition of carcinogenesis compared to placebo-treated controls. These studies, demonstrating the retention of cancer-inhibitory activity when retinoid administration is delayed, are of critical significance for possible clinical use of retinoids in cancer prevention.

CANCER OF THE RESPIRATORY TRACT

Saffiotti and coworkers (23) were the first to describe an inhibitory effect of retinoids on respiratory carcinogenesis. However, studies of the inhibition of chemically induced tumorigenesis of the respiratory tract by retinoids have been equivocal and, in some cases, contradictory. In the study by Saffiotti et al., tumors were induced in hamsters by the intratracheal instillation of benzo[a]pyrene adsorbed onto ferric oxide particles (3 mg benzo[a]pyrene plus 3 mg ferric oxide suspended in 0.2 ml saline), once a week for 10 weeks. Treatment with retinyl palmitate markedly reduced both the incidence and number of respiratory tumors. However, retinyl acetate was ineffective in inhibiting development of lung tumors induced by the Saffiotti technique. Nettesheim et al. (24), on the other hand, showed that retinyl acetate inhibited metastatic lung nodules induced in rats by 3-methylcholanthrene. Bronchial carcinoma induced by the Saffiotti procedure was effectively inhibited by 13-cis-retinoic acid. However, enhancement of MNU-induced tracheobronchial carcinogenesis has been reported with 13-cis-retinoic acid, ethyl retinamide, and N-(4-hydroxyethyl)retinamide (25). In an early study, 4-HPR neither enhanced nor inhibited tracheobronchial carcinogenesis induced with MNU (26). More recently, however, we have found that 4-HPR is an effective inhibitor of DEN-induced lung carcinogenesis in the hamster, but has little effect on MNU-induced tracheobronchial carcinogenesis in this species. A combination of 4-HPR, selenium, and vitamin E was more effective than when the agents were administered alone (27).

The experiments described in the preceding paragraphs demonstrate that several natural and synthetic retinoids are highly effective in inhibiting carcinogenesis induced with a variety of chemical carcinogens. It is also apparent that, in most cases, the synthetic retinoids are more efficacious than the natural retinoids and are considerably less toxic. In those experimental systems (mammary, skin) which exhibit definite initiation and promotion stages of carcinogenesis, the retinoids have proven to be highly effective chemopreventive agents. However, if a definitive promotional phase is absent in an experimental tumor system, or is ill defined (tracheobronchial, lung), ambiguous results as to the chemopreventive effectiveness of the retinoids have been obtained; and in isolated cases, the compounds may even promote carcinogenesis. Nevertheless, the overwhelming evidence indicates that retinoids inhibit carcinogenesis in such experimental tumor model systems.

REFERENCES

1. Hicks, R.M. The scientific basis for regarding vitamin A and its analogues as anti-carcinogenic agents. Proc. Nutr. Soc., 42: 83-93, 1983.
2. Rogers, A.E., Herndon, B.J., and Newberne, P.M. Induction by dimethylhydrazine of intestinal carcinoma in normal rats fed high and low levels of vitamin A. Cancer Res., 33: 1003-1009, 1973.

3. Cohen, S.M., Wittenberg, J.F., and Bryn, G.T. Effect
    of avitaminosis A and hypervitaminosis A on urinary
    bladder carcinogenicity of N-[4-(5-nitro-2-furyl)-2-
    thiazolyl]formamide. Cancer Res., 36: 2334-2339,
    1976.
4. Sporn, M.B., Dunlop, N.M., Newton, D.L., and Smith,
    J.M. Prevention of chemical carcinogenesis by vitamin
    A and its synthetic analogs (retinoids). Fed. Proc.,
    35: 1335-1338, 1976.
5. Moon, R.C., McCormick, D.L., and Mehta, R.G.
    Inhibition of carcinogenesis by retinoids. Cancer
    Res., 43: 2469s-2475s, 1983.
6. Lotan, R. Effects of vitamin A and its analogs
    (retinoids) on normal and neoplastic cells. Biochem.
    Biophys. Acta., 605: 33-91, 1980.
7. Moon, R.C., Grubbs, C.J., and Sporn, M.B. Inhibition
    of 7,12-dimethylbenz(a)anthracene-induced mammary
    carcinogenesis by retinyl acetate. Cancer Res., 36:
    2626-2630, 1976.
8. McCormick, D.L., and Moon, R.C. Influence of delayed
    administration of retinyl acetate on mammary
    carcinogenesis. Cancer Res., 42: 2639-2643, 1982.
9. Moon, R.C., Thompson, H.J., Becci, P.J., Grubbs, C.J.,
    Gander, R.J., Newton, D.L., Smith, J.M., Phillips,
    S.R., Henderson, W.R., Mullen, L.T., Brown, C.C., and
    Sporn, M.B. N-(4-hydroxyphenyl)retinamide, a new
    retinoid for prevention of breast cancer in the rat.
    Cancer Res., 39: 1339-1346, 1979.
10. McCormick, D.L., Sowell, Z.L., Thompson, C.A., and
    Moon, R.C. Inhibition by retinoid and ovariectomy of
    additional primary malignancies in rats following
    surgical removal of the first mammary cancer. Cancer,
    51: 594-599, 1983.
11. Maiorana, A., and Gullino, P. Effect of retinyl
    acetate on the incidence of mammary carcinomas and
    hepatomas in mice. J. Natl. Cancer Inst., 64: 655-
    663, 1980.
12. Welsch, C.W., Goodrich-Smith, M., Brown, C.C., and
    Crowe, N. Enhancement by retinyl acetate of hormone
    induced mammary tumorigenesis in female GR/A mice. J.
    Natl. Cancer Inst., 67: 935-938, 1981.
13. Welsch, C.W., DeHoog, J.V., and Moon, R.C. Inhibition
    of mammary tumorigenesis in nulliparous C3H mice by
    chronic feeding of the synthetic retinoid, N-(4-
    hydroxyphenyl) retinamide. Carcinogenesis, 4: 1185-
    1187, 1983.

14. Ratko, T.A., Detrisac, C.J., Dinger, N.M., Thomas, C.F., Kelloff, G.J., and Moon, R.C. Chemopreventive efficacy of combined retinoid and tamoxifen treatment following surgical excision of a primary mammary cancer in female rats. Cancer Res., 49: 4472-4476, 1989.

15. Welsch, C.W., Brown, C.K., Goodrich-Smith, M., Chiusano, J., and Moon, R.C. Synergistic effect of chronic prolactin suppression and retinoid treatment in the prophylaxis of N-methyl-N-nitrosourea-induced mammary tumorigenesis in female Sprague-Dawley rats. Cancer Res., 40: 3095-3098, 1980.

16. Bertram, J.S. Inhibition of neoplastic transformation in vitro by retinoids. Cancer Surveys, 3: 243-262, 1983.

17. Thompson, H.J., Meeker, L.D., and Becci, P.J. Effect of combined selenium and retinyl acetate treatment on mammary carcinogenesis. Cancer Res., 41: 1413-1416, 1981.

18. Ip, C., and Ip, M.M. Chemoprevention of mammary tumorigenesis by a combined regimen of selenium and vitamin A. Carcinogenesis, 2: 915-918, 1981.

19. McCormick, D.L., Becci, P.J., and Moon, R.C. Inhibition of mammary and urinary bladder carcinogenesis by a retinoid and a maleic anhydride-divinyl ether copolymer (MVE-2). Carcinogenesis, 3: 1473-1477, 1982.

20. Sporn, M.B., Squire, R.A., Brown, C.C., Smith, J.M., Wenk, M.L., and Springer, S. 13-cis-retinoic acid: inhibition of bladder carcinogenesis in the rat. Science, 195: 487-489, 1977.

21. Moon, R.C., McCormick, D.L., Becci, P.J., Shealy, Y.F., Frickel, F., Paust, J., and Sporn, M.B. Influence of 15 retinoic acid amides on urinary bladder carcinogenesis in the mouse. Carcinogenesis, 3: 1469-1472, 1982.

22. Becci, P.J., Thompson, H.J., Grubbs, C.J., Brown, C.C., and Moon, R.C. Effect of delay in administration of 13-cis-retinoic acid on the inhibition of urinary bladder carcinogenesis in the rat. Cancer Res., 39: 3141-3144, 1979.

23. Saffiotti, U., Montesano, R., Sellakumar, A.R., and Bork, S.A. Experimental cancer of the lung, inhibition by vitamin A of the induction of tracheobronchial metaplasia and squamous cell tumor. Cancer, 20: 857-864, 1967.

24. Nettesheim, P., Cone, M.W., and Snyder, C. The influence of vitamin A on the susceptibility of the rat lung to 3-methylcholanthrene. Int. J. Cancer, 17: 341-357, 1976.

25. Stinson, S.P., Reznik, G., and Donahoe, R. Effect of three retinoids on tracheal carcinogenesis with N-methyl-N-nitrosourea in hamsters. J. Natl. Cancer Inst., 66: 947-951, 1981.

26. Grubbs, C.J., Becci, P.J., and Moon, R.C. Characterization of 1-methyl-1-nitrosourea (MNU)-induced tracheal carcinogenesis and the effect of feeding the retinoid N-(4-hydroxyphenyl)retinamide (4-HPR). Proc. Am. Assoc. Cancer Res., 21: 102, 1980.

27. Mehta, R.G., Rao, K.V.N., Detrisac, C.J., Kelloff, G.J., and Moon, R.C. Inhibition of diethylnitrosamine-induced lung carcinogenesis by retinoids. Proc. Am. Assoc. Cancer Res., 29: 129, 1988.

SELENIUM AND VITAMIN E IN CANCER PREVENTION

Raymond J. Shamberger

Senior Project Scientist

Ciba-Corning Diagnostics
132 Artino St.
Oberlin, Ohio 44074

INTRODUCTION

In the mid-1960's the interesting phenomenon of initiation and promotion had been established, but very little was known about the chemopreventive approach to carcinogenesis. Many investigators thought that a free radical mechanism was involved. Free radicals would cause tissue damage and peroxidation. Tissue damage also seemed to be related to the cancer process. The greater the tissue damage, the higher the number of cancers in many experiments.

One serious difficulty at that time and even today was to analytically detect a single early cancer cell in the midst of millions of normal cells containing similar biochemical components. Detection of microgram quantities by a gas chromatograph or through visible or ultraviolet spectroscopy was possible in the mid-1960's. There is an issue of very practical importance. Avogadros number is 1×10^{26} molecules/mole and with detection limits of 1×10^{-8} mole, one could detect 1×10^{18} molecules. This amount is a far greater number than one single cancer cell. Even today the most advanced enzyme-linked-amplified analytical method will detect about 1000 molecules with about a 10% variance or 1000 ± 100 molecules. The variance itself today in the best analytical method is still 100 times the single molecular event that needs to be detected.

Because of the analytical difficulties in detecting a singular molecular event, we decided to add components to the 7, 12-dimethylbenzantracene-croton oil tumor system to alter the number of tumors. In this way some insight might be gained into the mechanism of tumor formation.

Furthermore, if a free radical mechanism was involved, leading to an important peroxidation, the antioxidants might alter the number of tumors formed. In the initial experiments sodium selenide and vitamin E were applied to the skin at the same time as the tumor promotor, croton oil. Both sodium selenide and vitamin E reduced the number of tumors (1,2). The mechanism of this inhibition is still unkown. Dietary selenium has been found to inhibit carcinogen-induced cancer in numerous organ systems. Several possible mechanisms of this inhibition have been postulated.

INHIBITION OF CARCINOGEN INDUCED ANIMAL CANCER BY SELENIUM

Medina and Morrison (3) have summarized about 60 experiments and found that the vast majority of the experiments showed an inhibitory effect of selenium supplementation in 10 of 11 organ systems. Eight experiments showed no effect and four experiments showed enhancement. These experiments are summarized and updated in Table 1. Selenium inhibited tumor development in epithelial tissues of colon, mammary gland, liver, skin, stomach and esophagus (3). Tumors were induced by several types of carcinogens, ultraviolet light, and mouse mammary tumor virus. Because of the chemopreventive effect by selenium of the colon, mammary and stomach cancer, selenium has interest because of its possible value against human cancer. Colon, mammary and stomach cancer are major causes of cancer death in humans. It is also interesting that selenium prevented cancer induced by carcinogens, virus and ultraviolet irradiation. Therefore, selenium may inhibit cancer through the same molecular mechanism. The key steps of viral, carcinogen and irradiation induced cancer that is inhibited by selenium may be the same for all three types of carcinogenic stimulus. These observations may be ultimately important in identifying the key steps of cancer inhibition.

Most of the experiments used sodium selenite at dietary levels of 0.5 and 1.0 ppm. These levels should be considered supranutritional because the rodent requirement for selenium is about 0.1 ppm. Selenium in the organic forms are also effective inhibitors of tumorigeneses but are usually utilized at greater dietary levels than the inorganic forms. Selenomethionine and p-methoxybenzeneselenol inhibit mammary and stomach tumorigeneses (3).

Table 1. Effect of Selenium Supplementation on Tumorigenesis (3).

Organ	Species	Carcinogen	Effect on tumorigenesis		
			decrease	increase	no effect
Liver	rat	DAB,AAF, DEN,AFB1	8	2	0
Colon	rat	DMH,MAM, AOM,BOP	10	0	0
Colon	mouse	DMH	1	0	0
Mammary gland	rat	DMBA, MNU,Ad-9	13	1	0
Mammary gland	mouse	DMBA. MMTV	11	0	3
Skin	mouse	DMBA,UV	5	1	0
Stomach	mouse	BP	1	0	1
Stomach	rat	MNNG	1	0	0
Esophagus	rat	MBN	2	0	0
Oral Cavity	hamster	DMBA	2	0	0
Trachea	hamster	MNU	1	0	2
Pancreas	hamster	BOP	1	0	1
Kidney	rat	AOM	1	0	0
Lung	mice	urethan	1	0	1

DAB = 3-methly-4-diaminoazobenzene; AAF = 2-acetylaminofluorine;
DEN = diethylnitrosamine; AFB1 = aflatoxin B1; DMH = 1,2-dimethylhydrazine;
MAM = methylazoxymethanol acetate; AOM = azoxymethane;
BOB = bis(2-oxopropyl)nitrosamine; DMBA = 7,12-dimethylbenzanthracene;
MNU = methylnitrosourea; Ad-9 = adenovirus type 9; MMTV = mouse mammary tumor
virus; BP = benzo(a)pyrene; MMNG = N-methyl-N'-nitro-N-nitrosoguanidine;
MBN = methylbenzylnitrosamine.

There have been several studies investigating the effects of selenium deficient diets on carcinogenesis. In general, a selenium deficiency does not affect carcinogenesis in the colon or liver of the rat (4). Selenium deficiency enhances carcinogenesis in mouse skin and rat mammary glands.

EFFECT OF SELENIUM ON SKIN, COLON, LIVER AND MAMMARY CANCER IN ANIMALS

The chemopreventative effect of selenium has been primarily studied on the skin, colon, liver and mammary gland in animals. The greatest effects have been observed in colon and mammary tumorigenesis. This may indicate that the effect is related to fat metabolism because the colon and mammary gland are fat responsive organs in regard to the cancer process.

Skin

Topical sodium selenide and vitamin E (1,2) significantly reduced the number of tumors in mice initiated with 7,12-dimethylbenzanthracene and promoted with croton oil (Table 2). Selenium-deficient diets and selenium-supplemented diets also reduced the number of benzopyrene induced tumors. Thorling et al (5) has added selenium to the drinking water and was able to inhibit development of skin hyperplasia and pigmentation induced by ultraviolet light in hairless mice.

Table 2. Influence of Selenium on Chemical Carcinogens on Skin

Level in diet		Species of animal	Chemical carcinogen and reference	% Tumor reduction by selenium
Se	Diet			
.0005%[a]	commercial	mice	DMBA*-croton oil (1,2)	26
.0005%[a]	commercial	mice	3-methylcholanthrene (2)	22
1.0ppm	torula yeast	mice	benzopyrene (2)	40
1.0ppm	torula yeast	mice	DMBA-croton oil (2)	32

a   applied to skin.
*   DMBA-7,12-dimethylbenzanthracene

Liver

The influence of chemical carcinogens on rat liver is summarized in Table 3.

Marked effects of dietary selenium were observed on liver carcinogenesis (6-12). In some experiments selenium was placed in the diet and in others selenium was added to the drinking water. Some of the carcinogens used were 3-methy-4-dimethylaminobenzene, 2-acetylaminofluorene and azoxymethane. The form of selenium used was usually sodium selenite, but in the experiments of Tanaka et al (11) 50.0 ppm of methoxybenzeneselenol was added to the diet. Le Boeuf et al (13) have found that dietary selenium significantly decreased the development of gamma-glutamyltranspeptidase-positive liver foci (GGTP foci) induced by diethylnitrosamine. In addition, Baldwin, et al (14) have also found that dietary selenium also decreased the development of GGTP foci induced by aflatoxin in rats.

Table 3. Influence of Selenium on Chemical Carcinogens on Rat Liver

Level in diet		Species of animal	Chemical carcinogen and reference	% Tumor reduction by selenium
Se	Diet			
5 ppm	Casein-based	rat	DAB* (6)	48
6 ppm [a]	Commercial	rat	DAB (7)	40
0.5 ppm	torula yeast	rat	AAF** (8)	83
4 ppm [a]	Commercial	rat	AAF (9)	48
1.0 ppm	***	rat	Aflatoxin B_1 (10)	80
50.0 ppm	Commercial	rat	AM**** (11)	47
4 ppm [a]	Commercial	rat	Aflatoxin B_1 (12)	36

DAB*   3-methly-4-dimethylaminobenzene
AAF** 2-acetylaminofluorene
Methoxbenzeneselenol***
AM**** Axoxymethane****
[a]   Drinking water

Colon

Chemopreventative effects of dietary selenium have also been observed when 1,2-dimethylhydrazine, bis (2-oxopropyl) nitrosamine and azoxymethane were used as the carcinogenic stimulus (Table 4) (15-20).

Soulier et al (19) have observed a significant reduction in tumor incidence in the proximal half of the colon in contrast to the distal part of the colon. When selenium was measured in the proximal and distal colon the level of selenium was greater in the proximal part of the colon in contrast to the distal part of the colon (21). The difference in selenium in levels may relate to the difference in the carcinogenic response of the proximal and distal colon to carcinogens.

Table 3. Influence of Selenium on Chemical Carcinogens on Rat Colon

Level in diet		Species of animal	Chemical carcinogen and reference	% Tumor reduction by selenium
Se	Diet			
4 ppm [a]	Commercial	rat	DMH* (15)	54
4 ppm [a]	Commercial	rat	DMH (16)	56
4 ppm [a]	Commercial	rat	DMH (16)	43
4 ppm [a]	Commercial	rat	DMH (17)	18
1.0 ppm	Casein-based	rat	BOP** (18)	45
2 ppm a	Casein-based	rat	AM**** (19)	15
2 ppm a	Casein-based	rat	AM (20)	7

DMH*   1,2-dimethylhydrazine
BOP**   bis-(2-oxopropyl) nitrosamine
AM***   Azoxymethane
[a]   Drinking water

Mammary Cancer

The greatest number of chemopreventative experiments have been done with the mammary gland. In general, several reductions of mammary tumorigenesis has been observed with dietary selenium (Table 5).

Table 3. Influence of Selenium on Chemical Carcinogens or Virus on Mammary Glands

Level in diet		Species of animal	Chemical carcinogen and reference	% Tumor reduction by selenium
Se	Diet			
6 ppm [a]	Commercial	mice	MMTV*(22)	88
6 ppm [a]	Commercial	mice	DMBA** (23)	62
1 ppm	Torula yeast (5% unsat. fat)	rat	DMBA (24)	25
1 ppm	Torula yeast (25% unsat.fat)	rat	DMBA (24)	38
1 ppm	Torula yeast (25% unsat.fat)	rat	DMBA (24)	17
1.5 ppm	Torula yeast (5% oil)	rat	DMBA (25)	28
1.5 ppm	Torula yeast (25% oil)	rat	DMBA (25)	21
0.1 ppm	Torula yeast (25% oil)	rat	DMBA (26)	38
5 ppm	Commercial	rat	MNU*** (27)	11
1.0 ppm	Torula yeast	rat	MNU (27)	0
4 ppm [a]	Commercial	mice	DMBA (28)	52

MMTV* Mouse mammary tumor virus
DMBA** 7,12-dimethylbenzanthracene
MNU*** N-methyl-N-nitrosourea
[a]   Drinking water

Tumorigenesis induced by mouse mammary tumor virus, DMBA and MNU were inhibited by dietary selenium. This particular type is similar to colon cancer in that mammary cancer is fat responsive and of special interest to humans.

Ip, et al (29) have also studied the effect of varying the timing of feeding sodium selenite to animals dosed with DMBA. Experimental groups were supplemented with 5 ppm for various periods of time: -2 to 24 weeks; -2 to +2; +2 to +24; +2 to +12; +12 to +24; and -2 to +12. Selenium inhibited tumorigenesis to various degrees at all time periods, but selenium fed throughout the experiment exhibited a maximal inhibition.

Schrauzer and Ishmael (22) have found that selenite and arsenite lowered the incidence of mouse mammary tumor virus induced mammary cancer, but the growth of transplanted mammary tumors was greatly enhanced by arsenite. Ip and Ganther (30) found that arsenite reduced the chemopreventative effect of selenium in the DMBA-induced rat mammary cancer system, but together with trimethylselenonium metabolite also had a chemopreventative effect. Arsenite may be blocking the methyltransferase step, but when fed with 40 ppm of trimethylselenonium instead of 3 ppm selenite, may enhance demethylation and make a metabolic return to a more active methylated form such as dimethylselenide. Ip (31) has also found that by feeding a high level of methionine that greater amounts of selenium can be fed to rats. In this way higher amounts of selenium could be fed to animals without toxicity, thereby enhancing the chemopreventative effect of selenium.

Sodium selenite has inhibited the transformation of mammary cells in organ culture of the whole mammary glands from BABL/c female mice (32). Selenium may act by preventing progression of the transformed cells to potentially neoplastic lesions in the glands "in vitro".

CASE-CONTROL STUDIES

Coates et al (33) has summarized several of the prospective case-control studies with serum selenium and they are summarized in Table 6. In these types of studies serum is stored years in advance and cancer cases are compared to controls.

Results of Published Prospective Case-Control Serum Selenium Studies (33)

Study and location	Cancer site(s) and reference	No. of cases	Mean selenium level (ug/liter) for controls	Relative risk
Willett et al., 1983 14 US locations	All (33)	111	136	2 LQ/HQ [a]
Salonen et al., 1984 Finland	All (33)	128	54	3 LT/R [b]
Salonen et al., 1985 Finland	All (33)	51	61	5 LT/R
Peleg et al., 1985 Georgia	All (33)	130	115	1 LQ/HQ
Menkes et al., 1986 Maryland	Lung (33)	99	110	0.7 LQ/HQ
Kok et al., 1987 The Netherlands	All (33)	69	137	2 LQ/HQ
Coates et al., 1988 NW Washington	All (33)	156	162	1 LQ/HQ
Knekt et al., 1988 Finland	GI (34)	150	61	3.3 LQ/HQ

[a] LQ/HQ   Low quintile/high quintile
[b] LT/R   Low tertile/remainder

In five of eight studies there was a positive relative risk factor of 2 or more. All three studies from Finland were positive with a relative risk of three or more. The investigations were based on small numbers of cases of specific sites (33,34). There was wide confidence limits around site-specific case control differences and relative risk estimates. Inconsistencies of these results by study, sex, site and level of serum selenium may indicate the serum selenium levels may not represent cancer risk. The low selenium levels may reflect a general low nutrient status. In addition to a low serum selenium there could be low levels of many other nutrients which are more representative of the cancer process than selenium. Vitamin A and carotene could be important in this regard.

The animal experiments seems to indicate that a supra-nutritional level is required to have a chemopreventative effect on cancer and deficient dietary levels or dietary levels at 0.1 ppm may not have much chemopreventative effect. The human dietary levels probably reflect on animal dietary equivalent of 0.1 ppm, a level at which not much effect should be expected. Further research is needed with large sample sizes to resolve this question.

MECHANISMS OF SELENIUM CHEMOPREVENTION

DNA Effect

Wortzman, et al. (35) has found that dietary selenium reduces the appearance of DNA fragments induced by aminoacetylfluorene (AAF) as determined by sucrose gradient centrifugation. These breaks were repaired 24 hours after injection of AAF, but under the same conditions, AAF failed to damage the DNA in the livers of selenium-suppplemented rats. Lawson and Birt have found that 5 ppm selenium helped reduce single strand breaks induced by N-Nitroso(2-oxopropyl)amine (36). Human chromosome breakage induced by 7,12-dimethylbenzanthracene has been reduced in the cultures with incubated selenium (27). Peroxidation may increase damage to DNA. Shamberger (38) and Ip (26) have shown there is an association between an increase of peroxidation and skin and mammary tissue carcinogenesis especially when dietary fat is increased. Lipid peroxidation may be the primary mechanism by which dietary fat increases cancer development.

Frenkel et al (39) have found that DNA and RNA polymerases were inhibited by 1mm selenotrisulfide.

Medina has examined the effect of selenium on DNA synthesis in a mammary cell line grown in vitro (40). Low doses of selenium stimulated cell growth and high doses inhibited cell growth. When cell growth was decreased, there was also a decreased cell number, reduced uptake of ^{3}H-thymidine into DNA, decreased DNA labeling index and decreased DNA synthesis. A delay in the G_2 and 5-phase of the cell cycle was observed by flow cytofluorometry of selenium treated mammary cells. The biochemical basis for this effect remains to be determined.

Amino Acid Synthesis

Vernie et al (41) have observed the reaction products of selenite and thiols have an inhibitory effect on protein synthesis in intact P815 and LI210 cells. Some of the inhibition may be attributed to toxicity, but it is also possible that selenium at nutritional levels might inhibit protein synthesis and cellular growth.

Effect on Carcinogen Metabolism

High -performance liquid chromatography analyses have shown that selenium supplemented animals dosed with AAF excreted less N-hydroxy-AAF but more 5-hydroxy-AAF. Dietary selenium may be protecting against AAF induced hepatogenesis by at least inpart to its ability to inhibit the in vivo production of N-hydroxyl-AAF, which is the proximate carcinogenic metabolite of AAF (42). Milner et al (43) have found that sodium selenite inhibits the binding of DMBA to DNA in tertiary cultures of fetal mouse cells. Sodium selenite seems to be selective in inhibitng the anti-dihydro-diol-epoxide product formation at certain times in the presence of an induction of a DMBA-activating enzyme system. Once induction has occured, sodium selenite seems to be no longer capable of inhibiting the DMBA-DNA binding.

Other Mechanisms

Selenium dioxide, selenious acid, and selenic acid have been found to inhibit protein kinase C from acute myelocytic leukemia cells (44). Protein kinase C has been shown to play an important role in tumor promotion, cell regulation and in membrane signal transduction.

Sodium selenite, GSH and vitamin E all decreased phorbol ester induced ornithine decarobxylase activity and increased glutathione peroxidase activity in mouse epidermis in vivo (45). The ornithine decarboxylase step is a key step in tumor promotion and reducing the enzyme level seems to also reduce the carcinogenic effect.

Dietary supplementation and injections of selenium have been shown to enhance production of IgG and IgM anti-sheep red blood cell (SRBC) antibodies in immunized mice (46). Selenium supplementation has been observed to cause the enhanced expression of spontaneous killer cell cytotoxicity in spleen cells and of specific cytotoxic T-lymphocyte cytotoxicity in peritoneal exudate cells (48).

VITAMIN E AND CANCER

It is apparent from the proceedings of this symposium and the literature that vitamin E has a greater effect in tissue culture. Chemopreventative effects by vitamin E on solid tumors do not seem to be as great as those by selenium. Large amounts of vitamin E are usually needed to have much effect. Some of the chemopreventative effects of vitamin E on solid tumors are summarized in Table 7 (48).

In general, large or milligram quantitites of vitamin E are required to chemoprevent cancer in animals in contrast to microgram quantities for selenium in regard to solid tumors. However, in the case of tissue culture vitamin E seems to much more effective than in the solid tumor system. Prasad (50) has observed a marked inhibition of the growth of neuroblastoma cells in tissue culture. In the proceedings of this conference he has presented evidence that vitamin E is acting through the inhibition of adenyl cyclase in neuroblastoma cells.

Selenium and vitamin E have been found to inhibit the UV-induced and chemically induced transformation of C3H1OT 1/2 cells (51). Vitamin E may be acting through the prostaglandin system.

Overall, more research is needed with vitamin E in regard to its mechanism of action and the reasons for the differences in its action in solid tumors and its action in tissue culture.

Table 7. Summary of the Influence of Vitamin E on Chemical Carcinogenesis (48)

Site	Species and reference	Agent	Vitamin E route (dosage)	Effect
Skin	mouse (1)*	DMBA** + Croton Oil	Topical	↓
Skin	mouse (49)*	DMBA + TPA***	Topical (7 mg/week)	↓
Skin	mouse	DMBA + TPA***	Topical (17mg 2Xwk)	↓
Skin	mouse	DBP****	Diet (25-50g/kg)	NE
Cheek pouch	hamster	DMBA	Oral (7 IV 2Xwk)	↓
			Oral (10 IV 2Xwk)	↓
Forestomach	mouse	DMBA	Diet (10g/kg)	↓
Colon	mouse	DMH*****	Diet (0.6g/kg)	↓
	mouse	DMH	Diet (40 g/kg)	↑
	rat	DMH	Vit. E def.	↑ or ↓
Mammary gland	rat	DMBA	ig (unclear)	↓
	rat	DMBA	Diet (30mg/kg)	NE (low fat) ↓ (high fat)
	rat	DMBA	Diet (50mg/kg)	NE (low SE) ↓ (high SE)
	rat	DMBA	Diet (2g/kg)	NE

```
*        added to list (48)
DMBA**   7,12-dimethylbenzanthracene
TPA***   tetradecanoyl-phorbol-acetate
DMP****  dibenzpyrene
DMH***** 1,2-dimethylhdrazine
```

REFERENCES

1. Shamberger, R.J. and Rudolph, G. Protection against cocarcinogensis by antioxidants. Experientia. 22: 116, 1966.

2. Shamberger, R.J. (1970). Relationship of selenium to cancer. I. Inhibitory effect of selenium on carcinogenesis. J. Nat. Cancer Inst. 44: 931-936, 1970.

3. Medina, D. and Morrison, D.G. Current ideas on selenium as a chemopreventative agent. Pathol. Immunopathol. Res. 7: 187-199, 1988.

4. Combs, Jr., G.F. and Clark, L.C. Can dietary selenium modify cancer risk? Nutr. Rev. 43:325-331, 1985.

5. Thorling, E.B., Overvad, K., and Bjerring, P. Oral selenium inhibits skin reactions to UV light in hairless mice. Acta. Path Microbiol. Immunol. Scand. Sect. A. 91:81-83, 1983.

6. Clayton, C.C. and Bauman, C.A. Diet and azo dye tumors. Effects of diet during a period when the dye is not fed. Cancer Res. 9: 575-582, 1949.

7. Griffin, A.C. and Jacobs, M.M. Effects of selenium on azo dye hepatocarcinogenesis. Cancer Lett. 3: 177-181, 1977.

8. Harr, J.R., Exon, J.H., Weswig, P.H., and Whanger, P.D. Relationship of dietary selenium concentration; chemical cancer induction; and tissue concentration of selenium in rats. Clin. Toxicol. 8:287-295, 1972.

9. Marshall, M.V., Arnott, M.S., Jacobs, M. M., and Griffin, A.C. Selenium effects on the carcinogenicity and metabolism of 2-acetylaminofluorene. Cancer Lett. 7: 331-338, 1979.

10. Grant, K.E., Conner, M.W., and Newberne, P.M. Effect of dietary sodium selenite upon lesions induced by repeated small doses of aflatoxin B_1. Toxicol. Appl. Pharm. 41: 166, 1977.

11. Tanaka, T., Reddy, B.S., and El-Bayoumy, K. Inhibition by dietary organo-selenium p-methoxybenzeneselenol of hepatocarcinogenesis induced by azoxymethane in rats. Jpn J. Cancer Res. (GANN) 76: 462-467, 1985.

12. Yu, S.Y., Chu, Y.J., and Li, W.G. Selenium chemoprevention of liver cancer in animals and possible human applications. Biol Tr. Elem. Res. 15: 231-241, 1988.

13. LeBoeuf, R.A., Laishes, B.A., Hoekstra, W.G. Effects of dietary selenium concentration on the development of enzyme-altered liver foci and hepatocellular carcinoma induced by diethylnitrosamine or N-acetylaminofluorene in rats. Cancer Res. 45: 5489-5495, 1985.

14. Baldwin, S., Parker, R.S. Influence of dietary fat and selenium in initiation and promotion of aflatoxin B_1-induced preneoplastic foci in rat liver. Carcinogenesis 8: 101-107, 1987.

15. Jacobs, M.M., Jansson, B., and Griffin, A.C. Inhibitory effects of selenium on 1,2-dimethylhydrazine and methylazoxymethanol acetate induction of colon tumors. Cancer Lett. 2: 133-138, 1977.

16. Jacobs, M.M, Forst, C.F., and Beams, F.A. Biochemical and clinical effects of selenium on dimethylhydrazine-induced colon cancer in rats. Cancer Res. 41: 4458-4465, 1981.

17. Ankerst, J., and Sjogren, H.O. Effect of selenium on the induction of breast fibroadenomas by adenovirus type 9 and 1,2-dimethylhdrazine-induced bowel carcinogenesis in rats. Int. J. Cancer 29: 707,710, 1982.

18. Birt. D. F., Lawson, T.A., Julius, A.D., Runice, C.E., and Salmasi, S. Inhibition by dietary selenium of colon cancer induced in the rat by bis(2-oxopropyl)nitrosamine. Cancer Res. 42: 4456-4459, 1982.

19. Soulier, B.K., Wilson, P.S., and Nigro, N.D. Effect of selenium on azoxymethane-induced intestinal cancer. Cancer Lett. 12: 343-348, 1981.

20. Nigro, N.D., Bull, A.W., Wilson, P.S., Soullier, B.K., and Alousi, M.A. Combined inhibitors of carcinogenesis. Effect on azoxymethane-induced intestinal cancer in rats. J. Nat. Cancer Inst. 69: 103-107, 1982.

21. Banner, W.P., DeCosse, J.J., Tan, Q.H., and Zedeck, M.S. Selective distribution of selenium in colon parallels its antitumor activity. Carcinogenesis. 5: 1543-1546, 1984.

22. Schrauzer, G.N. and Ishmael, D. Effects of selenium and of arsenic on the genesis of spontaneous mammary tumors in inbred C_3H mice. Ann. Clin. Lab Sci. 4: 411-417, 1974.

23. Medina, D. and Shephard, F. Selenium-mediated inhibition of 7,12-dimethylbenzanthracene-induced mouse mammary tumorigenesis. Carcinogenesis 2: 451-455, 1981.

24. Ip, C. and Sinha, D.K. Enhancement of mammary tumorigenesis by dietary selenium deficiency in rats with a high polyunsaturated diet. Cancer Res. 41: 31-34, 1981.

25. Ip, C. Factors influencing the anticarcinogenic efficacy of selenium in dimethylbenzanthracene-induced mammary tumorigenesis in rats. Cancer Res. 41: 2683-2686, 1981.

26. Ip, C. Modification of mammary carcinogenesis and tissue peroxidation by selenium deficiency and dietary fat. Nutr. Cancer 2: 136-142, 1981.

27. Thompson, H.J. and Becci, P.J. Selenium inhibition of N-methyl-N-nitrosourea-induced mammary carcinogenesis in the rat. J. Nat. Cancer Inst. 65: 1299-1301, 1980.

28. Welsch, C.W., Goodrich-Smith, M., Brown, C.K., Greene, H.D.., and Hamel, E.J. Selenium and the genesis of murine mammary tumors. Carcinogenesis 2: 519-522, 1981.

29. Ip, C. Prophylaxis of mammary neoplasia by selenium supplementation in the initiation and promotion phases of chemical carcinogenesis. Cancer Res. 41: 4386-4390, 1981.

30. Ip, C. and Ganther, H. Efficiacy of trimethylselenonium versus selenite in cancer chemoprevention and its modulation by arsenite. Carcinogenesis 9: 1481-1484, 1988.

31. Ip, C. Differential effect of dietary methionine on the biopotency of selenomethionine and selenite in cancer chemoprevention. J. Nat. Cancer Inst. 80: 258-262, 1988.

32. Chatterjee, M. and Banerjee, M.R. Selenium mediated dose-inhibition of 7,12-dimethylbenzanthracene-induced transformation of mammary cells in organ culture. Cancer Lett. 17: 187-195, 1982.

33. Coates, R. J., Weiss, N. S., Daling J.R., Morris, J.S. and Labbe, R.F. Serum levels of selenium and retinol and the subsequent risk of cancer. Amer. J. Epidemiol. 128: 515-523, 1988.

34. Knekt, P., Aromaa, A., Maatela, J., Alfthan, G., Aaran, R., Teppo,L. and Hakama, M. Serum vitamin E, serum selenium and the risk of gastrointestinal cancer. Int. J. Cancer 42: 846-850, 1988.

35. Wortzam, M. S., Besbris, H.J., and Cohen, A.M. (1980). Effect of dietary selenium on the interaction between 2-acetylaminofluorene and rat liver DNA in vivo. Cancer Res. 40: 2670-2676, 1980.

36. Lawson, T. and Birt, D. BOP induced damage of pancreas DNA and its repair in hamsters pretreated with selenium. Proc. Am. Assoc. Cancer Res. 22: 93,1981.

37. Shamberger, R.J., Baughman, F.F., Kalchert, S.L., Willis, C.E., and Hoffman, G.C. Carcinogen-induced chromosomal breakage decreased by antioxidants. Proc. Natl. Acad. Sci. 70: 1461-1463, 1973.

38. Shamberger, R.J. Increase of peroxidation in carcinogenesis. J. Nat. Cancer Inst. 48: 1491-1497, 1972.

39. Frenkel, G.D., Walcott, A and Middleton, C. Inhibition of RNA and DNA polymerases by the product of the reaction of selenite with sulphydryl compounds. Molec. Pharmacol. 31: 112-116, 1987.

40. Medina, D. Selenium and murine mammary tumorigenesis. In Volume II, Diet, Nutrition and Cancer: A critical Evaluation. CRC Press, Boca Raton, Fla. 23-42, 1986.

41. Vernie, L. N., Vries, M.D. Karreman, L., Topp, R.J., and Bont, W.S. Inhibition of amino acid incorporation in a cell-free system and inhibition of protein synthesis in cultured cells by reaction products of selenite and thiols. Biochem. et Biophys. Acta 739: 1-7, 1983.

42. Besbris, H.J., Wortzman, M.S., and Cohen, A.M. Effects of dietary selenium on the metabolism and excretion of 2-acetylaminofluorene in the rat. J. Toxicol. Environ. Health 9: 63-76, 1982.

43. Milner, J.A., Pigott, M.A. and Dipple, A. Selective effects of sodium selenite on 7,12-dimethylbenzanthracene DNA binding in fetal mouse cell cultures. Cancer Res. 45: 6347-6354, 1985.

44. Su, Huai-De, Shoji, M., Mazzei, G.J., Vogler, W.R., and Kuo, J.F. Effects of selenium compounds on phospholipid/Ca2+-dependent leukemic cells. Cancer Res. 46: 3684-3687, 1986.

45. Perchellet, J.P., Abney, N.L., Thomas, R.M., Guislain, Y.L., and Perchellet, E.M. Effects of combined treatments with selenium, glutathione and vitamin E on glutathione peroxidase activity, ornithine decarboxylase induction, and complete and multistage carcinogenesis in mouse skin. Cancer Res. 477-485, 1987.

46. Spallholz, J.E., Martin, J.L., Gerlach, M.L. and Heinzerling, R.H. Immunological responses of mice fed diets supplemented with selenite selenium. Proc. Soc. Exp. Biol. Med. 143: 685-689, 973.

47. Petrie, H.T., Klassen, L.W, Klassen, P.S., O'Dell, J. R. and Kay, H.D. Selenium and the immune response: 2. Enhancement of murine cytotoxic T-lymphocyte and natural killer cell cytotoxicity in vivo. J. Leuk. Biol. 45: 215-220, 1989.

48. Birt, D.F. Update on the effects of vitamins A,C and E and selenium on carcinogenesis. Proc. Soc. Expt. Biol. Med. 183: 311-320, 1986.

49. Slaga, T.J. and Bracken, W.M. The effects of antioxidants on skin tumor initiation and aryl hydrocarbon hydroxylase. Cancer Res. 37: 1631-1635, 1977.

50. Prasad, K.N., Ramanjam, S. and Gaudreau, D. Vitamin E induces morphological differentiation and increases the effect of ionizing radiation on neuroblastoma cells in culture. Proc. Soc. Exp. Biol. Med. 161: 570-573, 1979.

51. Borek, C., Ong, A., Mason, H., Donahue, L., and Biaglow, J.E. Selenium and vitamin E inhibit radiogenic and chemically induced transformation in vitro via different mechanisms. Proc. Natn. Acad. Sci. 83: 1490-1494 1986.

Nutrients and Cancer Prevention K. N. Prasad and F. L. Meyskens, Jr., eds. © 1990 The Humana Press

VITAMIN B₆ AND CANCER

Hans P. Fortmeyer

TVA des Klinikum der J.W.Goethe Universität

Theodor Stern Kai 7, D-6000 Frankfurt/Main, F. R. G.

The title of the invited paper asks for reviewing the role of vitamin B6 in cancer under all aspects, strictly spoken. The available space, however, is limited. It will be impossible to cover all the possible facets of this subject here. But in case of this vitamin true relevance seems to be more or less restricted to tumor proliferation. Vitamin B6 apparently plays not such a significant role in cancerogenesis as vitamin A does, for instance. The general consequences of vitamin B6 availability for the state of immunity should not be totally neglected, of course. A satisfactory state of immunity may be helpful in the control of metastatic formation. But at the present the dominating field of interest in vitamin B6 seems to be the metabolism of this vitamin in established tumor tissues and its possible influences on tumor proliferation. Therefore this review will be restricted on some interesting and maybe promising findings in this regard. Our research team contributed to them. A comparably new animal model was available to us. It allows completely new approaches to the problem of human tumor and nutrition. This model are athymic rodents, the so-called nude mice and rats, nu/nu resp. rnu/rnu. The immune system of such animals is unable to identify foreign tissues. This characteristic is due to a hereditary aplasia of functional thymus tissues and cells. Therefore human tumor tissue can be xenotransplanted and subsequently passaged into such immune deficient animals. Rejection of grafts never will take place in nude mice. The model of human tumor transplants into nude mice is widely used in oncology now (1). From the beginning on we were of opinion that the model could be a helpful tool in nutritional oncology also. We were right. In course of time we were able to gather a lot of information on interesting relationships between proliferation of human tumor tissue and vitamin B6 availability (2,3).

225

Vitamin B6 responsive growth is well known in certain animal tumors for a long time (4). Vitamin B6 dependence of proliferation had been observed in hepatomas of rat (5,6) and in other neoplasms of laboratory animals (7), either induced or passaged ones. The underlying metabolic peculiarity had been investigated in detail by TRYFIATES, THANNASSI and other researchers (8,9). Such dependences of tumor proliferation on vitamin B6 had never been described in malignomas of human patients. But nevertheless vitamin B6 depending growth of not so few animal tumors stimulated early attempts to treat tumor diseases in man by vitamin depleting measurements. In view of our present knowledge these early attempts were condemned to fail. The investigators mainly treated tumors, in which such dependences seem to occur very rarely or not at all, in lymphomas, for instance. Secondly, the authors used such high doses of a certain vitamin antagonist, 4-deoxy-pyridoxine, that treated patients suffered from serious symptoms of vitamin deficiency after shortest time and the therapeutic trials had to be stopped immediately (10).

But meanwhile we learned that there exist not so few human tumors in which proliferation is clearly dependent on the supply of vitamin B6. We were able to demonstrate such dependences in human tumor xenografts into athymic nude mice. Our research work originally started with general screening procedures. We treated tumor grafted mice with high doses of a multivitamin B preparation (BVK Roche). Increased vitamin supply led to distinct enhancement of tumor proliferation in certain human tumor lines (11). It became obvious that a competition for certain nutrients took place between the grafted tumor specimens and their host organisms. We had to find out which components of the used vitamin preparation were responsible for the observed enhancement of transplant growth. Therefore, we turned about and commenced with defined deficient diets. All of them belonged to the series of ALTROMIN (Lage/Lippe, FRG) special semisynthetic diets. Control animals were fed ALTROMIN C 1000, which represents the control diet of the series. It fully meets the demands of laboratory mice in every respect. Control animals were counterfaced by groups of grafted mice which were supplied with special deficient diets, i. e. with diets which are missing or deficient in one specific component of C 1000. We used ALTROMIN diets deficient in vitamin B1, poor of vitamin B2, deficient in vitamin B6, poor in vitamin B12, and short in nicotinamide. One human breast cancer showed distinct nicotinamide dependent growth behaviour (12). But it was an exception more or less. All other tumor lines, in which enhanced proliferation was observed under multivitamin treatment, developed retardation of growth in pyridoxine deficiency only. In course of time 6 out of 14 investigated breast cancers proved to be vitamin B6 responsive ones (13).

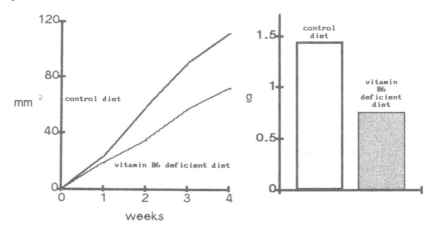

<u>Figure 1:</u>   Human breast cancer CH, 18 passages into nude mice - Mean of transplant growth and tumor weights at postmortem.

Figure 1 demonstrates the typical growth behaviour of a pyridoxine responsive breast cancer line, proliferation primarily depending on the dietary supply of vitamin B6. We usually started feeding of the specific experimental diets one week before transplantation was performed. Vitamin B6 gradually decreased in poorly supplied mice, as shown by the amount of xanthurenic acid in the urine of mice after tryptophane load. It should be emphasized, however, that clinical symptoms of pyridoxine deficiency never developed. Nevertheless tumor growth in poorly supplied mice dropped off compared to the controls.

The difference in tumor size continuously increased in course of such an experiment. The two columns in figure 1 represent the mean tumor weights at the end of the experiment. The animals were sacrificed and postmortems were performed 28 days after transplantation. Mean size and mean weight of the tumor grafts widely differed between the two feeding groups. The differences were highly significant as it was common in such experiments.

It had been mentioned above that vitamin B6 responsive growth was observed in six of 14 human breast cancer lines. But it was demonstrable in quite other tumor types also. Table 1 compiles those 37 different human tumor lines, which were investigated in respect to possible vitamin B6 responsive growth behaviour up to this day. 21 of them showed vitamin B6 dependent growth anew. They belonged to quite different types of tumor. They were carcinomas of the thyroid or sarcomas of soft tissue, lung cancers or neuroblastomas etc. All of them showed the same dependence of tumor proliferation on the supply

Table 1
Vitamin B6 Dependent Growth of Human Malignant
Tumors, Xenotransplanted and Subsequently Passaged
into Athymic Nude Mice.

	+/ -
Breast Cancer	6/8
Lung Cancer	3/4
Neuroblastoma	1/0
Anaplastic Cancer of the Thyroid	4/2
Cancer of the Stomach	2/2
Cancer of the Colon	3/0
Sarcoma of Soft Parts	1/0

with dietary vitamin B6, which have had been seen in the breast cancers before.

It has to be emphasized that tumors with such vitamin response have nothing common in histological appearance obviously. They are of quite different types, but vitamin B6 responsive growth is also not restricted to certain morphological appearances within the same type of tumor. One of the lung cancers with positive findings was a parvicellular one, for instance. But the three other lung tumors were not. We found either medullary and scirrhous tumors among the positive breast cancers.

The high-grade vitamin B6 dependence of certain individual tumor tissues seems to be based on metabolic peculiarities on the cellular level. Different researchers investigated it in animal tumors biochemically. Their favored tools were hepatomas of the rat. The results seem to be partially contradictory at the present. A complete insight in the tumor specific pathways of vitamin B6 respectively of its metabolites is not yet achieved. But meanwhile we know many interesting fragments, like the highly reduced or even missing availability of pyridoxine-5'-phosphate oxidase, for instance (14). Best approach to the matter is achieved by studying the original publications (6 ,8 ,9 , 14 , 15, 16, 17, 18, 19, 20, 21, 22, 23, 24). Summarizing it seems that tumor cells or animals with hepatomas resp. with certain other tumors developed additional abilities for the utilization of vitamin B6, which normal animals or normal cells lack, maybe in connection with a highly increased demand. New pathways are created here. This assumption is supported by new tumor associated metabolites of vitamin B6, which were described by TRYFIATES (25, 26, 27).

Two interesting observations, which were made by us, should be mentioned here, because they indicate apparently altered metabolic conditions in vitamin B6 responsive tumors. The content of tryptophan was significantly lowered in sera of mice, which were grafted with vitamin B6 responsive tumors, see table 2. The tryptophan lowering effect was seen either in animals, which fed on the fully supplied control diet (ALTROMIN C 1000), and in poorly supplied ones (ALTROMIN C 1023).

We transplanted such vitamin B6 responsive tumors not only in nude mice, but sometimes in nude rats also. The latter ones, grafted with a special technique, which was described by us in detail some years ago (28), enabled us to measure the arterial input and venous output values of a graft. In vitamin B6 responsive tumor lines we found deviations from normal in serine mainly, see fig.2. Four tumor specimens were not vitamin B6 responsive ones. They showed a positive serine balance toward output. Two other ones, however, represent responsive tumors. Here the venous release is much more smaller than the arterial uptake had been. In this connexion it may be of interest that TRYFIATES, SHULER & MORRIS (29) found nearly no serine dehydratase, a pyridoxal phosphate requiring enzyme, in a rat hepatoma with vitamin B6 responsive growth.

At the Tucson Conference of '82 HELSON (30) reported on growth promotion of vitamin B6 in human neuroblastomas and retinoblastomas. He described the effect either in cell culture and in nude mice. Vitamin E-succinate was toxic to cells in culture. In the book with the Conference papers (31) and in subsequent other publications (32), however, neither he nor other investigators mentioned vitamin B6 again. The authors only described the adverse effect of vitamin E on tumor cells. It was noticed either in vitro and in vivo. The researchers used comparatively high doses of vitamin E in their animals.These high doses

.

Table 2
Human Breast Cancers Xenotransplanted and Subsequently Passaged into Nude Mice. Tryptophan levels (mean) of the mouse sera.

Breast Cancer (passage)	response to vitamin B6	content of tryptophan *	
		C1000	C1023
S T (48)	yes	6.98	4.81
J E (20)	yes	6.70	5.78
W O (10)	no	9.21	11.27
S C (26)	no	7.96	8.47
*)nmol per o.1 ml	(n = 10)		

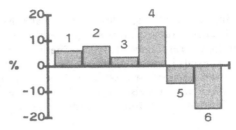

Figure 2
Human breast cancer xenografts, passaged into rnu/rnu rats by using
the so-called pouching technique. Content of serine in venous release,
compared with arterial input. 1 - 4 not vitamin B6 responsive tumors, 5
and 6 responsive ones. n = 10

led to a temporary toxic reduction of body weight in treated mice. We
tried to reproduce these results with some of our tumor lines (33). But
bearing in mind the fact that in hyposomic nude mice tumor
proliferation normally decreases or is even stopped at all (34), we tried
to avoid any toxic effects of vitamin E, i.e. losses of weight primarily,
by using smaller doses. We gave EPHYNAL i.p., 50 mg per kg BW a
day only. We were not able to produce any adverse effects on transplant
growth in nude mice at all. Sometimes we even experienced a certain
enhancement of tumor growth by EPHYNAL treatment (2). The reason
for it apparently was a roborant effect of vitamin E on nude mice with
heavy tumor burdens. It was concluded from a considerable rise in
mean of body weight (3 g) in vitamin E treated animals. On the other
hand, the addition of EPHYNAL to cell cultures of the same tumor
lines was followed by a distinct reduction in the number of cell indeed.
This effect was dose dependent. The addition of vitamin B6, however,
has had a promoting effect on cell numbers in the same tumor lines
(33). We are of opinion that the partially contradictory findings in vivo
and in vitro verify the experience that results from cell cultures cannot
be simply transfered to living organisms. Organisms own regulatory
mechanisms, which are missing in cell culture.

A clear dividing line between responders and not responsive tumors
existed in our experiments. Responsive tumors, however, showed a
remaining growth of not inconsiderable extent even in animals, which
were supplied with diets practically free of pyridoxine for very long
periods. This was true even after 5 months of deficient feeding. There
were at least two possible reasons for this persisting tumor proliferation.
It showed that both of them contributed to it.

From a loss of response in course of subsequent passages into
athymic nude mice and from other observations it can be definitely

concluded that so-called responders consist of a mixed population of vitamin B responsive and not responsive cells usually. The sometimes very adverse relation in size between tumor recipient mice and their grown grafts favors the selection of not responsive clones in course of numerous nude mouse passages.

But another reason plays a role also. It showed that it may be the more important one. Certain components of the intestinal flora produce considerable amounts of pyridoxine. PETUELY (35) suggests that this factor may not play a role in man. But in rodents resorption is favoured by their coprophagic habits. Resorption of vitamin B6, produced by the intestinal flora, seems to be the reason why even long lasting application of a deficient diet was well tolerated by our tumor bearing mice.

Various substances or drugs are effective antagonists to vitamin B6. Therefore we decided to extent our experimental design in order to determine whether additional application of such antagonists ist followed by further reduction of vitamin B6 levels and additional diminuation of transplant growth as a result of it. This therapeutic principle had been successfully used in vitamin B6 responsive tumors of rodents by others (36, 37). 4-deoxy-pyridoxine is a reliable antagonist to vitamin B6, for instance. The combined use of the deficient diet C 1023 and 4-deoxy-pyridoxine produced stronger inhibiting effects on proliferation of responsive breast cancers than deficient feeding alone (38). But 4-deoxy-pyridoxine is not a licensed drug. On the other hand, there exist some registered and approved drugs, which are known antagonists to vitamin B6 also. We tested D-penicillamine, in which this side-effect had been described also. The drug was given intraperitoneally. We used daily doses of 120 to 160 mg per kg BW in our tumor grafted mice.

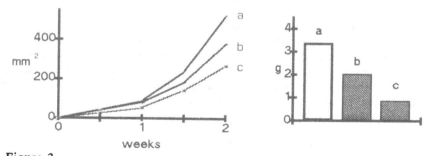

Figure 3

Human breast cancer R E, 19 passages into nude mice. Mean of transplant growth and tumor weights at postmortem. a - control diet, b - deficient diet, c - deficient diet and D-penicillamine intraperitoneally.

The results, which we gained with a fast growing human breast cancer, are illustrated by figure 3. Tumor grafts grew less in nude mice, which fed on deficient diet C 1023. But this adverse effect on tumor growth was considerably enhanced by additional therapy with D-penicillamine. The observed differences in mean tumor size proved to be highly significant. All mice were sacrificed two weeks after transplantation. The final weights of their tumor grafts at postmortem are given in figure 3 also. They corresponded the intravital measurements in principle. But the differences between the three groups were more pronounced here. The mean of tumor weight in penicillamine treated mice was less than one third of tumor weight in fully vitamin supplied control mice.

We got similar results in all those vitamin B6 responsive tumor lines, which we treated with penicillamine. Penicillamine successfully reduced tumor proliferation in each case. The effect was not only seen in mice, which fed on the deficient diet. But it was observed in fully supplied animals also. Impressive results were obtained, inspite of the fact that not a single mouse showed any symptoms of vitamin deficiency or losses of weight only. An always well tolerated but nevertheless efficient dose had been around 3 mg per animal a day. The adverse effect on tumor growth was enhanced, if the dose of penicillamine was doubled. But in this situation first clinical symptoms of vitamin deficiency became obvious. Beyond a distinct reduction of animal weight alterations of skin were observed.

The results of our experiments seem to be clear and convincing. The question arose whether our experimental findings on vitamin B6 responsive growth of human tumors may have certain consequences for afflicted human patients. Are possibilities for palliative or therapeutic use appearing in outlines at least? The answer to this question seems to be urgent. We also believe that the number of human tumors, in which proliferation is primarily depending on their supply with vitamin B6 is a considerable one. The presumption is not only based on own experimental results with xenotransplants into nude mice, but also on certain observations of lowered vitamin B6 levels in human patients. Most of the literature on corresponding clinical findings is reviewed by LEKLEM et al. (39). We should interpret the reduced vitamin B6 levels in human tumor patients in a new way. Some authors of the past (39,40) were of opinion that it would be beneficial to cancer patients with lowered levels of vitamin B6 to return their values to normal by substitution of vitamin B6. However, such attempts seems to be dangerous and should be avoided in view of our experimental findings. Otherwise a distinct enhancement of tumor proliferation may be expected. The aim of any clinician should be a controlled restriction of vitamin B6 availability or the avoidance of a shifting supply at least.

We suppose that those human tumors which have had shown vitamin B6 responsive development are congruent with the clinical case material, in which low serum levels of vitamin B6 had been observed. LEKLEM and co-authors (39), for instance, observed increased urinary excretion of tryptophan metabolites after tryptophan load in 5 of 18 breast cancer patients. On the other hand, we found vitamin B6 responsive growth in 6 out of 14 breast cancers, passaged into athymic nude mice. Iit is nearly the same rate in both cases..

A moderate reduction of pyridoxine supply did not provoke any clinical symptoms of vitamin deficiency in our laboratory animals. Nevertheless, in cases of such limited reduction of vitamin B6 availability distinct inhibitory effects on tumor proliferation were observed. Therefore, it seems to be a good policy and poor of risks to initiate suitable dietary measurements and guidance, which avoid a shifting dietary supply of vitamin B6 at least, as a first step.

Our experiments on nude mouse transplants gave evidence of the fact that nutrition, which merely avoids vitamin B6 uptake, is not quite sufficient for our purposes. The intestinal flora may contribute to the total supply very often. As mentioned before, PETUELY (35) is of opinion, that its share is less in man than in rodent species and may be ignored here totally. The coprophagic habits of rodents facilitate resorption of substances, which are produced by the flora of the large intestine, without any doubt. In man, however, a certain degree of vitamin supply by intestinal bacteria cannot be excluded in advance. Symptoms of deficiency are apparently very rare in man, even after comparatively extended periods of vitamin B6 free nutrition. KOLB (41), in contrast to PETUELY, explains this fact by a certain resorption of enterally formed vitamin B6. Beyond it, it seems difficult to force a diet, which is consequently deficient in vitamin B6, on many patients. Corresponding dietary measurements and prescriptions will not be accepted in many cases. This counts for ambulatory patients especially.

For all these reasons, additional but careful use of vitamin B6 antagonists in human patients should be kept in mind at least. Antagonists would be able to counteract either a shifting dietary supply and a possible supply from quite other sources. At present, D-penicillamine seems to be the substance of choice. It is an approved and well-known drug. However, approximate knowledge of the actual state in respect to vitamin B6 availability seems to be an unalterable precondition for such treatment. The extent of further antagonistic or dietary efforts could be prescribed, if the vitamin values are above a desired level. On the other hand, vitamin depleting measurements should be avoided at all or reduced if the actually available vitamin B6 is

found to be below a critical value. All symptoms of clinical vitamin
deficiency have to be strictly avoided.

REFERENCES

1.) FORTMEYER, H. P.: Thymusaplastische Maus (nu/nu) -
Thymusaplastische Ratte (rnu/rnu) - Haltung, Zucht, Versuchsmodelle.
P. Parey, Berlin & Hamburg, 1981.

2.) TIMM, C.: Entwicklung menschlicher Tumore auf Nacktmäusen
(NMRI-nu/nu) in Abhängigkeit vom Vitamin B6. Inaug. Diss. Vet.
Med. Berlin, 1985.

3.) FORTMEYER, H. P., TIMM, C., BLUM, U., WENISCH, H. J. C.,
& FÖRSTER, H.: Vitamin B6 responsive growth of human tumors.
Anticancer Res., 8, 813-818, 1988.

4.) BISCHOFF, F., INGRAHAM, L. P., RUPP, J. J.: Influence of
vitamin B6 and panthotenic acid on the growth of sarcoma 180. Arch.
Path., 35, 713-716, 1943.

5.) TRYFIATES, G. P., LARSON, L., MORRIS, H. P.: Effect of
pyridoxine dose on the growth of transplantable MORRIS hepatoma
7288 Ctc. J. Nutr., 108, 417-420, 1978.

6.) TRYFIATES, G. P.: Vitamin B6 effects on the growth of MORRIS
hepatomas and the development of enzymatic activity. In: H. P.
MORRIS & W. E. CRISS (eds): MORRIS Hepatomas: Mechanisms of
Regulation, pp. 607-642. Plenum, New York, 1978.

7.) MIHICH, E., ROSEN, F., NICHOL, C. A.: The effect of pyridoxine
deficiency on a spectrum of mouse and rat tumors. Cancer Res., 19,
1244-1248, 1959.

8.) TRYFIATES, G. P. & BISHOP, R.: Pyridoxine metabolism in rats
with 7777 hepatoma. J. Nutr. Growth Cancer, 2, 229-241, 1985.

9.) THANASSI, J. W.: Vitamin B6 metabolism in relation to MORRIS
hepatomas. In: K. N. PRASAD (ed): Vitamins, Nutrition and Cancer,
pp. 251-265. Karger, Basel & New York, 1984.

10.) GAILANI, S. D., HOLLAND, J. F., NUSSBAUM A. & OLSON,
K. B.: Clinical and biochemical studies of pyridoxine deficiency in
patients with neoplastic diseases. Cancer, 21,975-988, 1968.

11.) FORTMEYER, H. P.: Untersuchungen zu den besonderen nutritiven Bedürfnissen thymusaplastischer Mäuse (nu/nu) wie zur Bedeutung einer standardisierten Ernährung für die Ergebnisse onkologischer Arbeiten an diesen Versuchstieren. Habil. Med. Frankfurt/Main, 1982.

12.) TESSERAUX, M., TIMM, C., BASTERT, G. & FORTMEYER, H. P.: The growth behaviour of human breast cancers on nude mice, which were poorly supplied with nicotinamide. Zsch. Versuchstierk., 28, 99, 1986.

13.) RUSE, M.,: Zur wachstumsbeeinflussenden Wirkung von D-Penicillamin auf Vitamin B6 abhängig wachsende Mammakarzinome des Menschen im Nacktmaustransplantat. Inaug. Diss. Med. Frankfurt/Main, 1988.

14.) NUTTER, L. M., MEISLER, N. T., & THANASSI, J. W.: Absence of pyridoxine (pyridoxamine) 5'-phosphate oxidase in MORRIS hepatoma 7777. Biochemistry, 22, 1599-1604, 1983.

15.) TRYFIATES, G. P. & MORRIS, H. P.: Effect of pyridoxine deficiency on tyrosine transaminase activity and growth of four MORRIS hepatomas. J. Nat. Cancer.Inst., 52, 1259-1262, 1974.

16.) TRYFIATES, G. P., SHULER, J. K., HEFNER, M. J. & MORRIS, H. P.: Effect of B6 deficiency on hepatoma 7794 A growth rate: activities of tyrosine transaminase and serine dehydratase before and after induction by hydrocortisone. Eur. J. Cancer, 10, 147-154, 1974.

17.) TRYFIATES, G. P., SAUS, F. L. & MORRIS, H. P.: Hormonal induction of tyrosine transaminase in host liver and hepatoma No. 7777 of normal and cofactor depleted animals. J. Nat. Cancer Inst., 55, 839-841, 1975.

18.) TRYFIATES, G. P.: Effect of pyridoxine on the growth of MORRIS hepatoma No. 7288 Ctc and encyme activity. Oncology, 33, 209-211, 1976.

19.) SHULER, J. K. & TRYFIATES, G. P.: Expression of hormonally induced tyrosine aminotransferase in host liver and MORRIS hepatoma No. 7777 during cofactor depleting. Oncology, 35, 73-75, 1978.

20.) THANASSI, J. W., NUTTER, L. M., MEISLER, N. T., COMERS. P. & CHIU, J-F.: Vitamin B6 metabolism in MORRIS hepatomas. J. Biol. Chem., 256, 3370-3375, 1981.

21.) TRYFIATES, G. P., MORRIS, H. P. & SONIDIS, G. P.: Vitamin B6 and cancer (review). Anticancer Res., 1, 263-268, 1981.

22.) MEISLER, N. T., NUTTER, L. M. & THANASSI, J. W.: Vitamin B6 metabolism in liver and liver-derived tumors. Cancer Res., 42, 3538-3543, 1982.

23.) THANASSI, J. W., MEISLER, N. T. & KITTLER, J. M.: Vitamin B6 metabolism and cancer. In: R. D. REYNOLDS & J. E. LEKLEM (eds): Vitamin B-6: its Role in Health and Disease, pp. 319-336, A. R. Liss, New York, 1985.

24.) MEISLER, N.T. & THANASSI, J. W.: Vitamin B6 metabolism in McA-RH 7777 cells. Cancer Res., 48, 1080-1085, 1988.

25.) TRYFIATES, G. P.: Metabolic interconversions of pyridoxine by MORRIS hepatoma No. 7777 cells. Synthesis of a novel metabolite. Anticancer Res., 3, 53-58, 1983.

26.) TRYFIATES, G. P., BISHOP, R. & SMITH, R. R.: Novel vitamin B6 tumor metabolites. In: A. Evangelopoulos et al (eds): Chemical and Biological Aspects of Vitamin B6 Catalysis: Part A, pp 21-29, A. R. Liss, New York, 1984.

27.) TRYFIATES, G. P. & BISHOP, R. E.: Tentative structure of a novel vitamin B6 tumor product. In: TRYFIATES, G. P. & K. N. PRASAD (eds): Nutrition, Growth and Cancer, pp. 295-305, A. R. Liss, New York, 1988.

28.) STEINAU, H. U., BASTERT, G., EICHHOLZ, H., FORTMEYER, H. P. & SCHMIDT-MATTHIESEN, H.: Epigastric pouching technique: human xenografts in rnu/rnu rats. In: G. BASTERT, H. P. FORTMEYER & H. SCHMIDT-MATTHIESEN (eds): Thymusaplastic Nude Mice and Rats in Clinical Oncology, pp. 531-542, G. Fischer, Stuttgart & New York, 1981.

29.) TRYFIATES, G. P., SHULER, J. K. & MORRIS, H. P.: Enzyme activities in vitamin B6-deficient, normal, and tumor-bearing animals: effect of hydrocortisone. Proc. Soc. Exp. Biol. Med., 145, 1363-1367, 1974.

30.) HELSON, L.: Vitamins B-6 and human neuroblastoma (NB). In: 1st Intern. Conf. Modulation and Mediation of Cancers by Vitamins, Tucson, Abstract volume, 1982.

31.) HELSON, L., VERMA, M. & HELSON, C.: Vitamin E and human neuroblastoma. In: F. L. MEYSKENS & K. N. PRASAD (eds): Modulation and Mediation of Cancer by Vitamins, pp. 258-265, S. Karger, Basel & New York, 1983.

32.) VERMA, M., HELSON, C., TRAGANOS, F. & HELSON, L.: Effect of vitamin E compounds on human neuroblastoma in vitro and in nude mice. J. Exp. Cell Biol., 52, 379-384, 1984.

33.) FORTMEYER, H. P. & BUSSE, E.: Vitamin B6 dependent growth of human tumors, xenotransplanted and passaged into athymic nude mice. J. Cancer Res. Clin. Onc., 113, Suppl. S1, 1987.

34.) KÜSTERS, G.: Menschliche Tumoren auf Nacktmäusen (NMRI-nu/nu) im Energiedefizit. Inaug. Diss. Vet. med. München, 1984.

35.) PETUELY, F.: Die Darmflora und ihre Bedeutng beim Menschen. In: A. HOCK (ed): Vergleichende Ernährungslehre des Menschen und seiner Haustiere. G. Fischer, Stuttgart, 1966.

36.) LITTMAN, M. L., TAGUCHI, T. & SHIMIZU, Y.: Acceleration of growth of sarcoma 180 with pyridoxamine and retardation with penicillamine. Proc. Soc. Exp. Biol. Med., 113, 667-674, 1963.

37.) TRYFIATES, G. P.: Control of tumor growth by pyridoxine restriction or treatment with an antivitamin agent. Cancer Detect. Prevent., 4, 159-164, 1981.

38.) KNÖLL, L.: Zur wachstumsbeeinflussenden Wirkung von 4-deoxy-Pyridoxin auf vitamin-B6-abhängig wachsende Mammakarzinome des Menschen im Nacktmaustransplantat. Inaug. Diss. Med., Frankfurt/Main, 1989.

39.) LEKLEM, J. M., BROWN, R. R., POTERA, C. & BECKER, D. S.: A role for vitamin B6 in cancer. In: J. VAN EYS et al. (eds): Nutrition and Cancer. SP Medical & Scientific Books, New York & London, 1979.

40.) YOSHIDA, O, BROWN, R. R. & BRYAN, G. T.: Relationship between tryptophan metabolism and heterotopic recurrences of human urinary bladder tumors, Cancer, 25, 773-780, 1970.

41.) KOLB, E.: Die ernährungsphysiologische Bedeutung der Vitamine und die wichtigsten Vitaminmangelerkrankungen bei Mensch und Tier. In: A. HOCK (ed): Vergleichende Ernährungslehre des Menschen und seiner Haustiere, pp. 687-804, 1966.

Clinical Studies
in Cancer Prevention and Treatment

Nutrients and Cancer Prevention K. N. Prasad and F. L. Meyskens, Jr., eds. © 1990 The Humana Press

THE NUTRITIONAL CAUSES OF LARGE BOWEL CANCER

Data from the Melbourne Colorectal Cancer Study and
A 25 Year World Literature Overview, 1965-1989

Gabriel Kune, Susan Kune, Barry Field, Lyndsey Watson

University of Melbourne, Australia.

61 Erin Street, Richmond 3121, Victoria, Australia.

INTRODUCTION

Colorectal cancer is one of the commonest cancers in developed countries and worldwide, there are over 500,000 new cases each year [1] and over 300,000 deaths are directly attributable to this cancer. An understanding of the causes and the possibilities for prevention of this cancer are therefore of global interest and importance. This communication outlines "The Melbourne Colorectal Cancer Study" and the major findings of the study so far, focuses in detail on the nutritional findings of the study and then compares these to an overview of the literature during the previous 25 years, to conclude with our current understanding of the nutritional causes of large bowel cancer.

THE MELBOURNE COLORECTAL CANCER STUDY

Study Design

The Melbourne study is a large, comprehensive, population-based, epidemiological and clinicopathological investigation of colorectal cancer incidence, etiology and survival, with a unique study design [2,3] which allows for the simultaneous examination of the incidence pattern, all of the hypothesised causes and all of the survival determinants of colorectal cancer of a defined population in a single data set. The study has three principal parts,

namely the incidence study which examined the level and
pattern of colorectal cancer in Melbourne by age, sex,
site, subsite, country of birth, religion and occupation,
the case control study which examined all the previously
hypothesised causal and protective factors in the
development of colorectal cancer, and the survival study
which examined all the known survival determinants of the
cancer cases (Figure 1).

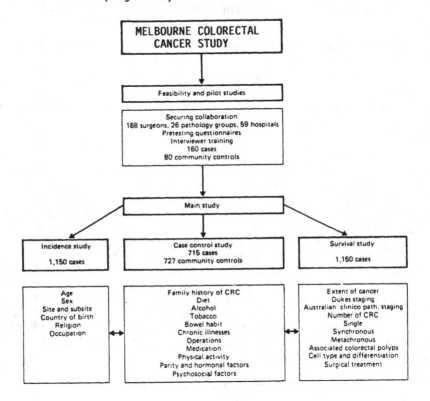

The study was population-based, confined to the City
of Melbourne, Australia (population 2.8 million) and
included all histologically confirmed new cases of
colorectal cancer first diagnosed during the 12 month
period April 1980 to April 1981 (1150 cases). For the case
control arm of the study, 715 of the 1150 colorectal cancer
cases were group matched by sex and age with 727 community
controls, also resident in Melbourne, using a random
sampling plan devised by the Australian Bureau of Statis-

tics, the Australian government agency which is responsible for the Australian Census and other Australian vital statistics.

Each respondent was administered two questionnaires by personal interview on two occasions, by two sets of interviewers. The first questionnaire included all the data needed for the incidence and case control study, with the exception of the dietary and alcohol data which formed the second interview.

Results of the Melbourne Study

For completeness, a brief description is given of the major non-nutritional findings of the Melbourne study. The incidence arm of the study indicated, as expected, that Melbourne has the characteristics of a population at high risk for the development of colorectal cancer [4]. The data on first generation migrants supported the general epidemiological concept that with migration from low risk to high risk countries for colorectal cancer, there is a transition of rates towards the risk levels of the new country. It was also found that those of Jewish background had rates double those of the Melbourne population [4].

A history of colorectal cancer in one or more first degree relatives was found to be a two to threefold risk for the subsequent development of colorectal cancer, indicating the importance of a hereditary predisposition [5]. Previous colorectal polypectomy for benign polyps was associated with a sixfold risk for the subsequent development of colorectal cancer when compared to those who did not give such a history [6]. Having children and having these children at an early age were both protective factors in the development of large bowel cancer and this protection applied to both females and males [7]. Chronic constipation, diarrhea and laxative use were not associated with the risk of large bowel cancer [8]. The use of oral contraceptives did not protect against bowel cancer [9], while the use of aspirin containing medications was protective [10]. Previous cholecystectomy was not a risk factor [11].

NUTRITIONAL FINDINGS OF THE MELBOURNE STUDY

Nutritional Methodology

Nutritional methodology needs to be detailed and accurate and this involves time, expertise and considerable expense, [2,3]. The strengths of the Melbourne study with respect to methodology, and particularly with respect to the nutritional methodology used are:

(1) The study is population-based for both cases and controls and this significantly minimises the problems of selection and exclusion bias [12].
(2) Community controls and not hospital controls were used. Hospital controls are inferior to community controls because the former are of necessity, already selected because of their hospital admission.
(3) Several pilot and feasibility studies were conducted before the main study [2,3]. The data obtained from these pilot studies were used to modify the final questionnaires, but the data themselves were not used in the main study.
(4) The cases were interviewed soon after diagnosis and therefore there was little time for them to reflect, thus minimising rumination bias. In this regard, self-administered questionnaires are likely to be inferior to questionnaires by personal interview.
(5) The dietary method used in the Melbourne study was accurate, albeit expensive [2]. The following were the important methodologic features of the dietary method:
i) The method was <u>quantitative</u> and involved a detailed diet history of all foods eaten during a period which was most representative of the previous 20 years. It involved a quantitative measurement of all foods eaten in Australia. It was <u>not</u> a frequency interview (either unquantified or semi-quantified), nor a 24 hour recall, as these methods are substantially less accurate than the complete diet history method [13-17].
ii) The dietary interview was administered by University qualified dietitians, all of whom had previous research experience in this area and who were specifically pretrained in the technique of interviewing. Thus the interview was <u>not</u> self-administered, nor was it administered by untrained or unqualified interviewers.
iii) Foods were quantified and placed into food groups. A computer program was used to convert food item data into nutrients, such as carbohydrate, fat, protein, fiber, beta

carotene, vitamin C etc. Nutrient composition data were obtained for almost 1000 food items, using Australian, US and UK food tables, as well as information from manufacturers [18]. For example, the fiber values represented the most accurate information available at the time of the study and allowed a measurement of fiber intake with greater accuracy than has been possible previously [18].

iv) Numerous reliability and validity tests were performed, such as testing interviewer bias, recall bias, the validity of the diet history method [16,18].

v) The dietitians were not aware of the hypotheses being tested and also their opinions regarding dietary causes of colorectal cancer were determined at the debriefing [16,18].

vi) The statistical analysis used was the most sophisticated available at the time of the study. Thus, apart from univariate analysis of food groups and nutrients, the analysis also involved multiple logistic regression analysis of the data as well as extensive statistical data modelling [18].

vii) As the study design allowed a simultaneous examination of all the dietary and non-dietary variables, it was possible to make corrections and adjustments for potential confounding factors, both within the dietary variables [18] and outside these variables, such as when examining the possible dietary component of positive family history of colorectal cancer [5].

Nutrition and Alcohol Results in the Melbourne Study

The principal findings of the nutrition and alcohol data have already been published in detail [18,19]. Since tnen, two further directly nutrition related publications one on sodium and potassium intake and a second on body mass index have appeared [20,21]. Apart from these, there are other significant diet related findings which will be also summarised here.

It is emphasised that the results which follow represent independent effects of foods and nutrients, because in all analyses the data were examined simultaneously. Also, the conclusions reached follow extensive data modelling representing almost a year of research activity by the investigators in which the main focus was the case-control diet analysis.

Nutritional Protective Factors

Several dietary factors were found to be statistically significantly protective against the development of large bowel cancer. The combination of a high fiber intake from any source (fruit, vegetables, cereals) and a high vegetable intake (potatoes excluded from vegetables) was uniformly protective for both males and females and for both colon and rectal cancer. A high fiber intake alone and a high vegetable intake alone was protective, but not as protective as the combination of high fiber/high vegetables intake [18]. Independently, a high intake of cruciferous vegetables was also found to be uniformly protective over and above their protective effect as a vegetable. Dietary vitamin C was protective for both colon and rectal cancer, for males and females and this was particularly so for dietary vitamin C intakes which were greater than 230 mg per day. A high fish intake was also uniformly protective, as was a moderate intake of milk and milk drinks (in the range of 200 ml of milk per day for males and about 150 ml of milk per day for females). A high dietary potassium/sodium ratio was also protective, especially for females [20]. The regular use of vitamin A and vitamin C supplements was highly protective for both males and females and for both colon and rectal cancer.

Nutritional Risk Factors

There were several nutritional risk factors in the Melbourne study. A high fat intake was a risk for both males and females. A high beef intake was a risk factor for both colon and rectal cancer in males. A low intake of milk and milk drinks below 100 ml per day for males and below 80 ml per day for females was a risk factor for both males and females. A high beer intake was a risk for rectal cancer. Interestingly, beer consumption was not a risk factor when modified by a high dietary vitamin C intake [19]. A high sodium intake was a risk for rectal cancer in both males and females [20]. A high body mass index, that is, being overweight or obese, was a risk factor for rectal cancer in males [21].

No Statistically Significant Association with Colorectal Cancer Risk

There were several foods and nutrients which had no statistically significant association with the risk of colorectal cancer or colon cancer or rectal cancer in either males or females. The food groups which had no statistically significant association with large bowel cancer risk included pulses, nuts and seeds, potatoes, cereals (bread, pasta, biscuits, breakfast cereals etc included), total meat intake, lamb, veal, poultry, rabbit, offal, eggs and milk products [18]. The nutrients which showed no statistically significant association with the risk of large bowel cancer included energy intake, protein, carbohydrate (fiber from any source excluded), phosphorus, iron, potassium, retinol, thiamine, riboflavin, niacin and alcohol expressed as ethanol [18,19]. Although beta carotene containing foods appeared to be protective in the initial analysis, when examined in the diet model this effect was totally explained by a high intake of vegetables, indicating that beta carotene containing foods did not have an independent and separate association with colorectal cancer risk and that it was the high vegetable intake which was the protective factor.

Nutritional Risk Score

The diet model was developed from the risk and protective factors found in the Melbourne study by assigning different coefficients of risk associated with large bowel cancer for each of the dietary variables. From this a "risk score" was calculated by adding the number of risk factors an individual had in their diet. Table 1 shows the number of cases and controls classified by their risk score and their risk relative to individuals with any four risk factors (this group was arbitrarily assigned a relative risk of 1.0). The risk score was strongly associated with colorectal cancer risk ($p < 0.0001$). Moreoever, the risk score has a statistically significant linear trend ($p < 0.0001$) and the risk is multiplied by 1.82 for each additional risk factor a person has. There is thus a monotonic relationship across the levels of the risk score with little departure from this trend [18]. A dietary risk score expresses the risk of a dietary pattern and is therefore a more realistic method of examining dietary risk in large bowel cancer than is an examination of individual food groups or nutrients, such as fiber or fat or energy intake alone. The concept of risk score has not so far been widely used in the presentation of dietary data and appears to be a useful analytic tool.

TABLE 1

Nutritional Risk Score in the Melbourne Colorectal Cancer Study

	Number of Risk Factors Present											
	0	1	2	3	4	5	6	7	8	9	10	11
Number of colorectal cancer cases	0	2	15	58	178	223	139	87	12	1	0	0
Number of controls	0	15	63	155	229	174	71	16	4	0	0	0
Relative risk age/sex adjusted	-	0.15	0.28	0.48	1.00	1.70	2.72	8.01	4.38	-	-	-

Other Nutrition Related Findings

There were several other important non-nutritional risk associations of large bowel cancer alluded to earlier in this presentation. Each of these statistically significant non-nutritional associations of large bowel cancer could have been confounded by diet and therefore for each, adjustments were made in relation to the dietary risk model.

Adjustment for the dietary risk factors did not significantly alter the family history risk and therefore it was considered that family history risk and dietary risks were two essentially different and independent variables [5]. Indeed, because of the design of the study and the sophistication of statistical analysis, this was the first investigation which showed that the dietary effects and the hereditary effects in the etiology of large bowel cancer were essentially separate and independent etiological factors.

Self-reported chronic constipation was found to be a marginally significant risk for large bowel cancer [8]. However, when adjusted for the previously described dietary risk factors, the constipation risk disappeared, indicating that it is the diet and not the constipation which is responsible for the actual risk observed. There was one notable exception to this, namely chronic constipation and a high dietary fat intake of greater than 100 g per day was found to be a highly statistically significant risk factor [8]. Finally, a particularly high relative risk of rectal cancer was found among those oral contraceptive users who were also beer drinkers [9].

WORLD LITERATURE REVIEW

Method

A world literature review was made of all case control studies relating nutritional factors to the development of large bowel cancer for the period 1965-1989. This included a Medlar search for this period, a search of international abstracts and any data that may have been published in a monograph or a multi-author book. This extensive search disclosed 40 studies [22-61].

Factors Examined. The demographic characteristics examined included country of study, whether it was hospital based or population-based, sites studied, the numbers and sources of cases and controls, and their method of matching. A careful examination was made of the dietary history obtained, and particularly whether it was a detailed quantitative diet history or merely a frequency questionnaire which may have been unquantified, semi-quantified or quantified, or just a 24 hour recall method. An examination was also made of the statistical analysis and particularly whether this was a univariate analysis only or whether it included corrections for other nutritional or confounding factors and whether it also included logistic regression and statistical modelling of the data.

Dietary Factors Examined. Dietary factors were examined as food groups and as individual food items, and also examined when classified as macronutrients and micronutrients. The food groups of animal origin included meat, fish and other seafood, dairy products and eggs; food groups of plant origin included vegetables, fruit, cereals and nuts; macronutrients as fats, protein, carbohydrate, fiber, alcohol and energy intake; micronutrients as vitamins and minerals. The effect of tea and coffee drinking and of the frequency of meals was also examined.

RESULTS

Methodology Used

The following is an overview and critique of the methodology used in the 40 case control studies examined: Almost half of the investigations studied males and females grouped together, one-quarter grouped colon and rectum sites together and did not investigate site separately, while one-fifth studied colon cancer only and one studied rectal cancer only. Only one-third of the studies were truly population-based, an important requirement of a modern case control study, while most studies were hospital based. The total number of cases was over 22,000 and controls over 32,000. There were eight studies with a small number of respondents (less than 400). A detailed quantitative dietary history was used in only one-quarter of the studies, while the much less accurate unquantified frequency method was used in almost half of the 40 studies. Most studies used univariate analysis only, and only one-fifth used multiple logistic regression analysis, while only one-quarter made statistical adjustments for other dietary variables. Only eight of the 40 studies (20%) incorporated the four aspects of methodology, which in the authors' view makes for a high quality, accurate nutritional case control investigation of cancer risk, namely, that the study is randomly selected and population-based, it has sufficient respondents to be able to make meaninful statistical calculations (500 or more), it uses a detailed quantitative diet history and employs multivariate analysis. Although 80% of the studies had major methodologic shortcomings, when the data were summarily expressed, a definite pattern of nutritional risk emerged.

Nutritional Results

The nutritional results are expressed in a summary form (Tables 2 and 3). The authors emphasise that some interpretations and approximations had to be made, particularly with the earlier studies, because in several instances, results were not clearly expressed, in others no calculations of statistical significance were made, while in some studies, data known to have been examined were just not published in the paper. Table 2 expresses the statistically significant foods and food groups, while Table 3 shows the results for macronutrients and micronutrients. In the interpretation of the results, less weight was placed on those studies which show no association and more on those which showed either a statistically significant protective or risk effect, as lack of association may merely mirror the lack of sensitivity of the method used.

Meat consumption, in particular beef intake and to a lesser extent lamb intake were risks, while pork and poultry consumption were not as obviously risk factors as was beef. Interestingly, three of 17 studies found fish consumption to be protective. Only a few studies showed milk and milk products to be a risk and most showed no association or else a protective effect. Eggs generally showed no association with the risk.

A high vegetable intake was almost uniformly a protective factor. Cruciferous vegetables appeared to be especially protective. Carrot consumption showed no association with the risk, in keeping with the finding of the Melbourne study that beta carotene consumption is unassociated with the risk of colorectal cancer. Potatoes were also not associated with the risk. String beans and fava beans appeared to be the only risk factors in the vegetable group. Fruit in general was a protective factor, in keeping with an inverse relationship between colorectal cancer and vitamin C consumption. Cereal intake was largely not associated with the risk of colorectal cancer. This is in keeping with the finding in the Melbourne Study that a high fiber intake is most protective when in association with a high vegetable intake [18]. Interestingly, increasing frequency of meals was a risk factor in both of the two studies which examined this effect.

Examining the data when expressed as nutrients, fats were a risk in several studies. Protective effects of fats were noted mainly when the fats consumed mainly consisted of vegetable oils. Saturated fatty acids were a risk,

TABLE 2

Statistically Significant Foods and Food Groups Found in
40 Colorectal Cancer Case-Control Studies

Food/Food Groups Examined	Number of Studies	Risk	Protection	No Association
MEAT	20	12 (6)	2 (1)	6
Beef	15	6 (3)	0	9
Lamb	12	6 (2)	0	6
Pork	13	3 (2)	2	8
Poultry	12	4 (2)	1 (1)	7
Rabbit	2	2	0	0
GAME	2	0	0	2
FISH AND SEAFOOD	17	3 (3)	3	11
DAIRY PRODUCTS	18	5 (5)	4 (2)	9
Milk Drinks	11	3 (3)	1	7
Cheese	9	0	1 (1)	8
Butter	10	1 (1)	1 (1)	8
Yoghurt	3	0	0	3
EGGS	12	2 (2)	1 (raw)	9
VEGETABLES	20	2 (2 beans)	13	5
Cruciferous	14	0	9 (5)	5
Leafy	2	0	1	1
Lettuce	6	0	2	4
Peppers	5	0	1 (1)	4
Carrots	4	0	1 (1)	3
Potatoes	10	1 (1)	0	9
String beans	10	2 (1)	0 (1)	8
Fava beans	1	1	0	0
FRUIT	18	1 (1)	6	11
CEREALS	16	3 (3)	2 (2)	11
White bread	4	0	0	4
Wholemeal bread	4	0	1 (1)	3
Oatmeal/oats	2	0	0	2
Rice	8	4 (1)	1 (1)	3
Pasta	3	2 (1)	0	1
TEA	5	0	1	4
COFFEE	8	1 (1)	2	5
FREQUENCY OF MEALS	2	2 (1)	0	0

Note: () indicate number of studies in which effect present for subsets
of cases only, such as males only or colon cancer only, etc.

TABLE 3

Statistically Significant Nutrients Found in 40 Colorectal
Cancer Case-Control Studies

Nutrient Examined	Number of of Studies	Risk	Protection	No Association
FATS	25	10 (5)	7 (4 veg oil)	8
Saturated fatty acids	8	4	1 (1)	3
Unsaturated	4	0	1 (1)	3
Cholesterol	5	2 (1)	0	3
High unsat/sat ratio oil	1	0	1	0
PROTEIN	12	4 (2)	1	7
CARBOHYDRATE	12	3 (1)	0	9
Starchy food	5	2 (1)	1 (1)	2
Oligosaccharides	3	1	0	2
FIBER	20	2 (1)	7 (2)	11
ALCOHOL	19	8	2 (spirits)	9
Beer	11	6 (5)	0	5
Wine	3	2 (1)	0	1
Spirits	4	1	2 (2)	1
ENERGY	9	4 (2)	0	5
VITAMINS	13	1	4 (1)	8
Vitamin A	9	1	0	8
Beta carotene	6	0	0	6
Vitamin C	11	0	3 (1)	8
Vitamin D	2	0	0	2
Vitamin E	1	0	0	1
Vitamin B1	3	0	1	2
Vitamin B2	3	1 (1)	1	1
Vitamin B6	2	0	2	0
Nicotinic acid	1	1 (1)	0	0
Vitamin supplements	1	0	1	0
CALCIUM	5	0	1 (1)	4
POTASSIUM	4	0	3	1
SALT	11	5 (2)	0	6

Note: () indicate number of studies in which effect present for subsets of cases,
such as males only or colon cancer only etc.

while unsaturated fatty acids may be protective. Protein intake and carbohydrate intake were more often found to be risk rather than protective factors. When an association was found, dietary fiber was usually protective, although a protective effect was less clear than that for vegetables and fruit. Alcohol, and particularly beer and particularly for rectal cancer, was a risk factor. When an association was found, a high energy intake was a risk factor.

Dietary vitamin C was protective in all three studies in which a statistically significant association was found, whilst dietary vitamin A, D, E and beta carotene were not associated with the risk of colorectal cancer. Vitamin supplements were highly statistically significantly protective for both males and females and for both colon cancer and rectal cancer, in the one study which examined this effect [18]. When an association was present, a high potassium intake was protective whilst a high salt intake was a risk factor.

CONCLUSION

Previous diet is an important etiological factor in the development of large bowel cancer. The Melbourne Colorectal Cancer Study, as well as other epidemiological research of the past 25 years indicates that it is the whole dietary pattern rather than merely individual foods or food groups which are important in the dietary etiology of this cancer. Expressed as a very broad generalisation, a high intake of foods of animal origin, particularly red meat and fat, and a low intake of foods of plant origin, particularly vegetables and fruit and to a lesser extent cereals, constitutes a high risk dietary pattern in the etiology of colorectal cancer.

REFERENCES

1. MUIR CS, PARKIN DSM. The world cancer burden: Prevent or perish. Br Med J 290:5-6, 1985.
2. KUNE GA, KUNE S. The Melbourne colorectal cancer study. A description of the investigation. University of Melbourne, Department of Surgery publication. ISBN 0 86839 569 X, pp 1-31, 1986.
3. KUNE GA, KUNE S. New design to examine colorectal cancer cause and survival. Dig Surg 4:156-159, 1987.

4. KUNE S, KUNE GA, WATSON LF. The Melbourne colorectal cancer study: Incidence findings by age, sex, site, migrants and religion. Int J Epidemiol 15:483-493, 1986.

5. KUNE GA, KUNE S, WATSON LF. The role of heredity in the etiology of large bowel cancer: Data from the Melbourne colorectal cancer study. World J Surg 13:124-131, 1989.

6. KUNE GA, KUNE S, WATSON LF. History of colorectal polypectomy and risk of subsequent colorectal cancer. Br J Surg 74:1064-1065, 1987.

7. KUNE GA, KUNE S, WATSON LF. Children, age at first birth and colorectal cancer risk. Data from the Melbourne colorectal cancer study. Am J epidemiol 129:533-542, 1989.

8. KUNE GA, KUNE S, FIELD B, WATSON LF. The role of chronic constipation, diarrhea and laxative use in the etiology of large bowel cancer. Data from the Melbourne colorectal cancer study. Dis Colon Rectum 31:507-512, 1988.

9. KUNE GA, KUNE S, WATSON LF. Oral contraceptive use does not protect against large bowel cancer. Contraception (submitted 1989).

10. KUNE GA, KUNE S, WATSON LF. Colorectal cancer risk, chronic illnesses, operations and medication: Case control results from the Melbourne colorectal cancer study. Cancer Res 48:4399-4404, 1988.

11. KUNE GA, KUNE S, WATSON LF. Large bowel cancer after cholecystectomy. Am J Surg 156:359-362, 1988.

12. SKEGG DCG. Potential for bias in case control studies of oral contraceptives and breast cancer. Am J Epidemiol 127:205-212, 1988.

13. HANKIN JH, NOMURA AMJ, LEE J. Reproducibility of a diet history questionnaire in a case control study of breast cancer. Am J Clin Nutr 37:981-985, 1983.

14. CHU S, KOLONEL LN, HANKIN JH. A comparison of frequency and quantitative dietary methods for epidemiological studies of diet and disease. Am J Epidemiol 119:323-334, 1984.

15. LEE J, KOLONEL LN, HANKIN JH. Cholesterol intake as measured by unquantified and quantified food frequency interview: Implications for epidemiological research. Int J Epidemiol 14:249-253, 1985.

16. KUNE S, KUNE GA, WATSON LF. Observations on the reliability and validity of the design and diet history method in the Melbourne colorectal cancer study. Nutr Cancer 9:5-20, 1987.

17. BOUTRON MC, GAIVRE J, MILAN C, LORCERIE B, ESTEVE J. A comparison of two diet history questionnaires that measure usual food intake. Nutr Cancer 12:83-91, 1989.

18. KUNE S, KUNE GA, WATSON LF. Case-control study of dietary etiological factors: The Melbourne colorectal cancer study. Nutr Cancer 9:21-42, 1987.

19. KUNE S, KUNE GA, WATSON LF. Case-control study of alcoholic beverages as etiological factors: The Melbourne colorectal cancer study. Nutr Cancer 9:43-56, 1987.

2U. KUNE GA, KUNE S, WATSON LF. Dietary sodium and potassium intake and colorectal cancer risk. Nutr Cancer (in press for December 1989).

21. KUNE GA, KUNE S, WATSON LF. Body weight and physical activity as predictors of colorectal cancer risk. Nutr Cancer (in press for January 1990).

22. HIGGINSON J. Etiological factors in gastrointestinal cancer in man. J Nat Cancer Inst 37:527-545, 1966.

23. WYNDER EL, SHIGEMATSU T. Environmental factors of cancer of the colon and rectum. Cancer 20:1520-1561, 1967.

24. WYNDER EL, KAJITANI T, ISHIKAWA S, DODO H, TAKANO A. Environmental factors of cancer of the colon and rectum. II. Japanese epidemiological data. Cancer 23:1210-1220, 1969.

25. BJELKE E. Case-control study of cancer of the stomach, colon, and rectum. Proc 10th Int Cancer Congress, Vol 5. Chicago:Year Book, pp 320-334, 1971.

26. HAENSZEL W, BERG JW, SEGI M, KURIHARA M, LOCKE FB. Large-bowel cancer in Hawaiian Japanese. J Natl Cancer Inst 51:1765-1779, 1973.

27. MODAN B, BARELL V, LUBIN F, MODAN M. Dietary factors and cancer in Israel. Cancer Res 35:3503-3506, 1975.

28. MODAN B, BARELL V, LUBIN F, MODAN M, GREENBERG RA, GRAHAM S. Low-fiber intake as an etiologic factor in cancer of the colon. J Natl Cancer Inst 55:15-18, 1975.

29. DALES LG, FRIEDMAN GD, URY HK, GROSSMAN S, WILLIAMS SR. A case-control study of relationships of diet and other traits to colorectal cancer in American blacks. Am J Epidemiol 109:132-144, 1978.

30. GRAHAM S, DAYAL H, SWANSON M, MITTELMAN A, WILKINSON G. Diet in the epidemiology of cancer of the colon and rectum. J Natl Cancer Inst 61:709-714, 1978.

31. JAIN M, COOK GM, DAVIS FG, GRACE MG, HOWE GR, MILLER AB. A case-control study of diet and colorectal cancer. Int J Cancer 26:757-768, 1980.

32. HAENSZEL W, LOCKE FB, SEGI M. A case-control study of large bowel cancer in Japan. JNCI 64:17-22, 1980.

33. VOBECKY J, CARO J, DEVROEDE G. A case-control study of risk factors for large bowel carcinoma. Cancer 51:1958-1963, 1983.

34. HOWE GR, MILLER AB, JAIN M, COOK G. Dietary factors in relation to the etiology of colorectal cancer. Cancer Detection & Prevention 5:331-334, 1982.

35. TUYNS AJ, PEQUIGNOT G, GIGNOUX M, VALLA A. Cancers of the digestive tract, alcohol and tobacco. Int J Cancer 30:9-11, 1982.

36. POTTER JD, McMICHAEL AJ, BONETT AZ. Diet, alcohol and large-bowel cancer: A case control study. Proc Nutr Soc Aust 7:123-126, 1982.

37. MacLENNAN R, CORREA P, HEILBRUN L, NEWELL G, POLLACK E. Report of a workshop: Cancers of the colon and rectum. Nat Cancer Inst Monograph 62:145-149, 1982.

38. WARD K, MORIARTY KJ, O'NEILL S, CLARK ML, DEAN G. Alcohol and colo-rectal cancer. Gut 24:A981, 1983.

39. MANOUSOS O, DAY NE, TRICHOPOULOS D, GEROVASSILIS F, TZONOU A, POLYCHRONOPOULOU A. Diet and colorectal cancer: A case-control study in Greece. Int J Cancer 32:1-5, 1983.

40. MILLER AB, HOWE GR, JAIN M, CRAIB KJP, HARRISON L. Food items and food groups as risk factors in a case-control study of diet and colo-rectal cancer. Int J Cancer 32:155-161, 1983.

41. MACQUART-MOULIN G, DURBEC J-P, CORNEE J, BERTHEZENE P, SOUTHGATE DAT. Diet and colorectal cancer. Gastroenterol Clin Biol 7:277-286, 1983.

42. PICKLE LW, GREENE MH, ZIEGLER RG, TOLEDO A, HOOVER R, LYNCH T, FRAUMENI JF Jr. Colorectal cancer in rural Nebraska. Cancer Res 44:363-369, 1984.

43. McMICHAEL AJ, POTTER JD. Diet and colon cancer: Integration of the descriptive, analytic, and metabolic epidemiology. Natl Cancer Inst Monogr 69:223-228, 1985.

44. HEILBRUN LK, NOMURA A, HANKIN JH, STEMMERMANN GN. Dietary vitamin D and calcium and risk of colorectal cancer. Lancet 20:925, 1985.

45. TAJIMA K, TOMINAGA S. Dietary habits and gastrointestinal cancers: A comparative case-control study of stomach and large intestinal cancers in Nagoya, Japan. Jpn J Cancer Res (Gann) 76:705-716, 1985.

46. BRISTOL JB, EMMETT PM, HEATON KW, WILLIAMSON RCN. Sugar, fat, and the risk of colorectal cancer. Br Med J 291:1467-1470, 1985.

47. BERTA J-L, COSTE T, RAUTUREAU J, GUILLOUD-BATAILLE M, PEQUIGNOT G. Alimentation et cancers recto-coliques. Resultats d'une etude (cas-temoin). Gastroenterol Clin Biol 9:348-353, 1985.

48. POTTER JD, McMICHAEL AJ. Diet and cancer of the colon and rectum: A case-control study. JNCI 76:557-569, 1986.

49. MACQUART-MOULIN G, RIBOLI E, CORNEE J, CHARNAY B, BERTHEZENE P, DAY N. Case-control study on colorectal cancer and diet in Marseilles. Int J Cancer 38:183-191, 1986.

50. LYON JL, MAHONEY AW, WEST DW, GARDNER JW, SMITH KR, SORENSON AW, STANISH W. Energy intake: Its relationship to colon cancer risk. JNCI 78:853-861, 1987.

51. TUYNS AJ, HAELTERMAN M, KAAKS R. Colorectal cancer and the intake of nutrients: Oligosaccharides are a risk factor, fats are not. A case-control study in Belgium. Nutr Cancer 10:181-196, 1987.

52. TUYNS A. Salt and gastrointestinal cancer. Nutr Cancer 11:229-232, 1988.

53. TUYNS AJ, KAAKS R, HAELTERMAN M. Colorectal cancer and the consumption of foods: A case-control study in Belgium. Nutr Cancer 11:189-204, 1988.

54. GRAHAM S, MARSHALL J, HAUGHEY B, MITTELMAN A, SWANSON M, ZIELEZNY M, BYERS T, WILKINSON G, WEST D. Dietary epidemiology of cancer of the colon in Western New York. Am J Epidemiol 128:490-503, 1988.

55. PHILLIPS RL. Role of life-style and dietary habits in risk of cancer among Seventh-Day Adventists. Cancer Res 35:3513-3522, 1975.

56. VLAJINAC H, ADANJA B, JAREBINSKI M. Case-control study of the relationship of diet and colon cancer. Arch Geschwulstforsch 57:493-499, 1987.
57. KABAT GC, HOWSON CP, WYNDER EL. Beer consumption and rectal cancer. Int J Epidemiol 15:494-501, 1986.
58. SLATTERY ML, SORENSON AW, FORD MH. Dietary calcium intake as a mitigating factor in colon cancer. Am J Epidemiol 128:504-514, 1988.
59. LYON JL, MAHONEY AW. Fried foods and the risk of colon cancer. Am J Epidemiol 128:1000-1006, 1988.
60. SLATTERY ML, SORENSON AW, MAHONEY AW, FRENCH TK, KRITCHEVSKY D, STREET JC. Diet and colon cancer: Assessment of risk by fiber type and food source. J Natl Cancer Inst 80:1474-1480, 1988.
61. MARTINEZ I, TORRES R, FRIAS Z, COLON JR, FERNANDEZ N. Factors associated with adenocarcinomas of the large bowel in Puerto Rico. Adv Med Onc Res Educ 3:45-52, 1975.

Nutrients and Cancer Prevention K. N. Prasad and F. L. Meyskens, Jr., eds. © 1990 The Humana Press

AN INTERMEDIATE EVALUATION OF THE NUTRITION

INTERVENTION TRIALS IN LINXIAN, CHINA

LI JUN-YAO

Cancer Institute

Chinese Academy of Medical Sciences

INTRODUCTION

Over the past several years, the Cancer Institute of Chinese Academy of Medical Sciences (CICAMS) has been collaborating with NCI, USA in the conduct of two randomized, double-blind and placebo-controlled intervention trials in Linxian, China to test the hypothesis that dietary supplementation with vitamins and minerals might reduce the incidence and mortality of cancer. With the great concern and support from the two governments and joint hard work of Chinese and American scientists, a great deal of research activities has been finished either in the Linxian field or in the laboratories since signing of the first contract No.NO1-CP-41019 in 1984. Although there have been some difficulties, overall, the collaborative project proceeded in a very smooth and efficient manner. So far, screening and recruitment of study subjects were successful, the number of individual recruited exceeded originally projected sample size. Pill compliance to date assessed by pill counts and biochemical tests has been excellent. Significant improvements were made for determination of intermediate and final endpoints and quality control procedures were established.

Experimental studies of cancer, such as the ongoing nutrition intervention trials in Linxian, China, represent a powerful approach in testing the diet-cancer hypothesis. Such studies, however, are long and expensive, typically

requiring 15 or more years (1) for obtaining the final
outcome, depending to the compliance, mode of carcinogenesis and sample size. The use of intermediate endpoints is
a new and exciting approach in the study of carcinogenesis.
The major advantage to studies of intermediate endpoints
is that, relative to trials using cancer as the endpoint,
they can be conducted with smaller numbers of subjects
over shorter periods of time. To date, only a few nutrition intervention studies using intermediate endpoints
have been reported (2-6). One involved assessment of esophageal abnormalities in 567 persons in a county near Linxian who in the preceding year had received weekly supplements of retinol, riboflavin, and zinc or placebo. No treatment differences were found, although those whose blood
retinol level improved showed a lower prevalence of esophageal lesions, and micronuclei and tritiated thymidine
labeling were found in a smaller percent of cells from esophageal smears of treated compared to placebo subjects (4-
6). A major disadvantage of these investigations is that
none of the proposed intermediate endpoints has yet been
studied in sufficient detail to know if they are truly predictive of the subsequent development of cancer. Nesting
studies of intermediate endpoints within ongoing intervention studies in which cancer is the final endpoint provides
an opportunity to simultaneously test the relationship of
the intermediate endpoints to the final endpoint as well
as the relationship of the intervention to both the intermediate and final endpoints.

STUDY PROGRESS TO DATE ON THE NUTRITION
INTERVENTION TRIALS IN LINXIAN, CHINA

A. Dysplasia Trial

In the Autunm of 1983, approximately 14,000 persons
from the three northernmost communes in Linxian (Yaocun,
Rencun, and Donggong) participated in mass balloon cytology examinations. 3656 subjects with severe dysplasia were
identified from these examinations and asked to participat
in the screening phase of this intervention study. 3399
(93%) agreed to participate in screening evaluations (whic
included a questionnaire to obtain baseline data on health
and suspected risk factors, a blood sample aliquoted for
long-term storage, and toe nail clipping for future assay)
in August/September 1984 and 3393 were subsequently randomized and enrolled as study subjects. All subjects starte

taking intervention agents on 1 May, 1985 after a 6 month placebo run-in period. Individuals receive 2 multi-vitamin/mineral tablets (Centrum tablets produced by Lederle Laboratories,Inc.) each containing from 1 to 1.5 times the U.S. RDA for 25 vitamins and minerals and one 15 mg beta-carotene capsuls (provided by Hoffmann-LaRoche,Inc.), or 3 look-alike placebos. The barefoot doctors count and record the number of unused pills in their monthly visit.

Subject compliance with the pill-taking regimens has been excellent to date. Pill counts indicate that more than 90% of the participants are taking greater than 90% of their pills. Nutritional biochemical assessments have been conducted quarterly on population samples which demonstrate distinct differences between active and placebo recipients for each of the factors being tested.

Systems were established for ascertaining death and cancer occurrences among the cohorts being followed, in part based on utilizing the Linxian Cancer Registry. Loss to follow-up is close to zero. As of early 1988 the death rate among participants averaged 1.4% per year and the cancer incidence rate 1.1% per year. Approximately 85% of all cancers have been esophageal or stomach cancers, with most of the latter reported in the gastric cardia.

The cancer rate observed thus far has been less than two-thirds that predicted prior to the start of the trial. That prediction, based on the assumption that persons with dysplasia experience 3 times the risk of cancer of Linxian residents without dysplasia, now appears to be an overestimate (cancer incidence in the Dysplasia Trial is 1.5 rather than 3 times higher than in the General Population Trial). Part of the loss of statistical power resulting from this short fall of events is offset by our enrolling nearly 3400 instead of the originally expected 2000 participants. Using the revised cancer incidence data and actual numbers of participants, a 5-year trial would have over 85% power to detect a 40% reduction in cancer incidence rates in the treated compared to placebo group, a figure close to the originally projected study power.

B. General Population Trial

Contacting of adults age 40-69 in 3 northern Linxian communes to determine eligibility and willingness to participate in a 5-year vitamin/mineral supplementation trial began in March 1985. Unlike the Dysplasia Trial, refusals were more common, and an additional commune was included. Altogether, among nearly 50,000 individuals screened in the spring of 1985, approximately 30,000 (66%) agreed to enroll. Baseline interview data were obtained and 10-ml blood samples were collected and serum aliquots stored for all participants.

NCI arranged for the purchase (from Hoffmann-LaRoche Inc.) of the pills for the General Population Trial in 1985. Eight types of pills have been prepared. Using the designations A,B,C,D, respectively for the nutrient factors retinol/zinc, riboflavin/niacin, ascorbic acid/molybdenum, and tocopherol/carotene/selenium, persons were randomized (by NCI) into groups receiving one of the following 8 combinations of nutrients: AB,AC,AD,BC,BD,CD,ABCD,none. Delivery of the pills to China was delayed for several months, so the participants did not begin taking pills untill March 1986. As in the Dysplasia Trial, compliance measured by both pill counting and biochemical tests has been extremely high. By the end of 1987, over 40,000,000 pills had been distributed in this trial, with only 4% returned unused.

The death rate thus far in the General Population has been 1.3% per year; the cancer incidence rate 0.8% per year. The latter rate is above that projected prior to entry in the study, so the power to dect small (20%) differences in cancer incidence at the end of 5 years of intervention between those receiving or not receiving each of the four nutrient groups (A,B,C,D above) now exceeds 90%.

INTERMEDIATE ENDPOINTS OF THE NUTRITION INTERVENTION TRIALS IN LINXIAN, CHINA

Intervention trials that use cancer as an endpoint require a large number of participants and last for a prolonged period of time, they are costly and difficult to control. The application of "intermediate endpoints" which may reveal the response to chemopreventive regimes within a short timespan, and which may act as surrogates for cancer, is an attractive idea worthy of in-depth exploration. Nesting studies of intermediate endpoints using this ongoing nutrition intervention trials in Linxian, China provides an unique opportunity to explore the relationship of the relationship of the intermediate endpoints to the final outcome as well as the relationship of the intervention to both the intermediate endpoints and final endpoints. In conjunction with the Dysplasia Trial, several markers have been examined in October and November of 1987, at about the halfway point of the trial.

A. Specific Aims

The primary objectives of this study are to compare the effects of supplementation with multi-vitamins/minerals (versus placebo) on:
1. Cytologic abnormalities of the esophagus;
2. DNA- content of esophageal epithelial cells;
3. Endoscopically-observed abnormalities of the esophagus;
4. Histologic changes in esophageal epithelium;
5. Proliferative activity and functional status of esophageal epithelium;
6. Immune function;
7. Nitrosamine formation.

A secondary objective includes evaluation of the concordance between these various intermediate endpoints.

B. Materials and Methods

Subjects for these evaluations were selected from 3393 participants in an ongoing nutrition intervention study, the Dysplasia Trial, being conducted in Linxian, China. All subjects were previously identified as having severe esophageal dysplasia.

All 3393 subjects had samples collected for cytologic morphologic evaluation, DNA-content determination, and for counting the frequency of micronucleated cells. Before the trial started, 520 subjects had a baseline endoscopic examination of the esophagus with multiple biopsies. Endoscopic examination with biopsies were repeated on these subjects to study histologic changes, proliferative activity measured by microautoradiography of vitro tritiated thymidine uptake in epithelial cells, and functional status measured by immunohistochemical stains or various keratins, lectins, and blood groups. Bruchings at or near the biopsy sites were examined for routine cytologic abnormalities as well as DNA content determined by quantitative fluorescent image analysis. In addition, blood samples were also collected for evaluating cellular and humoral immune function and gastric juice and urine were obtained for nitrosamine formation assays.

Evaluation of these subjects following approximately

30 months of intervention treatment will allow observation
of potential effects on endpoints considered intermediate
in the carcinogenesis process (e.g., changes in cytology,
histology, DNA-content, proliferative activity etc.) as
well as the concordance between these various intermediate
endpoints. It will also enable study of the influence of
this intervention on two potential mechanisms of action (
e.g., alteration in immune status and the metabolism of a
family of carcinogens (e.g., nitrosamines).

Results from cytologic and QFIA examinations will be
dichotomized using predetermined criteria for positivity.
Each test will then be compared by treatment group as the
difference between two proportions. Additional comparisons for concordance between cytologic and QFIA test results will also be conducted. Changes in individual cytologic status between this examination and the examination
conducted prior to the trial will be determined, and transition rates from Grade III (marked severe dysplasia-the
only diagnosis in the initial exam) to Grade I (normal),
Grade II (hyperplasia), Grade IV (near carcinoma), and
Grade V (early carcinoma) will be contrasted between the
treatment groups. With approximately 1700 subjects in
each of the two treatment groups and all having Grade III
marked severe dysplasia at entry into the trial, we will
be able to detect an absolute difference between treatment
groups in the proportion of subjects with improvement to
Grade I or II of 6%. The percent cells with micronuclei
present will be compared using a Wilcoxon rank test or student's test.

The Papanicoulaou stained slides, QFIA from the bru-
ching, microautoradiogrphic studies of epithelial cell
proliferation, immunohistchemistry studies, and immunologic function will be compared either parametrically (e.g.,
t-test) or nonparametrically (e.g., Wilcoxon rank sum test
depending on the distribution of the indies. Similar pa-
rametric or nonparametric tests will be applied to the
comparisons of the nitrosamine results. The vitamin analysis data will be used to stratify the nitrosamine test
results. With 250 subjects in each treatment group, we
will be able to detect improvement from cytologic class
Grade III in the active treatment group compared to the
placebo of 15%. Similarly, for the nitrosamine analyses,
assuming a mean of 5.7 ug of nitrosoproline excreted per
day and a variance of 45.8, we will be able to detect an ab-

solute decrease of 1.96 ug/day in the active treatment group (or relative decrease of 34%).

C. Data Management

To maintain the blind of the ongoing clinical trial which these evaluations are a part, treatment codes will be maintained in secret at the study data management center at Westat. Laboratory results from each of the different tests conducted as part of this study will be sent to the study data management center. In consultation with study coordinators of this project, the data management center will provide individual investigators whatever statistical analyses and graphical presentation of results they require, by treatment group, for presentation in the scientific literature.

D. Preliminary Results

Endoscopic examinations were performed prior starting intervention agents on a subset of 520 Dysplasia Trial participants in January 1985. Subjects were selected at random primarily from among those with severe dysplasia Type 2, from all 3 communes (Yaocun 25%, Rencun 40%, and Donggang 35%) to include both male (42%) and female (58%). To maintain the blind of the ongoing trials, the results of the intermediate evaluation are still waiting to open the treatment code for comparing the effects of supplementation. Therefore, full assessment of the numerous evaluations conducted as part of this examination is not yet available.

Triated thymidine labeling studies performed in biopsy samples collected at the baseline endoscopic examination in 1985 from 44 subjects showed a gradient of increased expansion in the basal layer of proliferating cells, which was twice as high in the epithelial cell lining among those with histologic evidence of dysplasia as in near-normal subjects(7).

Quantitation of the DNA content of epithelial cells using a semi-automated technique was initially developed for use in detecting hyperploid cells from the blader in urine(8). This quantitative flurescence imaging assay (QFIA) has subsequently been adapted for use with bronchial epithelial cells from sputum and for esophageal epithelial cells obtained using the Chinese balloon swallow technique.

During a pilot study among esophageal balloon swallow samples collected from 20 subjects undergoing evaluation for
esophageal cancer at Yaocun commune hospital, 11 of 12 reported or suspected malignancies were found to be positive
using QFIA when 1,000-2,000 cells were scanned following
staining with Hoechst dye. Quality of sample collection
and preservation was excellent. The use of the QFIA on
samples collected using this technique may be a particularly valuable diagnostic tool as the net-covered balloon co-
llects cells from the entire esophagus.

We are also assessing intervention group differences
in rates of transition between dysplasia, hyperplasia, and
normal esophageal status determined by cytologic examinations of cells collected at the beginning, middle, and end
of the trial, including determination of cells micronucleus
frequency.

Gastric juice and urine were analyzed for N-nitroso
compounds, including nitrosoproline, nitrososarcosine, ni-
trosothiozolidine-4-carboxylic acid, and nitroso-2-methyl-
thioazolidine-4-carboxylic acid in the laboratory of Dr.
Lu Shi-Xin at the CICAMS.

Several immune parameters of human peripheral blood
lyphocytes PBL) were tested and compared with this intervention by Drs. Li Shao-Guang & Zhang you-Hui. The results
are as follows:

1. PBL proliferation in response to PHA stimulation
and LAK cell activity were found lower in the group with
nutrition supplementation than in the group with placebo.
This is the first evidence that prolonged nutrition supplementation (2.5 years) might have deleterious effect on the
immune system.

2. The immune function level in Linxian's patients
with severe esophageal dysplasia was lower as compared to
that of the normal subjects in Beijing. Further analysis
demonstrated that the patients' immune function level was
higher in males than females, with smoking history than
without.

3. For the first time methylbenzylnitrosamine (NMBzA
was found to strongly inhibit immune functions in vitro,
including proliferation response of PBL to PHA, capacity
of IL-2 production and LAK cell activity. This inhibitory
effect of NMBzA could be achieved in the absence of S9,

but the effect was much stronger when enzymetically activated. There was a negative correlation between the degree of inhibition and the immune status, ie, the lower the proliferative capability of PBL, the higher the degree of NMBzA-induced inhibition. Since the PBL proliferation was weaker in nutrition supplemented group than in placebo group, the former group was seen to be sensitive to NMBzA treatment.

There is yet no good explanation why nutritional supplementation did not improve, but instead, deteriorate the immune functions. The possibility of inadequacy in dosage of vitamins for long period of time was considered. The impact on esophageal cancer incidence require years of follow-up observation to ascertain.

SUMMARY

In collaboration with NCI in the USA, two randomized double-blind and placebo-controlled nutrition intervention trials to prevent esophageal cancer are underway in Linxian, China. The first trial is conducted among 3393 subjects with cytologically-diagnosed dysplasia, using simple two-arm design. The second one is in 30,258 adults aged 40-69 years old of general population, using a fractional factorial design. Both trials have been providing the selected multi-vitamins and minerals (or placebo) at dosage levels ranging from 1-4 times of the US Recommended Daily Allowances for dysplasia trial subjects since May 1985, and for general population trial subjects since March, 1986.

So far, participant compliance in taking pill has been excellent in terms of pill counts and biochemical tests for both trials. Nesting studies of intermediate endpoints, including changes in cytology, histology, DNA-content, proliferative activity, frequency of micronucleated cells, genetic marker and nitrosation, are carried out after approximately 30 months of intervention treatment in dysplasia trial. The intermediate evaluation provides an opportunity to simultaneously test the relationship of the intermediate endpoints to the final endpoints as well as the relationship of intervention to both the intermediate and final endpoints. To maintain the blind of the ongoing trials, the results of the intermediate evaluation are still waiting to open the treatment code for comparing the effects of supplementation.

REFERENCES

1. Zelen M. Are primary cancer prevention trials feasible? JNCI 1988; 80(18):1442-1444.

2. Stich HF, Rosin MP, Vallejera MO. Reduction with vitamin A and Beta-carotene administration of proportion of micronucleated buccal mucosal cells in Asian betel nut and tobocco chewers. Lancet 1984;i:1204-6

3. Gouveia J, Mathe G, Hercend T, Gros F, Lemaigre G, Santelli G, Homasson JP, Gailard JP, Angebault M, Bonniot JP, Lededente A, Marsac J, Parrot R, Pretet S. Degree of bronchial metaplasia in heavy smokers and its regression after treatment with a retinoid. Lancet 1982;i: 710-2.

4. Munoz N, Wahrendorf J, Lu LJ, Crespi M, Thurnham DI, et al. No effect of riboflavine, retinol, and zinc on prevalence of precancerous lesions of esophagus. Lancet 1985; 2:111-4.

5. Thurnham DI, Munoz N, Wahrendorf J, Crespi M. Aetiology of oesophageal cancer. Lancet 1987;1:1450.

6. Munoz N, Hayashi M, Lu JB, Wahrendorf J, Crespi M, Bosch FX. Effect of riboflavin, retinol, and zinc on micronuclei of buccal mucosa and of esophagus: a randomized double-blind intervention study in China. JNCI 1987;79:687-691.

7. Yang GC, Lipkin M, Yang K, Wang GQ, Li JY, Yang CS, Winawer S, Newmark H, Blot WJ, Fraumeni JR,Jr. Proliferation of esophageal epithelial cells among residents of Linxian, China. JNCI 1987;79(6):1241-6.

8. Hemstreet GP,III, west SS, Weems WL, Echols CK, McFarland S, Lewim J, Lindseth G. Quantitiative flurescence measurements of AO-stained normal and malignant blader cells. Int J Cancer 1983;31:577-85.

Nutrients and Cancer Prevention K. N. Prasad and F. L. Meyskens, Jr., eds. © 1990 The Humana Press

VITAMIN D ANALOGS AND THE TREATMENT OF CANCER

Hector F. DeLuca

University of Wisconsin-Madison

Department of Biochemistry
Madison, WI 53706

INTRODUCTION

Vitamin D is well known among biological scientists as being required for mineralization of the skeleton (1). In its absence, the disease rickets is precipitated in the young and osteomalacia in the adult (1). No reports of increased incidence of cancer in vitamin D deficiency have yet appeared. Because of the mineral actions of vitamin D, its possible connection to cancer has been considered remote. With the discovery of the vitamin D endocrine system revealing its ultimate active form 1,25-dihydroxyvitamin D_3 (1,25-$(OH)_2D_3$) has come the realization that it acts analogously to the steroid hormones. The appearance of the receptor to 1,25-$(OH)_2D_3$ in a large number of tissues not previously appreciated to be target organs has suggested a more widespread role of this vitamin (2). A major new function of the vitamin was discovered when Abe et al. (3) and Tanaka et al. (4) found that this compound induced differentiation of promyelocytic cells, M1 and HL-60, into monocytes with a cessation of growth. Similarly, additions of this hormone to osteogenic sarcoma cells or breast cancer cells suppress their growth and induce a differentiation response (5,6). A potential interest, therefore, in the vitamin D compounds as possible therapeutic agents has been suggested. Unfortunately, 1,25-$(OH)_2D_3$ has a most pronounced action in elevating plasma calcium concentration by increasing intestinal calcium

absorption and bone mineral mobilization. The
doses of 1,25-(OH)$_2$D$_3$ that would be required to suppress
malignant growth would cause severe hypercalcemia and
death as a result of this latter response. Work was
initiated to develop vitamin D compounds which might
retain the ability to induce differentiation of malignant
cells while losing their activity in raising plasma
calcium concentration (7,8). This has now been largely
successful, giving forth an array of new compounds with
considerable promise as helpful agents in the treatment
of malignancies having significiant quantities of
receptor for 1,25-(OH)$_2$D$_3$. This report will bring into
focus these investigations.

The Vitamin D Endocrine System

The classical functions of vitamin D are to elevate
plasma calcium and phosphorus concentrations which result
in the mineralization of the skeleton, thus preventing
the classical disease of rickets in children and
osteomalacia in the adult (1). To elevate plasma calcium
and phosphorus to bring about mineralization, vitamin D
acts on the enterocytes of the small intestine (9), on
the distal renal tubule cells of the kidney (10), and on
osteoblasts and bone lining cells to increase the
transport of calcium from the lumen of intesine, from the
lumen of the distal renal tubule, and from the bone fluid
compartment into the plasma (11). This in turn supports
normal neurological and muscular function as well as
supporting normal mineralization of newly formed skeletal
matrix. Because the vitamin D hormone is a potent
substance, its production is very strongly feedback
regulated (12). As illustrated in Figure 1, low plasma
calcium stimulates the parathyroid glands to secrete
parathyroid hormone. This hormone in turn stimulates the
proximal convoluted tubule cells to produce 1,25-(OH)$_2$D$_3$
from its precursor (13,14). 1,25-Dihydroxyvitamin D$_3$
is then transported to the bone lining cells and
osteoblasts (15), to the enterocytes of the small
intestine (16), and to the distal renal tubule cells
(16). 1,25-Dihydroxyvitamin D$_3$ stimulates active calcium
and phosphorus transport in the enterocytes of the small
intestine (9). Together with parathyroid hormone, it
stimulates the mobilization of calcium from bone (17),
and stimulates the reabsorption of calcium in the distal

PLASMA CALCIUM REGULATION

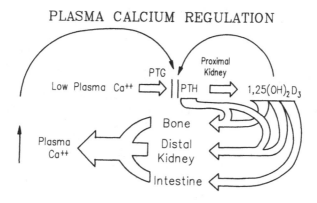

Figure 1. Diagrammatic representation of the regulation
of plasma calcium concentration involving the
vitamin D endocrine system. Low plasma calcium
concentration stimulates parathyroid glands to
secrete parathyroid hormone. This in turn
stimulates the production of $1,25-(OH)_2D_3$ in the
proximal convoluted tubule cells. This hormone
either by itself in the intestine or together with
the parathyroid hormone stimulates the mobilization
of calcium from bone and renal reabsorption of
calcium in the distal renal tubule. These three
sources of calcium raise plasma calcium to normal,
suppressing parathyroid hormone secretion.

renal tubule (10). The function in the distal renal
tubule and in the bone cells in terms of mobilizing
calcium requires the parathyroid hormone and vice versa
(10,11). Calcium, which is elevated in response to these
three actions, rises to a point where the parathyroids
are shut down which in turn shuts off production of the
vitamin D hormone. It is clear, therefore, that the
vitamin D hormone is primarily designed for regulating
plasma calcium concentration and is conversely regulated
by plasma calcium concentration in an indirect fashion.

Molecular Mechanism of Action of 1,25-(OH)$_2$D$_3$
in the Classical Target Tissues

1,25-Dihydroxyvitamin D$_3$ is a steroid and acts in a
fashion quite similar to other steroid hormones (18). A
receptor of 55,000 molecular weight in mammals (19) and
of 59,000-61,000 molecular weight in birds (20) has been
identified as a receptor for this hormone. It is found
entirely in the nucleus of the enterocytes, osteoblasts,
and renal tubule cells (15,16). The intestinal receptor
has been purified from porcine (21) and avian small
intestine (22,23) to a point where monoclonal antibodies
were generated (21,24). With monoclonal antibodies and
λgt-11 expression libraries, cDNAs encoding for the rat
kidney receptor (25) and the chick intestinal receptor
(26) were isolated and sequenced. Full length cDNA
encoding for the rat receptor (27) and the human receptor
(28) have been obtained and sequenced and hence the
entire structure of the 1,25-(OH)$_2$D$_3$ receptor is known.
The 1,25-(OH)$_2$D$_3$ receptor belongs to the superfamily of
steroid hormone receptors as illustrated in Figure 2.
The 1,25-(OH)$_2$D$_3$ receptor is the smallest of the group.

Homologous Regions

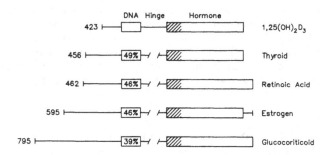

Figure 2.   Diagrammatic representation of the
        1,25-(OH)$_2$D$_3$ receptor as deduced from its cDNA.
        Included is a comparison of the structures of other
        steroid hormone receptors, illustrating that the
        1,25-(OH)$_2$D$_3$ receptor is a member of the steroid
        hormone superfamily of receptors.

It has two DNA binding zinc fingers (27,28). The human receptor is 427 amino acids in length, whereas the rat receptor is 423 amino acids in length. The porcine receptor has also been isolated in pure form by immunoaffinity chromatography and its partial sequence exactly agrees with the sequence deduced for the rat kidney receptor cDNA (29).

The genes that are activated by the $1,25-(OH)_2D_3$ receptor ligand complex are largely unknown. However, in the intestine, the calcium binding protein gene is believed to be a responsive gene to $1,25-(OH)_2D_3$ (30), while in the osteoblasts, the osteocalcin (31) and osteopontin (32) gene are believed to be D-responsive. Both the osteocalcin gene and the calcium binding protein gene have been cloned and the entire structures of these genes are known. So far a D-responsive element has been reported in the osteocalcin gene (33) and confirmed in this laboratory but a D-responsive element has not been located on the calcium binding protein gene. However, the actions and structures of the receptor suggest that indeed $1,25-(OH)_2D_3$ acts in a true steroid hormone fashion quite analogous to the glucocorticoid and estrogen systems.

Distribution of the $1,25-(OH)_2D_3$ Receptor Among Normal Tissue and Cancer Tissue

Nuclear localization of the radiolabeled $1,25-(OH)_2D_3$ and demonstration of the $1,25-(OH)_2D_3$ receptor have shown that the vitamin D hormone very likely has activities beyond calcium homeostasis. For example, it is located in many tissues, as shown in Table 1, suggesting that the vitamin D hormone may have biological functions at these sites (2). Certainly a silencer for the pre-proparathyroid gene that is $1,25-(OH)_2D_3$ activated has been reported (34). Furthermore, a requirement for $1,25-(OH)_2D_3$ to allow normal insulin secretion in response to glucose has been suggested (35). Very likely, therefore, the vitamin D hormone will be shown to have several functions not previously appreciated.

Of considerable interest is the demonstration by Eisman's group of the existence of the $1,25-(OH)_2D_3$

Table 1.   1,25-(OH)$_2$D$_3$ Receptor-Containing Tissues

Tissue	Nuclear Localization of 1,25-(OH)$_2$D$_3$	Receptor Major	Minor
Intestine (small)	X	X	
Kidney	X	X	
Bone	X	X	
Parathyroid Gland	X	X	
Colon	X		X
Pancreas	X		X
Placenta	X		X
Brain	X		X
Pituitary	X		X
Skin	X		X
Spleen	0		0
Stomach Endo Cells	X		?
Lymphocytes	0		0
Activated	0		X

receptor in many cancer cell lines (36,37) and in approximately 60% of fresh cancer tissue (38,39). We have recently been able to examine the receptor levels in 9 breast cancer samples taken at our University Hospital. We have used a new, sensitive and very accurate antibody sandwich assay using two monoclonal antibodies to the 1,25-(OH)$_2$D$_3$ receptor to determine total 1,25-(OH)$_2$D$_3$ receptor in these tumors. It was evident that there are appreciably larger amounts of the 1,25-(OH)$_2$D$_3$ receptor in the breast cancer tissue than estrogen as shown in Table 2. No progesterone receptor levels are presented but were found much lower than the estrogen receptor levels. It is clear, therefore, that at least breast cancer tissue has large amounts of a receptor which may make them responsive to the vitamin D hormone.

Table 2.   Breast Tumor Receptor Levels (in fmol/mg protein)

Sample	$1,25-(OH)_2D_3$	Estrogen
2	84.7	6
3	49.8	10
4	65.0	90
5	47.9	19
6	57.2	25
7	133.4	0
8	144.7	0
9	97.1	75
10	74.1	0

Estrogen receptor levels were determined by ligand binding. Progesterone levels not shown were similar to that of the estrogen receptor levels. The $1,25-(OH)_2D_3$ receptor levels were measured by a immunoradiometric assay involving two monoclonal antibodies directed to different epitope regions of the $1,25-(OH)_2D_3$ receptor. Fresh breast tumors were quickly frozen and then thawed, homogenized and high salt cytosols prepared. They were used immediately for measurement of receptor.

Response of Cancer Cells Lines to $1,25-(OH)_2D_3$

Suda and his colleagues were the first to clearly demonstrate that $1,25-(OH)_2D_3$ when added to cultures of promyelocytes cause their differentiation into monocytes with a consequent suppression of growth (3,4). We have confirmed this finding as illustrated in Figure 3. Similarly, differentiations of melanoma cells treated with $1,25-(OH)_2D_3$ have been shown and suppression of growth (40) in breast carcinoma cells in cultures have also been demonstrated (6,40). On occasion, a stimulation of growth with very low levels of $1,25-(OH)_2D_3$ have been found, and Eisman and his colleagues provided clear evidence that $1,25-(OH)_2D_3$ at low concentrations may stimulate growth of cancer cells

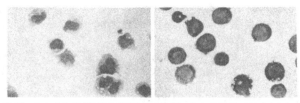

HL-60 cells treated with 100nM 1α,25(OH)$_2$D$_3$ HL-60 cells treated with vehicle only (ethanol)
(monocytes)   (promyelocytes)

Figure 3. Differentiation of the promyelocyte HL-60 cell
line to monocytes by incubation with 1α,25-(OH)$_2$D$_3$.

in culture but at higher concentrations will suppress
growth and cause differentiation (6). These important
findings have suggested that 1,25-(OH)$_2$D$_3$ might be
considered for the treatment of malignancies when the
cells show the presence of significant amounts of
1,25-(OH)$_2$D$_3$ receptor. Unfortunately the concentrations
of 1,25-(OH)$_2$D$_3$ required to suppress growth and cause
differentiation would most certainly cause hypercalcemia
and death to a patient being treated. One possible
solution is to place patients on low calcium intakes to
minimize the hypercalcemic effects of 1,25-(OH)$_2$D$_3$.
Eisman and his colleagues have used this approach and
have demonstrated in vivo that 1,25-(OH)$_2$D$_3$ can suppress
growth of transplantable cancer xenographs (41). The
feasibility, therefore, of suppression of cancerous
growths with 1,25-(OH)$_2$D$_3$ has been demonstrated in this
animal model.

In understanding the action of 1,25-(OH)$_2$D$_3$ in
inducing differentiation, we began to realize that the
activities of 1,25-(OH)$_2$D$_3$ on differentiation could be
separated from its actions in elevating plasma calcium
concentration through modifications of the molecule

(7,8). We previously reported that by modifying the side chain of 1,25-(OH)$_2$D$_3$, we could either increase or maintain the differentiative activities while at the same time decreasing the calcium mobilizing activities. Figure 4 illustrates the side chain modifications and the dose response curves of these analogs in inducing differentiation. We have learned that by adding carbons to the side chain at the 24-position, we could increase activity in causing differentiation while diminishing calcium mobilizing activity (42). We also observed that by increasing the carbon length in the 26- and 27-positions, we increased both calcium mobilizing activity and differentiative activity (7,8). We, therefore, prepared a series of 1,25-(OH)$_2$D$_3$ analogs, some of which are shown in Figure 5. In short, we have learned that by increasing the side chain length

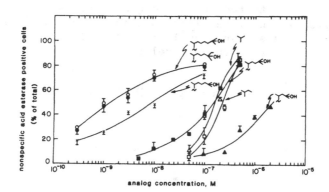

Figure 4. 1,25-(OH)$_2$D$_3$ analog response curves for HL-60 differentiation. The steroid nucleus is not shown but the side chain modifications are illustrated. Note that the homologated 1,25-(OH)$_2$D$_3$ compounds are 10 times more active than 1,25-(OH)$_2$D$_3$ itself. Of interest is the short isopropyl or isobutyl side chains which provide significant HL-60 differentiation activity while having no measurable calcium mobilizing activity.

chain by two carbons, we essentially eliminate the
calcium mobilizing activity while retaining a 10-fold
increase in differentiation of HL-60 cells (42). In this
Figure is illustrated the change in ratio of the two
biological activities. We have, therefore, clearly
designed compounds which have differentiative activity
and no calcium mobilizing activity. Similar reports have
appeared from the Chugai Pharmaceutical Company of Japan
with 22-oxa-1,25-(OH)$_2$D$_3$ and a side chain analog of
1,25-(OH)$_2$D$_3$ from Leo Pharmaceutical Company of Denmark
(43). We have tested the dihomo-1,25-(OH)$_2$D$_3$ analog in
the calcium mobilizing system and have found that this
compound will induce the 25-hydroxyvitamin
D-24-hydroxylase and will induce the intestinal calcium
binding protein but will not induce calcium transport
when administered in vivo (unpublished results). The
change in the activity ratio, therefore, applies in vivo
as well as in vitro. The Δ^{22}-24,24-dihomo-1,25-(OH)$_2$D$_3$
has also been tested in bone organ cultures and is
biologically inert in vitro in this system, while being
10 times more active than 1,25-(OH)$_2$D$_3$ in promoting
differentiation of the promyelocytes (44).

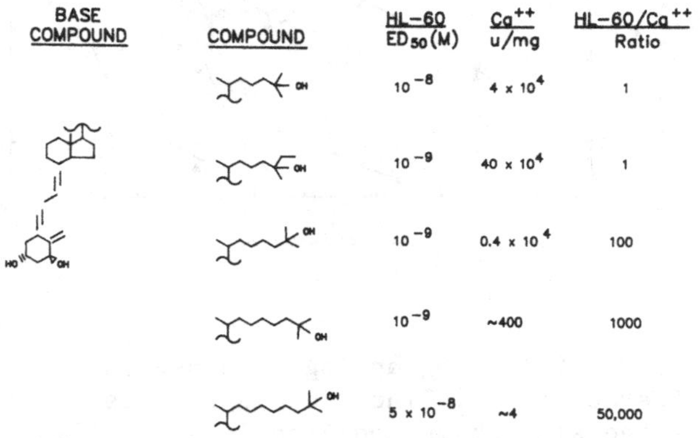

BASE COMPOUND	COMPOUND	HL-60 ED50(M)	Ca++ u/mg	HL-60/Ca++ Ratio
		10^{-8}	4×10^4	1
		10^{-9}	40×10^4	1
		10^{-9}	0.4×10^4	100
		10^{-9}	~400	1000
		5×10^{-8}	~4	50,000

Figure 5. Recently synthesized analogs of 1,25-(OH)$_2$D$_3$
    and their relative activities in causing HL-60
    differentiation or in mobilizing calcium in vivo.

To study these compounds more closely, we have learned how to prepare receptor from HL-60 cells (45) and have studied their binding affinity for the analogs. Of the analogs described above, $1,25-(OH)_2D_3$ is the tightest binder to the receptor and is closely followed by the $24-homo-1,25-(OH)_2D_3$. The dihomo compounds bind about 1/30 as well as the native hormone and the Δ^{22}-trihomo-$1,25-(OH)_2D_3$ binds about 1/130 as well as the native hormone. Since the trihomo compound has activity in causing differentiation approximately equal to that of $1,25-(OH)_2D_3$ but has no calcium mobilizing activity, it is clear that binding to the receptor is not the reason for this divergent activity. It is peculiar that by simply changing the ligand structure by lengthening the side chain we can eliminate calcium mobilizing activity while retaining differentiation activity, both of which are receptor-mediated. This suggests that the second step of receptor interaction with the ligand involving conformational change must be of critical importance in allowing binding to responsive elements in the promoter region of responsive genes. We have learned, for example, that the responsive element in the osteocalcin gene is not found in the calcium binding protein gene or in the promoter region of the $1,25-(OH)_2D_3$ receptor gene.

With the synthesis of $1,25-(OH)_2D_3$ analogs which no longer present hypercalcemia came the possibility of testing _in vivo_ suppression of cancerous growths. We have injected intravenously immune incompetent or Nude mice with 10^5 HL-60 cells per animal. We then provided to the positive controls, vehicle and to the other animals, the lengthened side chain $1,25-(OH)_2D_3$ derivatives. In preliminary results, death due to malignancy caused by HL-60 cells could be prevented on the short term by injection of the $1,25-(OH)_2D_3$ derivatives three times per week. Work is currently progressing on animal models of neoplasia and it is our belief that these compounds may prove useful in the treatment of at least some malignancies by suppressing their growth and causing differentiation.

SUMMARY AND CONCLUSIONS

Receptor to the $1,25-(OH)_2D_3$ hormone has been clearly demonstrated to be present in significant quantities in breast cancer cells and in a number of cancerous cell lines. These compounds when added to cancer tissue _in vivo_ and _in vitro_ can suppress growth and cause differentiation to non-malignant cells. However, the primary action of $1,25-(OH)_2D_3$ in causing hypercalcemia eliminates its possible use as an anti-cancer drug. Development of a series of analogs differing in the side chain has resulted in compounds which retain the differentiative activity and growth suppressing activity of $1,25-(OH)_2D_3$ while eliminating the calcium mobilizing activity. Results in normal animals reveal that these compounds function as predicted from the _in vitro_ models in _in vivo_ measurements. Additionally, preliminary results suggest that the vitamin D analogs which retain the differentiative activity can suppress malignant growth in Nude mice injected with human cancer cells, i.e. HL-60. These results suggest that therapy with vitamin D analogs may be useful for cancers characterized by significant amounts of receptor for $1,25-(OH)_2D_3$.

ACKNOWLEGMENTS

This work is supported by the National Institutes of Health DK-14881, by a grant from the National Foundation for Cancer Research, and by Unimed Corporation.

REFERENCES

1.   DeLuca, H. F. Vitamin D and its metabolites. In: "Modern Nutrition in Health and Disease" (Shils, M. E. and Young, V. R., eds.), Chapter 13, pp. 313-327. Lea & Febiger, Philadelphia, PA (1988).

2.   Link, R. and H. F. DeLuca. The vitamin D receptor. In: "The Receptors" (Conn, P. M., ed.), Vol. II, pp. 1-35. Academic Press, New York (1985).

3. Abe, E., C. Miyaura, H. Sakagami, M. Takeda, K. Konno, T. Yamazaki, S. Yoshiki, and T. Suda. Differentiation of mouse myeloid leukemia cells induced by 1α,25-dihydroxyvitamin D_3. Proc. Natl. Acad. Sci. USA 78, 4990-4994 (1981).

4. Tanaka, H., E. Abe, C. Miyaura, T. Kuribayashi, K. Konno, Y. Nishii, and T. Suda. 1α,25-dihydroxy-cholecalciferol and a human myeloid leukaemia cell line (HL-60). The presence of a cytosol receptor and induction of differentiation. Biochem. J. 204, 713-719 (1982).

5. Dokoh, S., C. A. Donaldson, and M. R. Haussler. Influence of 1,25-dihydroxyvitamin D_3 on cultured osteogenic sarcoma cells: Correlation with the 1,25-dihydroxyvitamin D_3 receptor. Cancer Res. 44, 2103-2109 (1984).

6. Frampton, R. J., S. A. Omond, and J. A. Eisman. Inhibition of human cancer cell growth by 1,25-dihydroxyvitamin D_3 metabolites. Cancer Res. 43, 4443-4447 (1983).

7. Ostrem, V. K., W. F. Lau, S. H. Lee, K. Perlman, J. Prahl, H. K. Schnoes, H. F. DeLuca, and N. Ikekawa. Induction of monocytic differentiation of HL-60 cells by 1,25-dihydroxyvitamin D analogs. J. Biol. Chem. 262, 14164-14171 (1987).

8. Ostrem, V. K., Y. Tanaka, J. Prahl, and H. F. DeLuca. 24- and 26-Homo-1,25-dihydroxyvitamin D_3: Preferential activity in inducing differentiation of human leukemia cells HL-60 in vitro. Proc. Natl. Acad. Sci. USA 84, 2610-2614 (1987).

9. DeLuca, H. F., R. T. Franceschi, B. P. Halloran, and E. R. Massaro. Molecular events involved in the 1,25-dihydroxyvitamin D_3 stimulation of intestinal calcium transport. Fed. Proc. 41, 66-71 (1982).

10. Yamamoto, M., Y. Kawanobe, H. Takahashi, E. Shimazawa, S. Kimura, and E. Ogata. Vitamin D deficiency and renal calcium transport in the rat. J. Clin. Invest. 74, 507-513 (1984).

11. Carlsson, A. Tracer experiments on the effect of
     vitamin D on the skeletal metabolism of calcium and
     phosphorus. Acta Physiol. Scand. 26, 212-220
     (1952).

12. DeLuca, H. F. The transformation of a vitamin into
     a hormone: The vitamin D story. The Harvey
     Lectures, Series 75, pp. 333-379. Academic Press,
     New York (1981).

13. Fraser, D. R. and E. Kodicek. Unique biosynthesis
     by kidney of a biologically active vitamin D
     metabolite. Nature 228, 764-766 (1970).

14. Brunette, M. G., M. Chan, C. Ferriere, and K. D.
     Roberts. Site of 1,25-dihydroxyvitamin D_3 synthesis
     in the kidney. Nature 276, 287-289 (1978).

15. Narbaitz, R., W. E. Stumpf, M. Sar, S. Huang, and H.
     F. DeLuca. Autoradiographic localization of target
     cells for 1α,25-dihydroxyvitamin D_3 in bones from
     fetal rats. Calcif. Tissue Int. 35, 177-182 (1983).

16. Stumpf, W. E., M. Sar, F. A. Reid, Y. Tanaka, and H.
     F. DeLuca. Target cells for 1,25-dihydroxyvitamin
     D_3 in intestinal tract, stomach, kidney, skin,
     pituitary and parathyroid. Science 206, 1188-1190
     (1979).

17. Garabedian, M., Y. Tanaka, M. F. Holick, and H. F.
     DeLuca. Response of intestinal calcium transport
     and bone calcium mobilization to 1,25-dihydroxy-
     vitamin D_3 in thyroparathyroidectomized rats.
     Endocrinology 94, 1022-1027 (1974).

18. DeLuca, H. F. The vitamin D story: A collaborative
     effort of basic science and clinical medicine.
     FASEB J. 2, 224-236 (1988).

19. Dame, M. C., E. A. Pierce, and H. F. DeLuca.
     Identification of the porcine intestinal
     1,25-dihydroxyvitamin D_3 receptor on sodium dodecyl
     sulfate-polyacrylamide gels by renaturation and
     immunoblotting. Proc. Natl. Acad. Sci. USA 82,
     7825-7829 (1985).

20. Mangelsdorf, D. J., J. W. Pike, and M. R. Haussler. Avian and mammalian receptors for 1,25-dihydroxyvitamin D$_3$: In vitro translation to characterize size and hormone-dependent regulation. Proc. Natl. Acad. Sci. USA 84, 354-358 (1987).

21. Dame, M. C., E. A. Pierce, J. M. Prahl, C. E. Hayes, and H. F. DeLuca. Monoclonal antibodies to the porcine intestinal receptor for 1,25-dihydroxyvitamin D$_3$: Interaction with distinct receptor domains. Biochemistry 25, 4523-4534 (1986).

22. Simpson, R. U., A. Hamstra, N. C. Kendrick, and H. F. DeLuca. Purification of the receptor for 1α,25-dihydroxyvitamin D$_3$ from chicken intestine. Biochemistry 22, 2586-2594 (1983).

23. Pike, J. W., and M. R. Haussler. Purification of chicken intestinal receptor for 1,25-dihydroxyvitamin D. Proc. Natl. Acad. Sci. USA 76, 5485-5489 (1979).

24. Pike, J. W., S. L. Marion, C. A. Donaldson, and M. R. Haussler. Serum and monoclonal antibodies against the chick intestinal receptor for 1,25-dihydroxyvitamin D$_3$. J. Biol. Chem. 258, 1289-1296 (1983).

25. Burmester, J. K., N. Maeda, and H. F. DeLuca. Isolation and expression of rat 1,25-dihydroxyvitamin D$_3$ receptor cDNA. Proc. Natl. Acad. Sci. USA 85, 1005-1009 (1988).

26. McDonnell, D. P., D. J. Mangelsdorf, J. W. Pike, M. R. Haussler, and B. W. O'Malley. Molecular cloning of complementary DNA encoding the avian receptor for vitamin D. Science 235, 1214-1217 (1987).

27. Burmester, J. K., R. J. Wiese, N. Maeda, and H. F. DeLuca. Structure and regulation of the rat 1,25-dihydroxyvitamin D$_3$ receptor. Proc. Natl. Acad. Sci. USA 85, 9499-9502 (1988).

28. Baker, A. R., D. P. McDonnell, M. Hughes, T. M. Crisp, D. J. Mangelsdorf, M. R. Haussler, J. W. Pike, J. Shine, and B. W. O'Malley. Cloning and

expression of full-length cDNA encoding human
vitamin D receptor. Proc. Natl. Acad. Sci. USA 85,
3294-4398 (1988).

29. Brown, T. A., J. M. Prahl, and H. F. DeLuca.
    Partial amino acid sequence of porcine
    1,25-dihydroxyvitamin D_3 receptor isolated by
    immunoaffinity chromatography. Proc. Natl. Acad.
    Sci. USA 85, 2454-2458 (1988).

30. Wasserman, R. H., and J. J. Feher. Vitamin
    D-dependent calcium-binding proteins. In: "Calcium
    Binding Proteins and Calcium Function" (R. H.
    Wasserman et al., eds.), pp. 292-302. Elsevier, New
    York (1977).

31. Price, P. A. and S. A. Baukol. 1,25-Dihydroxy-
    vitamin D_3 increases synthesis of the vitamin
    D-dependent bone protein by osteosarcoma cells. J.
    Biol. Chem. 255, 11660-11666 (1980).

32. Prince, C. W. and W. T. Butler. 1,25-Dihydroxy-
    vitamin D_3 regulates the biosynthesis of
    osteopontin, a bone-derived cell attachment protein,
    in clonal osteoblast-like osteosarcoma cells.
    Collagen Rel. Res. 7, 305-313 (1987).

33. Kerner, S. A., R. A. Scott, and J. W. Pike.
    Sequence elements in the human osteocalcin gene
    confer basal activation and inducible response to
    hormonal vitamin D_3. Proc. Natl. Acad. Sci. USA 86,
    4455-4459 (1989).

34. Russell, J., D. Lettieri, and L. M. Sherwood.
    Suppression by $1,25(OH)_2D_3$ of transcription of the
    pre-proparathyroid hormone gene. Endocrinology 119,
    2864-2867 (1986).

35. Chertow, B. S., W. I. Sivitz, N. G. Baranetsky, S.
    A. Clark, A. Waite, and H. F. DeLuca. Cellular
    mechanisms of insulin release. The effects of
    vitamin D deficiency and repletion on rat insulin
    secretion. Endocrinology 113, 1511-1518 (1983).

36. Eisman, J. A. 1,25-Dihydroxyvitamin D_3 receptor and
    role of $1,25-(OH)_2D_3$ in human cancer cells. In:

"Vitamin D" (R. Kumar, ed.), Chapter 14, pp. 365-382. Martinus Nijhoff, Boston, MA (1984).

37. Frampton, R. J., L. J. Suva, J. A. Eisman, D. M. Findlay, G. E. Moore, J. M. Moseley, and T. J. Martin. Presence of 1,25-dihydroxyvitamin D_3 receptors in established human cancer cell lines in culture. Cancer Res. <u>42</u>, 1116-1119 (1982).

38. Eisman, J. A., I. MacIntyre, T. J. Martin, R. J. Frampton, and R. J. B. King. Normal and malignant breast tissue is a target organ for 1,25-(OH)$_2$ vitamin D. Clin. Endocrinol. <u>13</u>, 267-272 (1980).

39. Eisman, J. A., L. J. Suva, and R. J. Frampton. 1,25-Dihydroxyvitamin D_3 receptor and breast cancer. A.N.Z.J. Surg. <u>54</u>, 17-20 (1984).

40. Eisman, J. A., and Frampton, R. J. Effects of 1,25-dihydroxyvitamin D_3 metabolites and analogues on human breast cancer and malignant melanoma cells. In: "Endocrine Control of Bone and Calcium Metabolism" (C. V. Colin, J. T. Potts, Jr., and T. Fujita, eds), pp. 237-238. Elsevier, Amsterdam (1984).

41. Eisman, J. A., D. H. Barkla, and P. J. M. Tutton. Suppression of <u>in vivo</u> growth of human cancer solid tumor xenografts by 1,25-dihydroxyvitamin D_3. Cancer Res. <u>47</u>, 21-25 (1987)

42. Perlman, K., A. Kutner, J. Prahl, C. Smith, M. Inaba, H. K. Schnoes, and H. F. DeLuca. 24-Homologated 1,25-dihydroxyvitamin D_3 compounds: Separation of calcium and cell differentiation activities. Biochemistry, in press (1989).

43. Calverley, M. J. Synthesis of MC 903, a biologically active vitamin D metabolite analogue. Tetrahedron Lett. <u>43</u>, 4609-4619 (1987).

44. Paulson, S. K., H. F. DeLuca, P. H. Stern, and K. Perlman. 24- and 26-Homo-1,25-dihydroxyvitamin D_3 analogs: Effects on <u>in vitro</u> bone resorption. J. Bone Min. Res., in press (1989).

45. Inaba, M. and H. F. DeLuca. Stabilization of
1,25-dihydroxyvitamin D_3 receptor in human leukemia
cell line, HL-60, with diisopropylfluorophosphate.
Biochim. Biophys. Acta <u>1010</u>, 20-27 (1989).

Nutrients and Cancer Prevention K. N. Prasad and F. L. Meyskens, Jr., eds. © 1990 The Humana Press

CONTROL OF HUMAN PRENEOPLASIA WITH RETINOIDS AND OTHER COMPOUNDS. Frank L. Meyskens, Jr., Clinical Cancer Center, University of California, Irvine, Orange, CA 92668

ABSTRACT

The understanding of carcinogenesis and early transformation events in human cancer is limited. Basic laboratory studies in animals suggests that the process of carcinogenesis can be divided into three distinct phases: initiation, promotion, and progression. Surprisingly, limited data suggests that the mechanisms involved in progression may be similar to those accompanying initiation and their control and modulation may be similar. However, we do not know whether progression is analogous to the process by which precancer in humans develops to cancer, but at a heuristic level the assumption seems reasonable. Compared to our understanding of the biologic properties of fully established cancers, the essential features of precancers have been remarkably little studied. The general accessibility of these lesions suggests that detailed investigation of their properties should be possible. An approach to a study of precancers in humans will be presented and the results of biologic and chemical trials updated for cervical dysplasia, oral leukoplakia, cutaneous precancers (dysplastic nevi, actinic keratoses, keratoacanthomas), Barrett's esophagus, and colon polyps.

INTRODUCTION

The best treatment of disease is prevention. Throughout medical history the prevalent overwhelming diseases of mankind have been controlled by the systematic application of prevention and control approaches utilizing basic laboratory discoveries and epidemiologic observations (Table 1). Such strategies are generally appreciated as effective by the medical profession and lay public for infectious diseases and other acute problems but only recently have similar tactics been used for the control of chronic diseases. The most notable early success of prevention approaches for chronic diseases has been the reduction of mortality from cardiovascular events, in large part a result of lowering cholesterol and blood pressure via dietary and pharmacologic means and smoking cessation and not through acute care management, such as high technology intensive care units.

Unknown is whether prevention and control strategies can reduce the mortality from cancer. Certainly, cessation of smoking, control of radon and decreased exposure to asbestis and ultraviolet light should reduce morality from cancer. Our society however has not in general been highly responsive to proscriptive practices when an individual's lifestyle is broached. Active intervention via prescription of chemopreventive compounds may well have wider acceptance, if the agent is simple and non-toxic.

CANCER FORMATION

A great deal has been learned about the process of cancer formation in the last two decades. Starting as early as the 1960's an appreciation of the development of cancer as a multi-step process was occurring. Refinement of our understanding of these events had led to an appreciation of the steps involved and the biologic changes effected (Table 2).

RETINOIDS AND PRENEOPLASIA

Vitamin A and B-Carotene have been of continuing interest to scientists and clinicians since their discovery and early characterization in the 1910's and 1920's. Vitamin A has been found to be essential for normal growth and development, reproductive capacity, fetal organ formation, vision, and bone maintenance as well as necessary but not sufficient for normal epithelial cell differentiation and maturation. The contribution of vitamin A to the latter function was largely ignored until the 1960's when a major interest in the use of the nutrient and synthetic derivatives as antiacne and antikeratizing agents was formulated. The introduction of the 13-cis form of vitamin A acid (Accutane, Isotretinoin) and the aromatic derivative Etretinate has profoundly impacted dermatologic practice.

In the early and mid 1970's interest in the use of retinoids as enhancers of epithelial cell differentiation and inhibitors of proliferation occurred (review, 1). Retinoids were experimentally assigned a function as antipromoters of the carcinogenesis process and until recently were relegated solely to that step. Recently three additional roles for retinoids have been recognized (2-4): immunological modifier, suppressor of progression (preneoplasia to neoplasia conversion), and cytostatic agent for some cancers (e.g. squamous cell cancer of the skin, mycosis fungoides).

Interest in the natural precursor to Vitamin A, B-carotene, has been much more recent, significantly sparked by an extensive review and analysis of the epidemiologic association identified between intake of B-carotene and risk for a number of cancers (5). Subsequently, several primary prevention trials were launched with B-carotene used as the major or sole intervention agent (review, 6). Development of supportive experimental laboratory data for B-carotene has been slow in coming since formulation of the compound is difficult and insolubility in biological media a problem. Nevertheless, in those animal studies which have been well done B-carotene has consistently inhibited tumor growth no matter what the type of carcinogen.

In the last several years a potential role for B-carotene, retinol, and the synthetic retinoids has been proposed for their use in the control and/or suppression of preneoplastic lesions (4). A summary of the supportive scientific data for this approach as well as a listing of ongoing and completed trials is provided in Table 3. Results from studies of the effect of these compounds on the preneoplastic process are just now accumulating (examples 7, 8). Although early in our understanding of the phenomena the following preliminary conclusions seem reasonable and can probably be safely made:

1. Oral leukoplakia is responsive to both retinoids and B-carotene. Long term trials will be needed to determine the optimal dosage and duration of therapy.

2. Bronchial metaplasia may be responsive to synthetic retinoids. Long term benefit in the setting of continued smoke exposure will be difficult to achieve.

3. Cervical dysplasia appears sensitive to retinoids. The result of an ongoing phase III trial of local retinoic acid will be a milestone and highly informative. Determination of the effect of B-carotene on this dysplastic lesion will be important, particularly since long term use of retinoids, which are known teratogens, in reproductively competent women will not be possible or ethical.

4. The measurement of various intermediate markers and their modulation by intervention agents should provide critical information to our understanding of the general and specific biological processes accompanying preneoplastic progression to established malignancy.

The inhibitory and/or suppressive effect of dietary and other compounds on the process of cancer formation seems well-established in animal models. The eventual role of the chemoprevention approach in human populations remains to be determined, but early results, particularly in reversal of preneoplastic disease appears highly promising.

REFERENCES

1. Bollag, W: Vitamin A and retinoids: from nutrition to pharmacology in dermatology and oncology. Lancet I:860-863, 1983.

2. Lotan, R: Immunolomodualtory effects of retionoids. J. Nut. Growth Cancer 3:57-65, 1986.

3. Lippman, S; Kessler, J; Meyskens, FL: Retinoids as preventive and therapeutic anticancer agents. Cancer Treat. Rep. Part I, Vol 71, No. 4:391-405, 1987. Part II, No. 5:493-515, 1987.

4. Meyskens, FL: Clinical trials of retinoids as differentiation inducers. In: The Status of Differentiation Therapy in Cancer, Waxman S, Rossi G.B. and Takaku F. (eds.), Raven Press, New York, PP. 349-359, 1987.

5. Peto, R; Doll, R; Buckley, J.D.; Sporn, M.D.: Can dietary beta-carotene materially reduce human cancer rates. Nature 290: 201-208, 1981.

6. Betram, JS; Kolonel, LN; Meyskens, FL: Rationale and strategies for chemoprevention of cancer in humans. Cancer Res. 47:3012-3031, 1987.

7. Hong, Wk; Endicott, J; Itri, LM, et al: 13-cis-retinoic acid in the treatment of oral leukoplakia. New Eng. J. Med 315:1501-1505, 1986.

8. Gouveia, J; Mathe, G; Hercend, T, et al: Degree of bronchial metaplasia in heavy smokers and its regression after treatment with a retinoid. Lancet 1:710-712, 1982.

9. Meyskens, FL; Gilmartin, E; Alberts DS; Levine NS; Brooks R; Salmon SE; and Surwit EA: Activity of Isotretinoin against squamous cell cancers and preneoplastic lesions. Cancer Treat. Rep. 66:1315-1319, 1982.

10. Levine, N; Miller, RC; and Meyskens, FL: Oral Isotretinoin therapy: Use in a patient with multiple cutaneous squamous cell carcinomas and keratoacanthomas. Arch Derm. 120: 1215-1218, 1984.

11. Alberts, DS; Coulthard, SW; Meyskens, FL: Phase I trial of topically applied trans-retinoic acid in cervical dysplasia-clinical efficacy. Invest. New Drugs 4:241-244, 1986.

12. Graham, V; Surwit, ES; Weiner, S; Meyskens, FL: Phase Ii trial of b-all-trans-retinoic acid for intraepithelial cervical neoplasia delivered via a collagen sponge and cervical cap. West Journal Med. 145:192-195, 1986.

13. Sampliner, RE; Garewal, HS; Meyskens, FL; Steinbronn, KK; Allen, VJ: Phase II trial of isotretinoin in Barrett's Esophagus. In press, 1989.

Table 1

Overwhelming Diseases of Mankind
Stopped by Systematic Application of Basic
Research to Prevention and Control

Disease	Basic Observations		Prevention and Control
	Epidemiologic	Laboratory	
Infections			
* Plague	X	NA	Sewage control
* Childhood diseases	X	X	Vaccine
Nutritional deficiencies			
* Scurvy (vitamin C)	X	NA	Supplementation
* Rickets (vitamin D)	X	X	Supplementation
* Blindness (vitamin A)	X	X	Supplementation
Trauma	X	X	Behavioral, culture
Chronic diseases			
*Cardiovascular	X	X	Diet and drugs (Lowering of cholesterol and blood pressure)
* Cancer	X	X	?

Table 2

Cancer Formation is a Multi-step Process

Stage	Initiation	Promotion	Progression
Biologic Level of Effect	Molecular/ genetic	Biochemical/ epigenetic	Molecular/ genetic
Preventive Strategy	Obviate exposure to carcinogen	antipromotion	Suppression with cytostatic agent, enhancement of differentiation immunological modification

Table 3

Summary of scientific evidence for role of B-carotene, vitamin A (retinol),
and synthetic retinoids in control of human preneoplasias.

Organ	Histology	Strength and Consistency of Evidence *			Ongoing phase I or phase II Trials***		Intermediate Markers ****
		Epidemiologic**	Laboratory	Clinical*	Agent	Location	
Oral	leukoplakia dysplasia	NA	NA	C,A,R	C C+A	U. Arizona, UC Irvine MD Anderson	EGFR
Bronchial	metaplasia	C	A,R	R	R C+A	MD Anderson U. Texas	EGFR, oncogenes
Esophagus • squamous • Barrett's	dysplasia metaplasia	C,A NA	NA no effect	no effect C,A no effect R			EGFR
Colon	polyps	A	NA	NA	C^a	Dartmouth	crypt labelling
Skin • actinic • dysplastic	hyperplasia melanocytic nevi	NA NA	A,R R	A,R R,?	C	Tanzania	oncogenes
Cervix	dysplasia	C,A	A,R	R	R	U. Arizona	HPV subtypes
Breast	hyperplasia	NA	R	NA	R^c	Milan	ER, PR receptors

Legend to Table 3 on next page

FIGURE 3 LEGEND

*   Symbols - C, B-carotene; A, retinol; R,
synthetic retinoids; NA -   no   available
data.

**   Epidemiologic/Clinical - symbol, strong
and/or consistent   associations.

*** Listed here are only those trials which
have regression of a preneoplasia an endpoint
or in which inhibition of preneoplastic
progression is probably occurring. There are
many other primary prevention trials using
these compounds as the intervention agent
(see 6).

**** Intermediate markers - generic markers
include measurement of changes in histology,
karyotype ploidy, and micronuclei. Markers
more specific to the organisms listed are shown
in the Table.

    Esophagus - squamous in a preliminary
trial no suppression of esophagitis was seen;
Barrett's, a phase II trial of 13 cis retinoic
acid was negative.

    Dysplastic nevi - local application of
retinoic acid consistently reversed dysplastic
nevi, but oral administration of 13 cis
retinoic acid had no effect.

a   B-carotene is used in conjunction with
vitamin C + vitamin E.

b   The endpoint is regression of skin changes
in albinos.

c   The endpoint is appearance of breast
cancer in contralateral breast of women with
early stage breast cancer.

CAROTENOIDS IN CANCER CHEMOPREVENTION AND SYNERGISM WITH RETINOL IN MASTALGIA TREATMENT

Leonida Santamaria, Amalia Bianchi Santamaria*, and Massimo dell'Orti

Camillo Golgi Institute of General Pathology, Centro Tumori; *Institute of Pharmacology II - University of Pavia, 27100 Pavia - Italy.

ABSTRACT

In 1980 beta-carotene (BC) and canthaxanthin (CX), carotenoids with and without pro-vitamin A activity, respectively, supplemented to female Swiss albino mice prevented at high extent benzo(a)pyrene (BP) - induced skin carcinogenesis in the dark and its photo-enhancement by UV (300-400 nm). The same experimental procedure adapted to 8-methoxypsoralen (8-MOP) photoinduction of breast carcinoma in mice (in 1984), and to gastric carcinogenesis induced by N-Methyl-N'-N-Nitrosoguanidine (MMNG) in rats (in 1985) showed the same antitumorigenic activity. These data suggested a rationale for human interventions to prevent, with carotenoid supplementation, second primary malignancies, when the first one is radically treated (surgery ± chemo/radiotherapy) in such organs as the lung, urinary bladder, breast, stomach, and colon-rectum. A first clinical case-report of 15 cases of this type of chemoprevention attempted during 1980-1989, produced results that, though certainly preliminary, are extremely encouraging as regards current intervention with randomized methods. None of the 15 cases recruited, on the basis of radical nature of treatment and patient adherence, showed any recurrence beyond their expected disease-free intervals. Recently, twenty five women, 23-41 year old, suffering from cyclical mastalgia associated or otherwise with benign breast disease (BBD) were treated with daily 20 mg BC supplementation and intermittent administration of retinol (retinyl palmitate) 300,000 IU per day for seven days before each menstrual period. After six months' treatment, the results revealed marked reduction in breast pain, and sometimes recovery, in 23-41 year old women with no toxic side effects, but healthy look because of a slight tanning of the skin. No such advantages in 5 older women with non-cyclical mastalgia treated as above were found. These data demonstrated a therapeutic synergism between BC and retinol, provided the above treatment scheme.

Key words: carotenoids/cancer chemoprevention/ breast pain disease/beta-carotene + retinol treatment.

BASIC ANIMAL EXPERIMENTS AND HUMAN INTERVENTIONS (LS, ABS)

The experimental demonstration of carotenoid antitumorigenesis properties preceded the epidemiological data referring to the inverse association between carotenoid intake or beta-carotene blood levels and cancer risk (1). Indeed, the latter was first reported in 1981, whereas, in 1980, beta-carotene (BC) and canthaxantin (CX), two carotenoids respectively with and without pro-vitamin A activity were found to prevent both (BP)-induced skin carcinogenesis in the dark and BP photocarcinogenic enhancement (BP-PCE) (UV 300-400 nm), when given as a diet supplement to female Swiss albino mice. The BP-PCE, apparently due to oxygen radicals generated by BP photodynamic action, was completely checked by BC or CX supplementation (2). In the same year, both carotenoids were found to delay UVB skin cancer and to prevent to a certain extent DMBA ± UVB carcinogenesis in hairless mice (3). In 1981, BC was found to be prophylactic and therapeutic against transplanted tumours (4).

The experimental procedure as in BP carcinogenesis adapted to 8-MOP photoinduction of mammary carcinoma in mice demonstrated, in 1984, the same antitumorigenic effect (up to 65%) by BC and CX (5). In this connection, it is worth reporting that 8-MOP photomutagenesis on *S. typhimurium* occurs through two steps: an anoxic mutagenic effect (an oxygen-independent DNA-8-MOP photoadduct) which is heavily enhanced by the presence of air, namely by an *in situ* generation of oxygen radicals, primarily singlet oxygen (6). Thus, both indirect BP and 8-MOP photocarcinogenesis appeared to be checked by carotenoids, likely because of an impairment of the ultimate carcinogen formation by scavenging or quenching oxygen radicals at the initiation and promotion phases.

In 1985, also the direct gastric carcinogenesis induced by MNNG in rats was prevented up to 70% by BC or CX diet supplementation. This anticarcinogenesis, however, occured at the progression phase (7). The anticarcinogenicity at the progression phase was likely due to scavenging of free radicals produced by gastric phlogosis. In fact, in the Ames' test carotenoids did not exert protective effect against MNNG direct mutagenesis, as expected (8). Later, in 1987, preventive effect of BC was found also against dimethyhydrazine (DMH) induced colon cancer in mice (9).

TABLE I BASIC REFERENCES OF CAROTENOID EFFECTS ON EXPERIMENTAL INDIRECT AND DIRECT CARCINOGENESES AND TUMOR TRANSPLANTATION

YEAR	AUTHOR	CAROTENOIDS		CARCINOGENIC MODEL	EFFECT	ASSUMED MECHANISM
		Type	Dosage (*)			
1973	DOROGOKUPLA A G ET AL (46)	RED CARROTS IN DIET	UNLIMITED	SKIN CANCER BY DMA IN MICE AND RATS (indirect)	PROTECTION DELAY	VITAMIN A
1977	EPSTEIN J (47)	BETA-CAROTENE I P	250 mg/Kg b w 3 TIMES/WEEK (100 mg/Kg b w /DAY)	UVB SKIN CANCER IN HAIRLESS MICE (indirect)	DELAY	UNDETERMINED
1980	MATHEWS - ROTH M M (3)	BETA-CAROTENE CANTHAXANTHIN P.O.	6680 mg/Kg b w /DAY idem	UV-B SKIN CANCER SKIN CANCER BY DMBA ± CROTON OIL OR ± UV-B IN HAIRLESS MICE (indirect)	DELAY PREVENTION	ANTIOXIDANT
1980	SANTAMARIA L ET AL (2)	BETA-CAROTENE (**) CANTHAXANTHIN supplemental P O	100 mg/Kg b w /DAY (DIETARY) + 100 mg/Kg b w /TWICE A WEEK (GAVAGE)	SKIN CARCINOGENESIS BY BP ± UVA IN MICE (indirect)	100% PREVENTION OF PCE 60% TOTAL	ANTIOXIDANT ACTING AT THE INITIATION STAGE
1980	SANTAMARIA L ET AL (2)	Idem	idem	UVA LONG TERM SKIN PHOTOCARCINOGENESIS IN MICE (indirect)	100% PREVENTION	ANTIOXIDANT
1981	SEIFTER R ET AL (4)	BETA-CAROTENE P O	1.8 mg/Kg b w /DAY	ADENO-CARCINOMA C3HBA IN MICE (transplantation)	DELAY/PREVENTION REGRESSION	VITAMIN A + IMMUNOSTIMUL.
1982	SEIFTER R ET AL (48)	BETA-CAROTENE P O	2.4 mg/Kg b w /DAY	M.Mu SV IN MICE (transplantation)	DELAY/PREVENTION/ > REGRESSION	VITAMIN A + IMMUNOSTIMUL.
1984	SANTAMARIA L ET AL (5)	BETA-CAROTENE CANTHAXANTIN SUPPLEMENTAL P O	Idem as above (1980)	BREAST PHOTO-CARCINOGENSIS BY 8-MOP (PUVA) IN MICE (indirect)	60% PREVENTION	ANTIOXIDANT ACTING AT THE PROMOTION STAGE
1985	SANTAMARIA L ET AL (6)	Idem	50 mg/Kg b w /DAY DIETARY + 100 mg/Kg b w /3 TIMES A WEEK (GAVAGE)	MULTIPHASIC GASTRIC CARCINOGENESIS BY MNNG IN RATS (direct)	BLOCKAGE OF PROGRESSION	ANTIOXIDANT ACTING AT THE PROGRESSION STAGE
1987	TEMPLE N J AND BASU T (32)	BETA-CAROTENE	4 mg/Kg b w /DAY	COLON CANCER BY DMH IN MICE (indirect)	50% ADENOMA 100% ADENOCARCINOM/ PREVENTION	ANTIOXIDANT + IMMUNOSTIMUL.

(*) The dosage of carotenoids was computed assuming that mice weighing 25 g eat about 5 g of pellets/day, whereas rats weighing about 250 g eat about 25 g of pellets/day

(**) All supplementaion, according to Santamaria et al started one month before carcinogenic treatments and continued throughout the experiments

These experimental findings allowed us to build up a rationale to prevent with carotenoid supplementation the onset of second primary malignancies in humans, when the first one is radically treated (surgery ± chemo/radiotherapy). This type of prevention was envisaged in such organs as the lung, the urinary bladder cancers, breast, stomach, and colon-rectum (7). At present, two controlled clinical trials are in progress to prevent recurrencies of lung and urinary bladder after radical excision. A pioneering first clinical case report of this type of chemoprevention was attempted, since 1980 in Pavia, when the very first clear-cut evidence of the antitumorigenesis properties of carotenoids was demonstrated. This produced an overall picture of results (at present 15 cases) that, though certainly preliminary, is extremely encouraging as regards the above current human intervention with randomized methods (10).

All these experimental findings together with those by others of basic significance, and human intervention data are reported here (Table I and II) in a comprehensive presentation that highlights their current state of development and prospects.

Table I gives the basic references of carotenoid effects on experimental indirect and direct carcinogeneses and tumor transplantation, computing the dosage of supplemented carotenoids and referring the type of the effect along with the assumed mechanism of action. Table I also clarifies that the antitumorigenic effect of carotenoid is independent of the pro-vitamin activity of beta-carotene since CX (with no pro-vitamin A activity) is antitumorigenic as well. The dosage of carotenoids employed in the different experiments is quite high (50-150 mg/Kg b.w./day), but it may be also relatively low (1.8 - 4 mg/Kg b.w./day), thus indicating the efficacy of the drug. In this connection, we may recall that BC up to the very high dosage of 1000 mg/Kg b.w./day is well tolerated by animals (14). We may also point out that supplementations according to Santamaria *et al.* started one month before carcinogenic treatments to produce a tissue "saturation" effect and continued throughout the experiments. The major fact in almost all this experimental work is that the mechanism of action of this antitumorigenic activity was due to the antioxidant property of carotenoids rather than to vitamin A production *in vivo*. Antioxidant property was likely able to inhibit the formation of the ultimate carcinogen (as in the indirect agents) and/or the endogenous synthesis of some carcinogens (as in direct agents, like nitrosoamine). In the first case the antitumorigenesis is exerted at the level of initiation (see BP skin carcinogenesis) or promotion (see 8-MOP breast cancer); in the second case, this action is shown at the progression phase. Nevertheless, the immunostimulating activity of this class of natural compounds, according to Seifter et al. (4,13) and Temple and Basu (9), certainly plays an important role. In this connection, it is worth reminding that the antioxidant activity counteracts the deterioration of the immune system induced by the radical reactions, thus stimulating the normal functions of T-lymphocytes (15).

As a support to the above animal experiments and their mechanisms of action, it is worth referring to *in vitro* findings as follows. Both BC and CX completely prevented the oxygen dependent step of photomutagenesis induced by 8-MOP + UVA in *Salmonella typhimurium* TA 102 (6, 8). Both BC and CX inhibited methycholantrene and X-ray induced neoplastic transformation of C3H/10T1 mouse fibroblast cultures; interestingly, in this model BC was more active, but with no conversion to retinol (27). Both BC and CX produced morphological differentiation in murine B 16 melanoma cell cultures, whereas retinol and buthylhydroxyanisole (BHA) produced in the model growth inhibition with no differentiation (28)

As far as human intervention (Tab. II) is concerned, it should be pointed out that our protocols for randomized trials to prevent second primary malignancies in humans (16), submitted for support as earlier as in 1983-86 to Italy and USA Government agencies, have been preceded independently by the following pioneering investigation.

The clear-cut results published in Pavia in 1980 on the antitumorigenesis of BC and CX, as demonstrated with regard to skin cancer induced by BP (2) stimulated immediate interest among GPs in a medical environment traditionally sensitive to scientific breakthroughs. This interest was particularly acute in one case, a classic story of a highly successful, highly professional middle-aged M.D. who decided to try out these findings on his family, himself and a few of his patients, naturally following ethical rules most scrupulously.

At that time, only experimental data provided a convincing theory as regards promising developments in the field of chemoprevention. In this connection, the authors were quite clear that oxygen radicals played a fundamental role in carcinogenicity whenever the balance in endogenous antioxidant systems is somehow impaired, especially by phlogistic processes which generate large amounts of active oxygen-excited species. This led the colleague mentioned above to co-operate actively in clinical attempts to prevent recurrences after radical treatment of epithelial tumours. He came to agree with our theory that complete removal of a malignancy with no lymph node involvement or even with the most accurate lymphadenectomy cannot reverse the already initiated state of all the remaining epithelial tissue of a particular anatomical

Table IIa. Clinical case report (1980-89). Cancer chemoprevention with BC (40%) + CX (60%) association (40 mg/day) against cancer recurrence after radical surgery ± chemo-radiotherapy (breast, lung, urinary bladder, large bowel, head and neck).

Patient	Sex	Age	Neoplasm surgery date	Chemotherapy and/or radio-therapy	Chemoprevention Initial date	Recurrences I II (up to 9/89)	Expected disease-free Interval
R.L.	F	47 (1980)	Breast ductal Infilt. Ca T2N0M0 Mastectomy 7/80	-	1980	- -	6/10
A.S.	F	57 (1980)	Breast mucoid Ca T2N1(5/5)M0 Mastectomy 3/80	1980 CMF 12 cycles	3/81; interrupted for 6 months In 1985 for car crash	- -	3/5 years
A.C.	M	60 (1985)	Lung epidermoid Ca right medium lobe T3N0 Lobectomy 7/85 II ep. Ca left upper lobe T3N0 Lobectomy 7/86	-	7/86	- -	1 year
C.B.	M	58 (1987)	Lung epidermoid Ca right lower lobe T3N0M0 Bilobectomy 8/87	Radiotherapy	9/87	- -	6 Mo/1 year
G.C.	M	58 (1987)	Lung adenoca. medium right lobe T3N0M0 G3 Pneumectomy Dx 10/87	-	3/88	- -	1 year
L.B.	M	60 (1983)	Urinary bladder Trans cell Ca G2 TUR 7/83	-	1985; interrupted 7-12/85 for car crash*	1985 TUR -	6 Mo./2 years
G.L.	M	63 (1986)	Urinary bladder Trans cell Ca G2 TUR 8/86	-	8/86	- -	6 Mo./2 years

During this period urinary bladder catheterism caused cystitis and subsequently cancer recurrence
After Santamaria et al. 1988, adapted and updated

Table IIb. Clinical case report (1980-89). Cancer chemoprevention with BC (40%) + CX (60%) association (40 mg/day) against cancer recurrence after radical surgery ± chemo- radiotherapy (breast, lung, urinary bladder, large bowel, head and neck).

Patient	Sex	Age	Neoplasm surgery date	Chemotherapy and/or radio-therapy	Chemoprevention Initial date	Recurrences I II (up to 9/89)	Expected disease-free interval
F.A.	M	49 (1986)	Urinary bladder Trans cell Ca G2 TUR 8/86	-	8/1986	- -	6 Mo./2 years
B.A.	M	60 (1984)	Urinary bladder Trans cell Ca G2 TUR 8/86	-	8/1986	- -	6 Mo./2 years
P.G.	F	60 (1984)	Urinary bladder Trans cell Ca G1 TUR 7/84	Adriblastin 20 mg/100 ml bladder washing 24 times/1 year	2/84 for one year then only vegetables and fruit enriched diet	- -	6 Mo./2 years
B.C.	M	59 (1984)	Larynx epid. Ca G1 T1aN0M0 Partial laryngectomy 1/84	-	2/1984	- -	2 years
L.P.	M	63 (1985)	Larynx epid. Ca G1 T1bN0M0 Partial laryngect. 6/85	-	7/1985	- -	2 years
A.C.	F	54 (1983)	Rhinopharynx undiff. Ca T2N2M0 1/83 lymphnode biopsy	radiotherapy 63+10 Gy 3/6/83	4/1983 plus vegetables and fruit enriched diet	- -	6 Mo./1 years
A.S.	F	37 (1982)	Colon adenocarcinoma T2N1(2/17)M0 5/1982	-	7/1982	- -	5 years
G.B.	F	60 (1988)	Colon-rectum adenoca. T3N+M+ (omentum) Resection 12/88	5-FU - folinic acid 5 cycles	12/1988	- -	3/6 Mo.

After Santamaria et al., 1988, adapted and updated

compartment. Any cells in this tissue were liable to undergo gene derepression by oxidation damage, thus giving rise to the expression of what is called a "second primary malignancy". Accordingly, the "saturation" dosage of carotenoids at the beginning of the treatment (as proposed elsewhere (16), i.e. 80 mg per day of carotenoids for 3 weeks) followed by a daily supplementation of 40 mg was adopted. The pharmaceutical preparation available in any pharmacy in nearby Switzerland or France, was a capsule containing 20 mg each of BC (40%) and CX (60%). This preparation originally made for the treatment of solar dermatosis was helpful in "sugaring the pill" i.e. in persuading patients to adhere to the treatment in that they found it produced a healthy look through the skin-tanning effect of carotenoids, especially CX. This clinical attempt was greatly encouraged by the fact, already known at that time, that BC was devoid of any toxicity (14). Later, it was reported that CX could store itself in the retina, with no functional impairment whatsoever, in about 20% of patients treated with high doses of BC + CX. (17)

A survey in 1988 of these clinical trials, begun 8 years ahead with a pioneering and somewhat brutal attempt, showed an apparent limitation as far as the number of cases (eleven) was concerned, but provided highly significant results owing to the strong evidence of the total preventive effects after radical treatment (surgery ± chemo- and/or radiotherapy) well beyond the expected disease-free intervals in pathologies affecting four different compartments. This study was, therefore, considered suitable for publication (10). Here the main features are reported in Table II even though no controls with placebos are envisaged. The only assessable parameter is the expected disease-free interval. In updating this Table II four more cases were added.

These findings demonstrated that supplemental BC and CX in association prevented of recurrences in *all* of the cases selected on the basis of radical tumour excision and adherence to treatment. One case (A.S.,F) had serious lymphnode involvement (5/5) and underwent high dosage chemotherapy (CMF) with an expectation of a 3 year disease-free interval. Another case (P.G.,F.) also had chemotherapy but at a very low local dosage. The A.C., M case is at present free from disease even though carotenoid supplementation was started after two subsequent lung lobectomies for two epidermoid cancers T3N0 (the second occurring 1 year after the first lobectomy). The L.B., M case is particularly significant: the patient suffering from superficial urinary bladder carcinoma G2, started chemoprevention soon after TUR in 1983, which was interrupted after two years for six months, because of a spine traumatic fracture (due to a car crash). During this period he underwent urinary bladder catheterism with concurrent cystitis. Two months later he suffered a tumour recurrence (trans. cell ca. G1), which was removed by TUR. This clearly confirmed the theoretical expectation that active oxygen radicals generated by a phlogistic process can trigger the expression of a second primary cancer. The most surprising, if not unexpected data relate to the A.C., M and A.C., F cases which had a severe prognosis. The G.B., F case was hopeless, nevertheless she was given carotenoids mostly for psychological relief. The surprising clinical results of this case are presently supported by the normalization of both CICA and CEA tumor marker levels. The patients suffering from lung, urinary bladder and head and neck cancers used to be heavy smokers. Apart from one (P.G.,F.) they have succeeded in abstaining from smoking.

The convincing results of this first clinical case report appeared to be confirmed by the history of a case personally reported to the authors by Correa in 1988. Five and a half years ahead a middle-aged patient underwent a kidney plus ureter removal due to three carcinomas in the calyx. Soon after surgery he adhered to BC supplementation, which would seem to explain his present good health. But the most interesting fact was that soon after surgery, dysplasias of bladder mucosa were detected, which completely disappeared after only two months. Similar to this case is that listed as C.B., M; soon after surgery, the patient adhered to BC + CX supplementation, he suffered cytological severe dysplasia, as observed in bronchial brushing, up to six months, afterwards it disappeared.

Last but not least, it should be noted that *all* the patients selected for our tentative no-recurrence cancer chemoprevention protocol are reported above, even those, such as A.C., M, A.C., and G.B., F, initially considered hopeless. At present, all fifteen cases display KB performance statuses equal to 100. They all work normally and no one suffered from side effects, not even CX deposit in the retina (17). There is no doubt that the overall picture emerging from these results, though certainly preliminary, is extremely encouraging as regards the current human interventions with randomized methods under the supervision of the Centro Tumori of the University of Pavia.

SYNERGISTIC THERAPEUTIC ACTIVITY OF BC AND RETINOL, AS FIRST OBSERVED IN THE TREATMENT OF MASTALGIA (LS, ABS, MDO)

Vitamin A was first used in the treatment of premenopausal patients with fibrocystic disease of the breast by Brocq et al. in 1956 (18) at a daily dose of 50,000 IU for 2 months. This led to symptomatic improvements consisting of a reduction in pain and some regression of breast masses.

Subsequently, increased knowledge regarding correlations between mammary trophic hormones (oestradiol, progesterone, testosterone, prolactin) and mastalgia associated or otherwise with benign breast disease (BBD) led to the current use of bromocriptine, danazol, dihydroprogesterone, norethisterone, phytohormone, etc. as more rational tools in the therapy of the above syndrome (19).

Nevertheless, the potential use of retinoids for chemoprevention of experimental breast carcinomas (20) restored interest in vitamin A and mastalgia using preparations of vitamin A both with and without vitamin E. Recently, vitamin A (all-*trans*-retinol) was administered at daily doses of 150,000 IU for 3 months in 12 high-risk patients with BBD, producing very encouraging results both with regard to complete or partial responses and pain reduction. But, in the majority of cases, these results were associated with toxic effects sometimes so severe that the treatment had to be discontinued or interrupted (21).

When we observed that carotenoids BC or CX greatly inhibit the incidence of breast cancer induced in female Swiss albino mice by 8-methoxypsoralen plus UVA light (320-400nm) (PUVA) (7), we thought that mastalgia might possibly be treated with BC as a vitamin A-precursor and as an antioxidant agent, the latter being a very useful tool in the phlogistic component of the syndrome. This approach proved to be unsuccessful. On the other hand, BC oral supplementation *plus* intermittent retinol administration produced the same favorable responses as mentioned above, but with no toxic side effects after 6 months' treatment (24). These results are reported and discussed below.

METHODS

Patient recruitment.
Patients were admitted to this study when the following clinical features were met: premenopausal, cyclical mastalgia with moderate or severe pain described with the terms "heaviness" and "tender to touch", present for at least 7 days before each menstrual period; often bilateral and not responsive to mild analgesics; with palpable but not measurable "normal" breast nodularity. These clinical features were those of the "cyclical pattern" according to the Cardiff system (22). Patients with the "non-cyclical pattern" in the Cardiff system, were also admitted. The patients with both "cyclical and non-cyclical patterns" admitted to the study had no signs other than those of BBD.

Clinical tests and evaluation criteria.

Prior to treatment, patients gave a complete history, and underwent physical examination, contact thermography (CT) of both breasts, complete blood counts (CBC), and liver function tests (LFT). CT, CBC, and LFT were repeated monthly; echotomography and mammography were carried out only as necessary. CT was adopted routinely, provided the evaluation was made by the same expert according to the Th_{1-5} classification (23) as follows: Th_1 = normal (symmetric hypervascularity in all quadrants); Th_2 = benign breast disease (marked asymmetric hypervascularity); Th_3 = suspicious lesions (vascular star or vascular amputation or vascular confluence); Th_4 = very suspicious lesions (vascular spot higher than 2° C); Th_5 = cancer (hot area spread all over a mammary quadrant). In this respect, patients admitted to this study had CT with Th_1 or Th_2 patterns only. All these tests made it possible to classify associated BBD as nodular, cystic or other dysplasias with the following grades: mild, moderate, severe, and as fibrocystic mastopathy (FCM). Pain and toxicity (headache, skin and lip dryness, nausea, dizziness, alopecia, etc..) were graded as follows: 0 = none; 1 = mild; 2 = moderate; 3 = severe. The subjective responses reported as complete or partial were defined respectively as a total disappearance of pain or a decrease in breast pain by at least one grade. The objective responses were defined as complete or partial with reference to all measurable or assessable lesions.

Beta-carotene supplementation associated with intermittent vitamin A administration.

Patients were treated with BC capsules (20 mg each) using Roche BC beadlets, containing BC in 10% within appropriate excipient, prepared so as to have 20 mg of active compound in a single capsule. The daily dosage of BC was 20 mg. This treatment was interrupted or otherwise during the administration of vitamin A. The latter in the form of palmitate ester (Arovit, Roche) was administered in pills at a dosage of 100,000 IU 3 times per day (300,000 IU) starting 7 days before each menstrual period and continuing for 7 days for each cycle. In this respect, it is recalled that 1 IU of retinol is equal to 0.30 µg; therefore 300,000 IU = 90 mg. The scheme of this therapeutical design is reported in Fig. 1.

RESULTS

Premenopausal women were recruited in this study according to the above admission criteria. Table III lists 25 patients in the 23-41 year age group, who were suffering from cyclical mastalgia and 5 older patients suffering from non-cyclical mastalgia. Combined BC and intermittent vitamin A supplementation induced a marked response in breast pain reducing or eliminating it after six months in the 23-41 year-old patients (average age 35). The results were less evident or absent in premenopausal patients over 41 years. These responses in pain degree as expressed in Fig. 2 made it possible to identify two sub-groups of patients according to initial pain degree 3 or 2 at the beginning. The reduction in pain in both sub-groups of the 23-41 year-old patients after

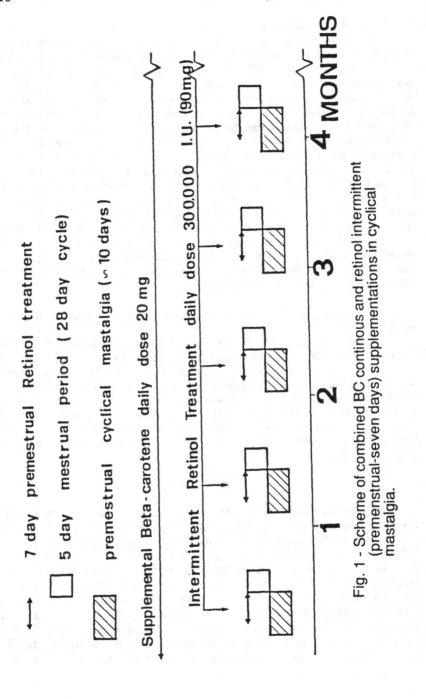

Fig. 1 - Scheme of combined BC continous and retinol intermittent (premenstrual-seven days) supplementations in cyclical mastalgia.

Table III. Characteristics of patients with mastodynia and effect of beta-carotene supplementation plus intermittent retinol administration

Patient No.	Age	Liver function initial & after 6mo.	Thermography initial R	initial L	after 6 mo. R	after 6 mo. L	Clinical examination initial & after 6 mo.	Echotomography	Mammography	Cyclical m. pain initial	Cyclical m. pain after 6 mo.	Side effects
1	23	normal	Th2	Th2	Th2	Th2	mild dy	mild dy		3	2	0
2	23	normal	Th1	Th1	Th1	Th1	moderate FCM (dy)			2	1	0
3	27	normal	Th2	Th2	Th1	Th1	mild dy			2	1	0
4	29	normal	Th2	Th2	Th1	Th1	mild dy	mild dy		3	1	0
5	29	normal	Th1	Th1	Th1	Th1	mild dy	cy dy		2	0	0
6	29	normal	Th2	Th2	Th1	Th1	FCM			2	1	0
7	30	normal	Th2	Th2	Th1	Th1	FCM	cy dy		2	2	0
8	31	normal	Th1	Th2	Th1	Th1	mild dy	mild FCM		3	1	0
9	35	normal	Th2-3	Th1	Th1	Th1	diffuse dy			2	1	0
10	35	normal	Th1	Th2	Th1	Th1	mild dy			2	1	0
11	37	normal	Th2	Th2	Th1	Th1	mild dy			2	2	0
12	39	normal	Th1	Th1	Th2	Th2	moderate FCM	mild dy	mild cy dy	3	2	0
13	39	normal	Th1	Th1	Th1	Th1	mild dy		mild dy	3	2	0
14	40	normal	Th2	Th2	Th2	Th2	FCM		FCM	3	2	0
15	40	normal	Th1	Th1	Th2	Th2	mild dy			2	1	0
16	41	normal	Th1	Th1	Th2	Th2	moderate dy			3	2	0
17	40	normal	Th2	Th2	Th1	Th1	moderate dy	FCM	fibrocystic dy	3	2	0
18	39	normal	Th1-2	Th1	Th1	Th1	mild dy	severe dy	dy	3	2	0
19	37	normal	Th1	Th2	Th2	Th2	mild dy	FCM	mild cy dy	2	1	0
20	39	normal	Th1	Th1	Th1	Th1	FCM	moderate dy		2	0	0
21	40	normal	Th2	Th2	Th1	Th1	mild dy			3	1	0
22	35	normal	Th1	Th1	Th2	Th1	mild dy			2	2	0
23	38	normal	Th1	Th1	Th1	Th1						0
24	34	normal	Th3	Th2	Th1	Th1						0
25		normal	Th2	Th2	Th2	Th2						0

Patient No.	Age	Liver function initial & after 6mo.	Thermography initial R	initial L	after 6 mo. R	after 6 mo. L	Clinical examination initial & after 6 mo.	Echotomography	Mammography	Non cyclical m. pain initial	Non cyclical m. pain after 6 mo.	Side effects
26	46	normal	Th2	Th2	Th2	Th2	mild dy		severe dy	3	3	0
27	47	normal	Th2	Th2	Th1	Th1	severe dy		mild dy	2	2	0
28	44	normal	Th2	Th2	Th1	Th1	mild dy		severe dy	2	2	0
29	45	normal	Th3	Th2	Th2	Th2	moderate dy		dy	3	3	0
30	45	normal	Th2	Th2	Th2	Th2	mild dy	FCM		3	3	0

dy = nodular dysplasia
cy = cystic
FCM = fibrocystic mastopathy

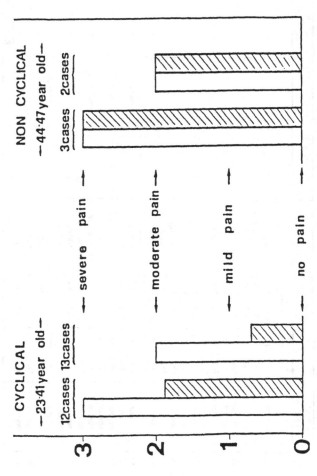

Fig. 2 - Responses in pain reduction after 6 month-treatment (BC + Retinol supplementation) in cyclical and non-cyclical mastalgia

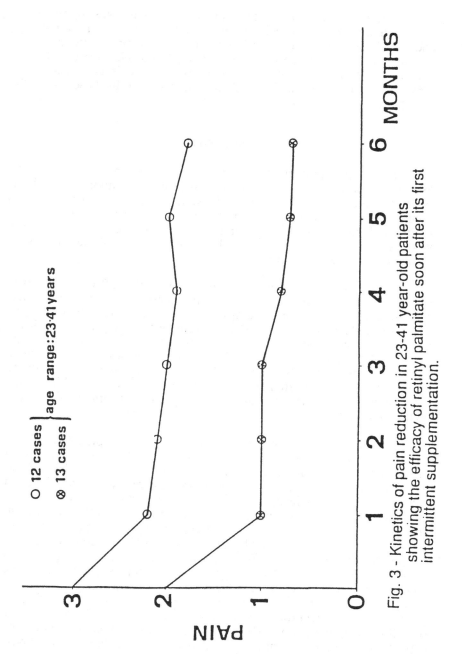

Fig. 3 - Kinetics of pain reduction in 23-41 year-old patients showing the efficacy of retinyl palmitate soon after its first intermittent supplementation.

one month was almost one degree, and after 6 months was slightly more, as shown in Fig. 3. The echotomography and mammography patterns, and physical examinations after six months' therapy were generally unchanged, but in some cases CT had improved. No increase in liver enzymes was observed. None of the toxic side effects, listed in the previous section, arose in any of the patients, even in those where the therapy was unsuccessful.

DISCUSSION

The current protocol for vitamin-A-alone treatment for mastalgia associated, or otherwise, with BBD, used in our Tumor Center is as follows: 300,000 IU daily for 30 days, interruption for 10 days, and vitamin A again for 30 days; this treatment over a total 70 days, was interrupted and repeated 2 or 3 times per year, unless toxic side effects were severe. The latter developed in the majority of the cases with different signs and in different degrees.

A first attempt to replace vitamin A with BC (20 mg per day) to obtain non toxic responses proved unsuccessful, as reported above. Subsequently, the combined therapy was tried with favourable responses. The most salient facts to consider in the above therapy are as follows: retinol produced positive responses in mastalgia whereas BC alone did not, although it is a provitamin-A substance and an anti-tumorigenic agent. This implies that vitamin A must be essential in maintaining normal epithelial differentiation, as it occurs when inhibiting the development of a variety of chemically-induced epithelial tumors including breast carcinomas in experimental animals (20).

The results of the combined treatment of BC plus intermittent retinol supplementation confirmed the efficacy of the therapeutic impact of vitamin A on the mastalgia syndrome and showed, for the first time to our knowledge, therapeutic association apparently synergistic in mechanism (24). Indeed, retinyl-palmitate's action in reducing or eliminating pain was evident soon after the first intermittent treatment, and was apparently maintained or enhanced by BC supplementation. Hence, the mechanism exerted by BC supplementation at low doses of 20 mg per day is presumably different from the mechanism arising from its provitamin-A property. This suggests that what is involved is the powerful antioxidant activity of BC in that this, most likely, is efficient in cutting down the oxygen radicals produced by the phlogistic component of the syndrome. It may also be the case that the better water solubility of retinyl palmitate plays a role since it may cross the oedema barrier faster than BC. Furthermore, it should be considered also the possible implication in the above treatment of the immune stimulating activity of BC (4,25). When tackling the above problem, it should be clear that BC functions as an antioxidant *in vivo*, whereas, under the same experimental conditions, retinol does not protect against oxygen radical damage (26), according to what years ago was experimentally demonstrated in cancer chemoprevention (2,7).

Apart from this difficulty in mechanism interpretation, the main advantage to be highlighted in these results after six months' treatment is the absence of undesirable side effects, except for a slight skin tanning giving, incidentally, a healthy look to the patients. Furthermore, the 23-41 year old patients with cyclical mastalgia in our limited survey may benefit from uninterrupted relief from pain and sometimes even total elimination of pain in contrast to the results obtained when the above vitamin-A-alone protocol was applied in our Tumor Center.

ACKNOWLEDGEMENTS

This work was supported by the Ministero della Sanità, Roma, Direzione Generale Servizi Medicina Sociale, Div.IV, contract N. 5OO.4/ RSC/57.3/T/1719, 1986 and 500/4/RSC/57.3/T/2128, 1987. The Ministero della Pubblica Istruzione, Roma, Direzione Generale Istruzione Universitaria, is acknowledged for providing research facilities with a special contribution (1987). It was also partially supported by the Lombardy Regional Government (1986). Hoffmann-La Roche Inc., Basel is acknowledged for providing the carotenoids. Dr. A. P. Baldry, is acknowledged for revising the English text.

REFERENCES

1) Shekelle, R.B., Lepper, M., Liu, S., Maliza, C., Raymor, W.J., and Rossof, A.H. Dietary vitamin A and risk of cancer in the Western Electric Study. The Lancet, November 28, 1981, 1185-1190.
2) Santamaria, L., Bianchi, A., Arnaboldi, A., and Andreoni, L. Prevention of the benzo(a)pyrene photocarcinogenic effect by beta-carotene and canthaxanthine. Preliminary study. Boll. Chim. Farm., 119: 745-748, 1980.
3) Mathews-Roth, M.M. Carotenoid pigments as antitumor agents. In: Nelson J.D. and Grassi, C. (Eds.) "Current Chemotherapy and Infectious Disease". The American Society for Microbiology, Washington, DC, pp. 1503-1505, 1980.

4) Seifter, E., Rettura, G. Stratford, F. and Levinson, S.M. C3HBA tumor prevention and treatment with beta-carotene. Fed. Proc. 40: 652-656, 1981.

5) Santamaria, L., Bianchi, A., Andreoni, L., Santagati, Arnaboldi, A.G., and Bermond, P. 8-Methoxypsoralen photocarcinogenesis and its preventiom by dietary carotenoids. Preliminary results. Med. Biol. Env., 12 (1): 533-537, 1984.

6) Santamaria, L., Bianchi, L., Bianchi, A., Pizzala, R., Santagati, G., and Bermond, P. Photomutagenicity by 8-methoxypsoralen with and without singlet oxygen involvement and its prevention by beta-carotene. Relevance to the mechanism of 8-MOP photocarcinogenesis and to PUVA application. Med. Biol Env., 12 (1): 541-549, 1984.

7) Santamaria, L., Bianchi, A., Arnaboldi, A., Andreoni, L., Santagati, G., Ravetto, C., Bianchi, L., Pizzala, R., and Bermond, P. Supplemental carotenoids prevent skin cancer by benzo(a)pyrene, breast cancer by PUVA, and gastric cancer by MNNG. Relevance in human chemoprevention. In: Meyskens, F.L., and Prasad, K.N. (Eds.) "Vitamins and Cancer-Human Cancer Prevention by Vitamins and Micronutrients". The Humana Press, Clifton, NY, pp. 139-159, 1985.

8) Santamaria, L., Bianchi, A., Arnaboldi, A., Ravetto, C., Bianchi, L., Pizzala, R., Andreoni, L., Santagati, G., and Bermond, P. Chemoprevention of indirect and direct chemical carcinogenesis by carotenoids as oxygen radical quenchers. Ann. N.Y. Acad. Sci., 534: 584-596, 1988.

9) Temple, N.J. and Basu, T.K. Protective effect of beta-carotene against colon tumors in mice. J. Natl. Cancer Inst. 78 (6): 1211-1214, 1987.

10) Santamaria, L. Benazzo, L., Benazzo, M., and Bianchi, A. First clinical case-report (1980-88) of cancer chemoprevention with beta-carotene plus canthaxanthin supplemented to patients after radical treatment. Med. Biol. Environn. 16: 945-950, 1988; and Boll. Chim. Farm. 127: 57-61 S., 1988.

11) Dorogokupla A.C., Troitzkaia, E.G., Adilgereieva, L.K., Postolnikov, S.F., Chekrigina, Z.P. Effect of carotene on the development of induced tumors . Zdravoor. Kazak. 10: 32-34, 1973.

12) Epstein, J. Effects of beta-carotene on UV-induced cancer formation in the hairless mouse skin. Photochem. Photobiol. 25: 211-213, 1977.

13) Seifter, E., Rettura, G., Padawer, J., Levenson, S.M. Moloney murine sarcoma virus tumors in CBA/J mice. Chemopreventive and chemotherapeutic action of supplemental beta-carotene. J.N.C.I., 68: 835-840, 1982.

14) Heywood, R., Palmer, A.K., Gregson, R.L. and Hummler, M. The toxicity of Beta-carotene. Toxicology 36: 91-100, 1985.

15) Feher, J., Csomos, G., and Vereckey, A. Free Radical Reactions in Medicine. Springer Verlag, Berlin, pp. 52-57, 1987.
16) Santamaria, L., Bianchi, A., Mobilio, G., Santagati, G., Ravetto, C., Bernardo, G., and Vetere, C. Cancer chemoprention by carotenoids. In: Tryfiates G.P. and Prasad K.N. (eds) "Nutrition Growth and Cancer" Alan. R. Liss Inc., New York, pp. 177-200, 1988.
17) Rousseau, A. Canthaxanthine deposits in the eye. J. Am. Acad. Dermatol. 8 (1): 123-124, 1983.
18) Brocq P., Stora C. and Bernheim L. De l'emploi de la vitamine A dans le traitement des mastoses. Ann. Endocrinol. 17: 193-200, 1956.
19) O'Brien P.M.S. The premenstrual syndrome: a review of the present status of therapy. Drugs 24: 140-151, 1982.
20) Editorial. Vitamin A, retinol, carotene, and cancer prevention. Brit. Med. J. 281: 957-958, 1980.
21) Band P.R., Deschamps M., Falardeau M., Ladoucerr J. and Cote J. Treatment of benign breast disease with vitamin A. Preventive Medicine, 13: 549-554, 1984.
22) Mansel R.E. Classification of mastalgia - the Cardiff system. In: Baum M. et al. (eds) Benign Breast Disease International Congress and Symposium Series N. 76, 33-41, The Royal Society of Medicine, London 1984.
23) Rocchi L. Termografia a contatto in senologia, Grafitart, Milano, pp.108-109,1985.
24) Santamaria, L., Dell'Orti, M., and Bianchi Santamaria, A. Beta-carotene supplementation associated with intermittent retinol administration in the treatment of pre-menopausal mastodynia. Boll. Chim. Farm., n.9, 1989, in press.
25) Roveta G., Bianchi A. and Santamaria L. Neutrophils in organ imprints of ß-carotene-supplemented ascites tumor bearing rats. Med. Biol. Environ. 15 (1): 463-468, 1987.
26) Blakely, S.R., Slaughter, L., Adkins, J., and Knight, E.V. Effects of ß-Carotene and retynil palmitate on corn oil-induced superoxide dismutase and catalase in rats. J. Nutr. 118: 152-158, 1988.
27) Pung, A., Rundhaug, J.E., Yoshizawa, C.N., and Bertram, J.S. Beta-carotene and canthaxanthin inhibit chemically- and physically-induced neoplastic transformation in 10T1/2 cells. Carcinogenesis: 9 (9), 1533-1539, 1988.
28) Hazuka, M.b., Edwards-Prasad, J., Newman, F. Kinzie, J., and Prasad, K.N. Beta-carotene induces morphological differentiation and decreases adenylate cyclase activity in melanoma cells in culture. J. Am. Coll. Nutr., 1989, in press.

Nutrients and Cancer Prevention K. N. Prasad and F. L. Meyskens, Jr., eds. © 1990 The Humana Press

ADJUVANT IMMUNOTHERAPY OF BREAST CANCER:

PROTOTYPIC OBSERVATIONS WITH ALPHA-TOCOPHEROL AND RETINOL

Maurice M. Black, M.D.,[1] Reinhard E. Zachrau, M.D.,[1] and

Monique F. Katz, M.D.[2]

[1]Department of Pathology, New York Medical College,

Valhalla, New York, and [2]Department of Radiology,

Columbia Presbyterian Hospital, New York, New York

Immune reactivity in cancer patients has been documented in terms of microscopically demonstrable lympho-reticuloendothelial (LRE) responses and by in vitro and in vivo tests of cell-mediated immunity (CMI) against autologous breast cancer. (1-5) Extensive studies, using a skin window (SW) test of such reactivity, indicate that the aggressive behavior of nuclear grade (NG)-characterized breast cancer is impeded by host CMI, directed against a determinant which is commonly expressed by the autologous cancer cells. (6) The prognostically significant CMI determinant of breast cancer is similar to a CMI determinant of gp55, the principal envelope glycoprotein of the murine mammary tumor virus of the RIII strain. (7-10) This determinant is more regularly expressed by preinvasive than invasive breast cancers. (11-14) Reactivity against the gp55-like immunogen also seems to impede the development of second invasive breast cancers. (15) According to these observations regarding the prognostic significance of spontaneous CMI, immunotherapeutic agents should have the ability to increase the intensity and/or duration of such specific immunity . Moreover, the treatment-related reactivity should show the same prognostic correlations, associated with spontaneous reactivity.
  Prompted by reports of immunostimulatory properties of high doses of retinoids and of alpha-tocopherol, (16-19)

we initiated, in 1981, a study of the effects of these
agents on CMI against autologous breast cancer and gp55.
These studies demonstrated that high doses of retinol in
the form of vitamin A (VA) could induce negative-to-
positive (N-P) changes in specific reactivity in breast
cancer patients, as judged by SW measurements. Similar
effects could be achieved by high doses of alpha-tocopherol in the form of vitamin E (VE). Moreover, the combination of VA and VE resulted in N-P changes in SW reactivity in some of the patients who were not responsive to
either agent alone. (20) We now update our observations
on the ability of VA and/or VE to induce and maintain
specific SW reactivity in breast cancer patients, and
report on the clinical significance of treatment-associ-
ated reactivity. It appears that, under controlled conditions, high doses of VA and/or VE satisfy the two basic
expectations of an adjuvant immunotherapeutic agent, i.e.,
that such treatment stimulates specific CMI against autologous breast cancer and that this, in turn, is associated
with the same prognostic significance as that of spontaneously occurring reactivity.

MATERIALS AND METHODS

SW tests were performed against autologous breast
cancer and against gp55 at various postoperative intervals. The details of the test procedure, including the
microscopic evaluation of SW's, have been described elsewhere. (10,15) The salient feature is the exposure of the
target, mounted on a glass coverslip, to an abraded area
of skin for approximately 30 hours. The coverslip is then
removed, stained with Wright's stain and examined microscopically for evidence of focal accumulations of lymphoid
and/or epithelioid cells, which is consistent with a CMI
response and was found to be prognostically favorable in
our prior studies.

All patients were free of recurrence and second
cancers at the times of treatment with retinol and/or
alpha-tocopherol. The influence of such treatment on SW
tests was evaluated in patients who had not developed
metastases or second primary breast cancers. In this
report, we shall use the abbreviation 'VE/VA' to refer
collectively to patients treated with one or both of these
agents. The daily dose of VE used was 1,200-1,600 IU,
while that of VA was 200,000-300,000 IU, in courses of 4-6

TABLE 1: Skin Window Reactivity against Gp55 in Relation
to VE/VA Treatment
(Treatment Started 6 Months to >10 Years Postoperatively)

Therapy Status	Total Number of Tests	Number of SW-1
Pre VE/VA	155	96(62%)[a]
On VE/VA		
VE	216	97(45%)
VA	46	18(39%)
VE+VA	47	16(34%)
Total	309	131(42%)[a,b]
Off VE/VA	263	143(54%)[b]

[a] $p<0.0005$; [b] $p<0.01$

weeks. The SW tests were graded as SW-1 = negative, SW-2 = intermediate and SW-3 = positive.

RESULTS

SW Reactivity against Gp55 in Relation to VE/VA Treatment

Table 1 lists the results of SW tests against gp55 before, during and after treatment with VE, VA or VE+VA. The VE/VA treatments were given over a wide range of postoperative intervals, i.e., 6 months to >10 years. Negative SW responses to gp55 were significantly less frequent among patients while taking VE/VA (42%), than among the same patients before initiation of the treatment (62%) and two to three months after its discontinuation (54%); $p<0.0005$ and $p<0.01$, respectively.

Further insight into the influence of VE/VA treatment on SW responses to gp55 are provided by examining the data in terms of the maximal SW response per patient before treatment and during the 24 months period after starting treatment. As seen in Table 2, VE/VA treatment was associated with an increase in the proportion of SW-3 and a reduction in SW-1 responses to gp55, $p<0.0005$ and $p<0.0001$, respectively. Thus, the VE/VA treatments, as administered in this study, were indeed associated with increases in SW reactivity against gp55.

TABLE 2: Influence of VE/VA Treatment on Skin Window
Responses of Breast Cancer Patients to Gp55, in Relation
to Prior Reactivity; Maximal Response / Patient / Interval

Pre-VE/VA SW Reactivity	Post-VE/VA SW Reactivity, <36 mpo			
	SW-3	SW-2	SW-1	Total
SW-3	13	1	--	14(35)[a]
SW-2	3	--	--	3
SW-1	19	3	1	23(58)[b]
Total	35(88)[a]	4	1(3)[b]	40(100)

a, b $p<0.0001$

SW Reactivity against Autologous Breast Cancer

As shown in Table 3, VE/VA treatment also increases
the SW reactivity against autologous breast cancer. Among
those patients who received VE/VA treatment, there were
significant differences in the pre- and post-treatment
proportions of patients with SW-1 responses, namely, 56%
and 5%, respectively; $p<0.0001$. Thus, it appears that the
VE/VA treatment <u>favors the augmentation of the specific
type of immune reactivity which is prognostically favorable when it occurs spontaneously</u>. It is, therefore, per-
tinent to determine whether the treatment-related reactivity has the same prognostic significance as spontaneous
reactivity.

Clinical Effects of VE/VA Adjuvant Treatment

Table 4 demonstrates that, among patients with NG I
or NG II breast cancers, the ratio of patients developing
metastases in <50 months postoperatively (mpo) / those
with no evidence of recurrent disease (NED) for >60 mpo
varies inversely with the maximal SW response to
autologous breast cancer. Thus, increased reactivity to
NG-characterized autologous breast cancer is associated
with a significantly reduced risk of early metastases.
While our series of VE/VA-treated patients is of limited
size, the prognostic significance of SW reactivity to

TABLE 3: Skin Window Reactivity against Autologous Breast Cancer, 1-36 Months Postoperatively, in Relation to VE/VA Therapy; Maximal Response / Patient / Interval

SW Response Intensity	Control Patients	VE/VA-treated Patients	
		Pre-Therapy	Post-Therapy
SW-3	82 (34)[a]	9 (23)[b]	25 (64)[a,b]
SW-2	18	8	12
SW-1	138 (58)[c]	22 (56)[d]	2 (5)[c,d]
Total	238 (100)	39 (100)	39 (100)

[a,b] $p<0.001$; [c,d] $p<0.0001$

TABLE 4: Survival Characteristics among Patients with NG I and NG II Invasive Breast Cancers, in Relation to the Maximal Skin Window Reactivity against Autologous Breast Cancer, 1-36 Months Postoperatively; VE/VA-treated and Untreated Patients

SW Response Intensity	Patients with Metast.<50 mpo / NED >60 mpo[a]	
	Untreated	VE/VA-treated
SW - 3	2/50 (0.04)[b,c]	2/13 (0.15)[d]
SW < 3	49/54 (0.91)[c]	2/ 5 (0.40)[d]

[a] All patients free of recurrence at the time of testing
[b] Numbers in parentheses, ratios
Corrected relative odds (SW-3/SW<3):

[c] 0.05 (p<0.0001) ; [d] 0.41 (N.S.)

NG-matched autologous breast cancer is similar in the VE/VA-treated and the control series.

As shown in Table 5, the prognostic significance of SW reactivity was maintained over extended postoperative intervals. Moreover, the prognostic significance of

TABLE 5: Survival Characteristics of NG I & NG II Breast
Cancer Patients, Subsequent to Defined SW Responses to
Autologous Cancer, 1-72 mpo; Control and VE/VA Series

SW Response Intensity	Patients with Metast.<50 mpo / NED >60 mpo[a]	
	Untreated	VE/VA-treated
SW-3	6/ 79 (0.08)[b]	2/ 6 (0.33)
SW<3		
Subsequent SW-3	7/103 (0.07)[c]	0/20[d]
Subsequent SW<3	135/214 (0.63)[c]	22/16 (1.34)[d]

[a] Time intervals between SW test and indicated event; all
patients free of recurrence at the time of testing
[b] Numbers in parentheses, ratios
Corrected relative odds (subsequent SW-3/SW<3):

[c] 0.11 (p<0.0001)   ;   [d] 0.02 (p<0.0001)

VE/VA-associated specific immunity was similar to that of
spontaneous reactivity.

SW Reactivity and Second Primary Breast Cancers

As indicated above, CMI which is capable of retarding
metastatic progression, should also reduce the risk of
second primary breast cancers. An impeded development of
subsequent breast cancers should also be a consequence of
CMI against gp55 since, characteristically, the CMI determinant in preinvasive breast cancer is similar to that of
gp55. Accordingly, procedures which can induce or maintain such reactivity, should impede the development of
second invasive breast cancers.

Twenty-one of our patients have developed a contralateral invasive breast cancer. Eleven of these patients
had SW-3 responses to gp55 and/or autologous breast
cancer, 1-24 mpo. In this group, none of the second
breast cancers occurred <40 mpo, and only 1 (9%) occurred
<60 mpo. In contrast, of the second breast cancers which

developed in 10 patients whose tests, were all less than
SW-3, 1-24 mpo, six developed <40 mpo and an additional
two developed <60 mpo. This difference is statistically
significant (p<.005).

Of the entire group of 21 patients who developed
second breast cancers, two had received VE/VA treatment.
One of these patients had a SW-3 response, <24 mpo. In
this patient, the second cancer did not appear until 62
mpo. In contrast, the other VE/VA-treated patient had no
SW-3 response, and in this patient the second cancer
appeared 18 mpo. Thus, in the control and the VE/VA
series, SW reactivity against gp55 and/or autologous
breast cancer appeared to impede the development of a
metachronous second primary invasive breast cancer.

In Table 6, we have indicated the relationship between
individual SW tests and the proportion of second primary
breast cancers that developed <40 months after various SW
responses. These tests were performed between one and 72
mpo on all 21 patients who subsequently developed second
cancers, 12-168 mpo. SW-3 responses to gp55 and/or
autologous breast cancer were uncommonly followed by
second breast cancers within the subsequent 40 months,
i.e., after only 2/22 tests (9%). Of 19 SW-1 and SW-2

TABLE 6: Proportion of Early (<40 Months) Metachronous
Second Invasive Breast Cancers in Relation to Prior SW
Reactivity against Gp55 or Autologous Breast Cancer, 1-72
mpo; VE/VA-treated and Untreated Patients

SW Response Intensity	Patients with Second BCa <40 mos/Total (%)[a]		
	Untreated	VE/VA-treated	Total
SW-3	1/18	1/ 4	2/22 (9)[b]
SW<3			
Subsequent SW-3	0/11	0/ 8	0/19 (0)[c]
Subsequent SW<3	26/36	11/11	37/47 (79)[b,c]

[a] Time interval between skin window test and diagnosis of
the second primary breast cancer; NED at time of testing
[b] p<0.005 ; [c] p<0.001

responses with a subsequent increase to a SW-3 response
within 30 months, none was followed by a second breast
cancer within 40 months. In contrast, a subsequent breast
cancer occurred within 40 months after 79% of those 47
SW<3 tests that were not followed by SW-3 responses. It
should be noted that the negative correlation between SW
reactivity against gp55 and/or autologous breast cancer
and the proportion of second invasive breast cancers that
occurred within the subsequent 40 months, were similar in
the control and the VE/VA-treated series.

COMMENTS

Our prior and current data provide compelling evidence
of the existence, dynamic variations and prognostic
significance of a specific type of CMI in breast cancer
patients. Accordingly, agents that can stimulate or
maintain such immune reactivity, should be therapeutically
and prophylactically important.

The present study has examined the immunotherapeutic
potential of high doses of alpha-tocopherol and retinol,
singly and together, in terms of these expectations. Our
observations support our initial findings which suggested
that alpha-tocopherol and retinol, administered in defined
doses and for defined intervals, are capable of stimulating specific CMI to gp55 and autologous breast cancer, as
judged by N-P changes in SW responses. Our current observations also demonstrate that such treatments favor the
maintenance of pre-existing postoperative positive responses. Most provocatively, it appears that VE/VA-associated
SW reactivity in breast cancer patients shows the same
types of relationships to metastatic progression and to
the proximate development of second primary breast cancers
as spontaneously occurring SW reactivity. Since the adjuvant use of high doses of alpha-tocopherol and/or retinol
favors the development and maintenance of a prognostically
favorable type of specific CMI, its use as a routine postoperative adjuvant treatment should be clinically beneficial.

We should also mention our observation that SW reactivity against autologous cancers of non-breast origin is
equally prognostically favorable. Moreover, VE/VA
treatment appears to exert a similar effect on SW reactivity in some postoperative patients with diverse types of
cancers, such as melanoma, pulmonary carcinoma, chondro-

sarcoma, lymphosarcoma and Hodgkin's disease. Thus, our present study provides a prototype for the evaluation of putative adjuvant immunotherapeutic agents in patients with diverse types of cancer.

If immunostimulation is clinically favorable in recognizable subpopulations, it should follow that immunosuppressive procedures might compromise such protective action. (6, 21) Thus, our present data justify our prior emphasis on the importance of the specific host CMI and of the nuclear grade of the cancer in the selection of the treatment of breast cancer patients. (2, 6)

REFERENCES

1. Black MM, Speer FD. Immunology of cancer. Surg Gynecol Obstet 1959; 109:105-116.
2. Black MM. Human breast cancer. A model for cancer immunology. Israel J Med Sci 1973; 9:284-299.
3. Black MM, Leis HP Jr, Shore B, Zachrau RE. Cellular hypersensitivity to breast cancer. Assessment by a leukocyte migration procedure. Cancer 1974; 3:952-958.
4. Black MM, Barclay THC, Hankey BF. Prognosis in breast cancer utilizing histologic characteristics of the primary tumor. Cancer 1975; 36:2048-2055.
5. Cannon GB, Dean JH, Herberman RB, Keels M, Alford C. Lymphoproliferative responses to autologous tumor extracts as prognostic indicators in patients with resected breast cancer. Int J Cancer 1981; 27:131-138.
6. Black MM, Zachrau RE. Immune mechanisms: Prognostic, therapeutic and preventive significance. In: Ariel, IM, Cleary, JB, eds. Breast Cancer: Diagnosis & Treatment. New York: McGraw-Hill, 1986; pp 128-142.
7. Black MM, Zachrau RE, Shore B, Moore DH, Leis HP, Jr. Prognostically favorable immunogens of human breast cancer tissue: Antigenic similarity to murine mammary tumor virus. Cancer 1975; 35:121-128.
8. Black MM, Zachrau RE, Shore B, Dion AS, Leis HP, Jr. Cellular immunity to autologous breast cancer and RIII-murine mammary tumor virus preparations. Cancer Res 1978; 38:2068-2076.
9. Zachrau RE, Black MM, Dion AS, Shore B, Williams CJ, Leis HP, Jr. Specificity of the simultaneous cell-mediated immune reactivity to RIII-murine mammary tumor virus glycoprotein 55 and human breast cancer tissues. Cancer Res 1978; 38:3414-3420.

10. Black MM, Zachrau RE, Ashikari RH, Hankey BF.
    Prognostic significance of cellular immunity to
    autologous breast carcinoma and glycoprotein 55. Arch
    Surg 1989; 124:202-206.
11. Black MM. Cellular and biologic manifestations of
    immunogenicity in precancerous mastopathy. Natl Cancer
    Inst Monogr 1972; 35:73-82.
12. Black MM. Structural, antigenic and biological
    characteristics of precancerous mastopathy. Cancer
    Res 1976; 36:2596-2604.
13. Black MM, Kwon CS. Precancerous mastopathie:
    Structural and biological considerations. Pathol Res
    Pract 1980; 116:491-514.
14. Black MM, Zachrau RE. Stepwise mammary carcinogenesis:
    Immunological considerations. In: Zander J, Baltzer
    J, eds. Advances in Early Detection and Treatment of
    Breast Cancer. New York: Springer, 1985; pp 64-72.
15. Black MM, Zachrau RE, Hankey BF, Wesley, M. Skin
    window reactivity to autologous breast cancer. An
    index of prognostically significant cell-mediated
    immunity. Cancer 1988; 62:72-83.
16. Cohen BE, Gill F, Cullen PR, Morris PJ. Reversal of
    postoperative immunosuppression in man by vitamin A.
    Surgery Gynec Obstet 1979; 149:658-662.
17. Patek P, Collin JL, Yogeeswaran G, Dennert G.
    Antitumor potential of retinoic acid: stimulation of
    immune-mediated effectors. Int J Cancer 1979; 24:624-
    628.
18. Beisel WR. Single nutrients and immunity. Am J Clin
    Nutr 1982; 35(Suppl):417-468.
19. Bellag W. Vitamin A and retinoids. From nutrition to
    pharmacotherapy in dermatology and oncology. Lancet
    1983; i:860-863.
20. Black MM, Zachrau RE, Dion AS, Katz M. Stimulation of
    prognostically favorable cell-mediated immunity of
    breast cancer patients by high dose vitamin A and
    vitamin E. In: Prasad KN, ed. Vitamins, Nutrition and
    Cancer. Basel: Karger, 1985; pp 134-146.
21. Strender LE,Blomgren H, Petrini B, et al. Immunologic
    monitoring in breast cancer patients receiving
    postoperative adjuvant chemotherapy. Cancer 1981;
    48:1996-2002.

Supported in part by a grant from the Cancer Research
Institute Inc., New York, New York

Nutrients and Cancer Prevention K. N. Prasad and F. L. Meyskens, Jr., eds. © 1990 The Humana Press

VITAMIN B-6 AND B-1 STATUS DURING

HORMONE THERAPY OF GYNECOLOGICAL CANCER

H.-A. Ladner[1] and R.M. Salkeld[2]

1 Department of Radiology, University Gynecology
Clinic, D-7800 Freiburg, Federal Republic of Germany
2 Section of Clinical Nutrition Research,
F. Hoffmann-La Roche Ltd, CH-4002 Basle, Switzerland

SUMMARY

The vitamin B-6 status (α-EGOT, PLP in erythrocytes) is impaired in patients with gynecological cancer
(cervix uteri, endometrium, ovary and breast), mainly in
patients with stage II and III uterine and ovarian
carcinomas. We compared the occurrence of 3 important
prognostic factors, undifferentiated malignant tumor
patients with oestrogen-progesterone-poor receptor status,
tumor grading, ploidy status and the epidermal growth
factor (EGF) in these patients with the vitamin B-6 status
before the beginning of therapy. We found that the low PLP
values before treatment were also a prognostic factor for
poor survival or the occurrence of distant metastases.
Similar to our findings about the lack of influence of
chemotherapy on vitamin B-6 and B-1 metabolism, we also
found no changes in the vitamin B-6 and B-1 values, (EGOT,
PLP and ETK) in 39 patients with gynecological carcinoma
during hormone therapy. Only tumor progression caused the
vitamin B-6 deficiency in these female tumor patients.

INTRODUCTION

Several studies show that the vitamin B-6 status is
impaired in patients with gynecological cancer (cervix,
endometrium uteri, ovary and breast). In studies with

329

patients who received radio- or chemotherapy we (LADNER and LIERSER 1972 (10), LADNER and SALKELD 1982, 1985 (11, 12) demonstrated that before the beginning of therapy about 30-40% of these cancer patients have a vitamin B-6 deficiency as measured by the erythrocyte glutamate-oxaloacetate transaminase (EGOT) activation test (22) and the pyridoxal 5'-phosphate (PLP) concentration in erythrocytes (PLP is the metabolically active form of vitamin B-6). These observations are comparable with the findings of other authors, who described pronounced changes in tryptophan metabolism, similar to those in vitamin B-6 deficiency, in Hodgkin's disease, bladder cancer and breast cancer. In the light of these findings we have to mention the observations of POTERA, LEKLEM, and DEVITA that the plasma PLP was reduced in cases of local recurrence and systemic metastases in breast cancer patients (13, 17) as well as in patients with advanced Hodgkin's disease (8).

During the course of our investigations we observed that the degree of vitamin B-6 and B-1 deficiency varied greatly from patient to patient because concomitant disease (e.g. diabetes mellitus, uremia and hyperthyroidism) caused more pronounced vitamin B-6 deficiency states after high-energy radiotherapy or after chemotherapy. Generally, a marked biochemical deficiency (α-EGOT, PLP in erythrocytes) of vitamin B-6 is provoked by radiation therapy (11). 65% of patients with stage II and III uterine carcinoma have a deficiency. In contrast, cytostatic agents impaired the vitamin B-6 status only in those subjects with a deficiency before treatment. We have no doubt that the vitamin B-6 deficiency during and after radio- and chemotherapy has an important influence on the prognosis of these patients. During our investigations we had the impression that all patients with endometrium and breast cancer, stage II and III, and with a pronounced vitamin B-6 deficiency status had a poor 5-year survival compared with the tumor patients without vitamin B-6 and B-1 deficiency. In the mean time we could demonstrate for breast and endometrium carcinoma patients that our impression is true: 1. the patients without vitamin B-6 deficiency have a 25% better prognosis than the patients with a deficiency status before the beginning of radiotherapy (11); 2. statistical analyses show that the cure rate in the group with pyridoxine supplementation (300 mg

daily only during the course of radiotherapy) was 15%
better (11).

In the light of new findings about the hormone
therapy of gynecological cancer we wish to draw your
attention to another important point in the oncology - the
possibility that certain cellular processes are influenced
by PLP: amino acid, lipid and carbohydrate metabolism and
in addition, the formation of niacin from tryptophan, the
functioning of erythrocytes and the expression of steroid
hormones. Now some specific remarks on the hormone
modulation:

1. PLP is a highly reactive molecule which LITWACK et al.
    1985 (14) have demonstrated binds to steroid recep-
    tors. These receptors are proteins and contain lysine
    residues that can interact with PLP. What are the
    implications of this research for humans and are there
    animal models which support the in vitro work? BENDER
    (4), and BUNCE and VESSAL 1987 (5) using rats have ob-
    served that compared to adequate vitamin B-6 intakes,
    a vitamin B-6 deficiency resulted in a greater accu-
    mulation of the hormone estradiol in the rat uterus, a
    target tissue for estradiol. Other animal studies have
    shown that the receptors for other hormones including
    androgens, progesterone and glucocorticoids also react
    with PLP. However, the known influence of steroids on
    both immune and reproductive systems suggests that
    vitamin B-6 status may be a contributing factor to the
    action of hormones on these systems.

2. Recent work in adult women suggests that an adequate
    vitamin B-6 status is necessary for proper immune
    function (21).

3. Indirect interactions, such as the effect of hormones
    on epidermal growth factor, shown in mice by
    PERHEENTUPA et al. 1987 (16), is a further factor
    which can play a role in tumor growth in the genital
    region.

Besides the interactions between vitamin B-6 status
and immune function described by many investigators in the
last 20 years new facts indicate that investigations
between hormone receptors and vitamin B-6 in patients with

gynecological cancers before and during therapy should be
given more attention than has previously been the case in
oncological vitamin B-6 research. With this background we
will give a short presentation of the results of our investigations during the hormone therapy of patients with
breast, endometrium and ovarian carcinoma.

RESULTS

1a. Correlation of 5-year Survival of Patients
with Endometrium and Breast Cancer with Low
PLP Values before Treatment

An extensive retrospective analysis was undertaken in
an attempt to identify prognostically significant pre-
treatment factors, above all: FIGO stage, histology and
hormonal receptors. PFLEIDERER et al. 1984 (15) found that
the receptor-negative cases were related to advanced
stages, earlier death, deep invasion, and more malignant
histological types. Of 36 patients with undifferentiated
malignant endometrium tumors, 23 were receptor-negative
and 9 others showed only a low progesterone receptor content of 30, 90 and 113 fmol/mg protein. 93% of these
patients had PLP levels less than 3.0 ng/ml before treatment. Similarly in 93 patients with breast cancer 63% were
receptor-negative and 96% had PLP levels less than 3.0
ng/ml. Among patients with carcinoma of endometrium or
breast, we found that those with undifferentiated malignant tumors had both a poorer 5-year survival rate and
lower pretreatment PLP values (<3.0 ng/ml) than those with
well-differentiated tumors.

In earlier investigations (11, 12) we could demonstrate that the extent of tumor-induced changes before
the start of chemo- or radiotherapy were dependent on the
stage of the tumor; the more the carcinoma had progressed,
the more pronounced was the impairment of the vitamin B-6
and B-1 activation tests. The retrospective analysis (Cox
regression, 90 patients) showed that the higher vitamin
B-6 activation test values (poorer vitamin B-6 status)
correlated with lower survival at 5 years in endometrium
cancer patients, especially in patients with pyometra, deep
invasion, or negative hormone-receptor status. Similar results were observed in 39 patients with breast cancer: the
low PLP values before treatment were a prognostic factor

for poor survival or the later occurrence of distant metastases.

Among the receptor-negative endometrium cancer cases, it is of interest that the number who were underweight, suffering from diabetes or had had preceding radiotherapy for cervical cancer was unproportionally high. In contrast those with receptor-positive (ER+, PR+) cancer were more frequently obese, had a preceding long term estrogen therapy or suffered from breast cancer as a second cancer.

1b. Correlation of ER/PR-negative Receptor Status in Endometrium, Ovarian and Breast Carcinoma with Low PLP Values before Treatment

The presence of estrogen and progesterone receptors in 40-70 % of ovarian cancers has led a number of investigators to suggest that they may help detect those patients with poor prognostic factors (e.g. tumor stage, histological subtype, and degree of differentiation) or identify those patients likely to respond to hormonal therapy (18). In our investigation (93 patients with ovarian carcinoma), serous and endometroid carcinomas were more likely to be receptor positive than the other histological subtypes (20). Therefore we observed the relationship of receptor status with stage, age, histological subtype, histological grade, and vitamin B-6 status. There was an association between age and receptor expression in the ER-rich/PR-rich group of tumors which were more common in women under 50 years of age. As others have also reported, there were conflicting data with respect to the association between tumor grade and receptor levels. This probably reflects the general lack of uniformity and poor reproducibility of the various grading systems currently in use (7). However, there was a relationship between the histological grade and the vitamin B-6 status (PLP in erythrocytes): 60 % of the moderately differentiated and 78 % of the poorly differentiated invasive epithelial ovarian cancer cases have low values (<3 ng/ml) of pyridoxal 5'-phosphate in erythrocytes. Up to 50 % of these patients tending to be ER-poor, but the numbers included in this study are too small to draw any definite conclusions about the relationship between histological grade and ER- or PR-status.

In the mean time, we (together with BAUKNECHT, GEYER and HILGARTH) determined DNA-histograms obtained from solid ovarian tumors analyzed by flow cytometry. 12 probes were analyzed in ovarian cancer patients with known receptor status, clinical stage, histological subtype, vitamin B-6 status (PLP), and grade. The numbers are however too small to allow meaningful assessment of the relationship between histological subtype, receptor expression and vitamin B-6 status, although it is interesting to note that 8 tumors with a low receptor level had also a poor vitamin B-6 status together with aneuploidy.

There is some evidence to suggest that patients with diploid prostatic cancers have a higher likelihood of responding to hormonal therapy than those with aneuploid tumors (23). A similar situation may exist in ovarian cancer (9). The aim of our prospective study was to determine the incidence of receptor (ER and PR) expression in a series of patients with ovarian epithelial tumors and to analyze their relationship with other determinants of biologic behavior including tumor ploidy and vitamin B-6 and B-1 status. 2 years after the beginning of this study we demonstrated that the patients with low PLP values before the start of therapy showed no changes in the PLP during the chemo- or hormone therapy. In 20 % of 12 cases with initial normal levels of PLP there was a slight decrease of PLP during the hormone therapy. As earlier reported, in 65 patients with metastasizing ovarian, endometrial or mammary carcinoma, there was no definite worsening of the deficiency during cytostatic treatment (12). A similar observation was made in 20 patients with metastasizing breast carcinoma during the hormone therapy.

1c. Correlation of Positive Tumor Epidermal Growth Factor in Ovarian Cancer with Low PLP Values before Treatment

Because of the controversial discussion about the value of prognostic factors in the treatment of gynecological carcinomas BAUKNECHT et al. 1988 (3) briefly described their preliminary results about the occurrence of a growth factor, a well-known polypeptide; together with BAUKNECHT we investigated its possible relationship to the vitamin B-6 status. The epidermal growth factor (EGF) intersets with specific cell-surface receptors (EGF- R), transducing intracellular signals to DNA synthesis and

cell division (6). EGF-R has been identified in ovarian
carcinomas and its predictive function for prognosis has
been described (1, 3); also in breast carcinoma (19).
Furthermore, Bauknecht et al. 1986 (2) recently published
the discovery of EGF-like factors (EGF-F) in tissue extract of ovarian carcinomas and their association with the
aggressive behavior of these tumors. For the adeno-
epithelial carcinoma, this association between the
presence of EGF-R and tumor prognosis qualifies also the
EGF-R as a prognostic marker (3). These findings support
the idea that the enhanced expression of EGF-R stimulates
the proliferation conditions of tumors, this being
clinically visible by its more aggressive behavior. Among
33 patients with the presence of EGF-R (advanced ovarian
and cervical cancer), we observed in 22 patients low
values of PLP in erythrocytes at the same time of investigation. The clinical follow-up of 42 patients with advanced ovarian, endometrium, breast and cervical carcinomas
showed a significant correlation of cases with tumor
progression and high EGF-F levels. 34 (81%) of these
patients had low PLP levels. With further investigations
we hope to understand better the regulation of the EGF
systems in tumors, specially the possible modulation of
EGF by hormones or vitamins.

2. Vitamin B-6 and B-1 Status before and during Hormone Therapy

In 39 patients with endometrium (9) or breast carcinoma (30) we determined the vitamin B-6 und B-1 status
(EGOT, PLP and ETK) before and during the hormone therapy.
In 28 cases we found no clear changes of the vitamin B-6
or B-1 status; in 9 cases we found a decrease of the PLP
values (7 less than 3 ng/ml) and an increase of α-EGOT
(6 greater than 2.0). In 7 of these 9 cases the vitamin
B-6 deficiency could be explained by tumor progression; in
2 cases by a deterioration of chronic renal disease or un-
stable diabetes. Among 9 breast cancer cases with low PLP
values we observed 6 cases with a vitamin B-1 deficiency.

The hormone therapy therefore did not appear to
change the vitamin B-6 status; the low PLP values were
signs of tumor progression or deterioration of concomitant
disease. These observations were similar to those during
the chemotherapy of patients with gynecological cancer but

in contrast to our observation during radiotherapy, that
radiation impaired vitamin B-6 status.

CONCLUSIONS

1. The vitamin B-6 status is impaired in patients with
   gynecological cancer (cervix uteri, endometrium, ovary
   and breast). Mainly patients with stage II and III
   uterine and ovarian carcinomas have a vitamin B-6
   deficiency (α-EGOT, PLP in erythrocytes).

   During our investigations we had the impression that
   all patients with advanced gynecological tumors and a
   pronounced vitamin B-6 deficiency status had a poor
   5-year survival. Therefore we compared the occurrence
   of other prognostic factors with the occurrence of high
   EGOT or low PLP values, especially in patients with:

   a. undifferentiated malignant tumor patients with ER-
      and PR-poor receptor status (endometrium / breast)
   b. tumor grade III and ER-poor receptor status; ploidy
      status (advanced ovarian cancer)
   c. presence of EGF-R and EGF-F (advanced ovarian and
      cervical cancer).

   Obviously these 3 factors indicate a poor 5-year survival. In the correlation with these 3 factors there is
   a high percentage of patients which a vitamin B-6 deficiency status before the beginning of therapy. Therefore, these findings support the idea that the vitamin
   B-6 deficiency - excluding concomitant disease - could
   be a poor prognostic factor. It is possible that the
   occurrence of vitamin B-6 deficiency also indicates a
   reduced immune status. Further investigation will try
   to elucidate more about these interactions between
   vitamin B-6 and certain tumor prognosis factors in
   connection with hormones and the immune mechanism.

2. Similar to our findings about the lack of influence of
   chemotherapy on vitamin B-6 and B-1 metabolism, we also
   found no changes in the vitamin B-6 and B-1 values
   (EGOT, PLP and ETK) in patients with endometrium and
   breast carcinoma during the hormone therapy. Only the
   tumor progression caused the vitamin B-6 deficiency in

these female patients, and sometimes also a vitamin B-1 deficiency.

REFERENCES

1 Bauknecht T, Rau B, Meerpohl H, Pfleiderer A. The prognostic value of the presence of EGF receptors in ovarian carcinomas. Tumor Diagn Ther 1984;5:62-66.
2 Bauknecht T, Kiechle M, Bauer G, Siebers J. Characterization of growth factors in human ovarian carcinomas. Cancer Res 1986;46:2614-2618.
3 Bauknecht T, Runge M, Schwall M, Pfleiderer A. Occurrence of epidermal growth factor receptors (EGF-R) in human adnexal tumors and their prognostic value in advanced ovarian carcinomas. Gynecol Oncol 1988;29:147-159.
4 Bender DA. Oestrogens and vitamin B-6 actions and interactions. World Rev Nutr Diet 1987;51:140.
5 Bunce GE, Vessal M. Effect of zinc and/or pyridoxine deficiency upon oestrogen retention and oestrogen receptor distribution in the rat uterus. J Steroid Biochem 1987;26:303.
6 Carpenter G, Cohen S. Epidermal growth factors. Ann Rev Biochem 1979;48:193-216.
7 Creasman WT, Sasso RA, Weed JC, McCartey KS. Ovarian carcinoma: histologic and clinical correlation of cytoplastic estrogen and progesterone binding. Gynecol Oncol 1981;12:319-327.
8 DeVita VT, Chabner BA, Livingston DM, Oliverio VT. Anergy and tryptophan metabolism in Hodgkin's disease. Am J Clin Nutr 1971;24:835-840.
9 Friedlander ML, Hedley DW, Taylor IW, Russell P, Coates AS, Tattersall MNH. Influence of cellular DNA content on survival in advanced ovarian cancer. Cancer Res 1984;44:397-400.
10 Ladner H-A, Lieser H. Zum Vitamin B-6-Stoffwechsel während der gynäkologischen Strahlentherapie. Radiologe 1972;12:240-242.
11 Ladner H-A, Salkeld RM. Vitamin B-6 status and administration during radiation therapy. In: Meyskens FL, jr, Prasad KN, eds. Vitamins and cancer. Clifton, New Jersey: Humana Press, 1986:429-437.
12 Ladner H-A, Salkeld RM. Vitamin B-6 status in cancer patients: Effect of tumour site, irradiation, hormones and chemotherapy. In: Tryfiates GP, Prasad KN, eds.

Nutrition, growth, and cancer. New York: Alan R Liss, 1988:273-281.

13 Leklem JE, Brown RR, Potera C, Becker DS. A role for vitamin B-6 in cancer. In: Van Eys et al, eds. Nutrition and cancer. New York: SP Medical and Scientific Books, 1979.

14 Litwack G, Miller-Diener A, DiSorbo DM, Schmidt TJ. In: Reynolds RD, Leklem JE, eds. Vitamin B-6: its role in health and disease. New York: Alan R Liss, 1985:177-191.

15 Pfleiderer A, Kleine W, König P, Geyer H. Hormonal receptors in endometrial cancer, analysis of clinical prognosis and risk factors. In: Wolff JP, Scott JS, eds. Hormones and sexual factors in human cancer aetiology. Amsterdam: Elsevier Science Publ BV, 1984:35-46.

16 Perheentupa J, Lakshmanan J, Hoath SB, Fisher DA. Hormonal modulation of mouse plasma concentration of epidermal growth factor. Acta encocrinol 1987;107:571-576.

17 Potera C, Rose DP, Brown RR. Vitamin B-6 deficiency in cancer patients. Am J Clin Nutr 1977;30:1677-1679.

18 Quinn MA, Pearce P, Rome R, Funder JW, Fortune D, Pepperell RJ. Cytoplasmic steroid receptors in ovarian tumours. Brit J Obstet Gynecol 1982;89:754-759.

19 Sainsbury J, Farndon J, Needham G, Malcolm A, Harris A. Epidermal growth factor receptor status as predictor of early recurrence and death from breast cancer. Lancet 1987;I:1398.

20 Schwartz PE, Livolsi VA, Hildreth N, MacLusky NJ, Naftolin FN, Eisenfeld AJ. Estrogen receptors in ovarian epithelial carcinoma. Obstet Gynecol 1982;59:229-238.

21 Talbott MC, Miller LT, Kerkvliet NI. Pyridoxine supplementation: effect on lymphocyte responses in elderly persons. Am J Clin Nutr 1987;46:659.

22 Vuilleumier JP, Keller HE, Rettenmaier R, Hunziker F. Clinical chemical methods for the routine assessment of the vitamin status in human populations. Part II: The water-soluble vitamins B-1, B-2 and B-6. Int J Vitam Nutr Res 1983;53:259-270.

23 Zetterberg A, Esparti PL. Prognostic significance of nuclear DNA levels in prostatic carcinoma. Scand J Urol Nephrol 1980;55(suppl):53-59.

Participants

WAYNE B. ANDERSON
National Cancer Institute
Building 36, Room 1D22
Bethesda, MD 20892

JOHN S. BERTRAM
University of Hawaii at Manoa
Cancer Research Center of Hawaii
1236 Lauhala Street
Honolulu, HI 96813

MAURICE M. BLACK
Department of Pathology
New York Medical College
Valhalla, NY 10595

CARMIA G. BOREK
Department of Radiological Research
College of Physicians and Surgeons
Columbia University
630 West 168th Street
New York, NY 10032

ANDRÉ CASTONGUAY
Laval University
Quebec City, Quebec
Canada, G1K7P4

HECTOR F. DeLUCA
Department of Biochemistry
University of Wisconsin
420 Henry Mall
Madison, WI 53706

HANS P. FORTMEYER
Klinikum der Johann Wolfgang
Goethe-Universitat
600 Frankfurt am Main 70, den
Federal Republic of Germany

HELEN L. GENSLER
Department of Radiation Oncology
and Cancer Center
University of Arizona
College of Medicine
Tucson, AZ 85724

MICHAEL J. HILL
PHLS Centre for Applied
Microbiology and Research
Bacterial Metabolism Research
Laboratory
Proton Down
Salisbury
Wiltshire SP4 OJG, England

LI JUN-YAO
Department of Epidemiology
Cancer Institute
Chinese Academy of Medical Sciences
Longtan Lake, Zuoanmenwai
Beijing, China

ANN R. KENNEDY
Department of Radiation Oncology
University of Pennsylvania Medical
School
Hospital of the University
of Pennsylvania
3400 Spruce Street
Philadelphia, PA 19104

GABRIEL A. KUNE
Surgical Department
Parkville,
The University of Melbourne
Victoria, Australia 3052

H.-A. LADNER
Department of Radiology
University Gynecology Clinic
D-7800 Freiburg,
Federal Republic of Germany

FRANK L. MEYSKENS, JR.
University of California
Irvine Medical Center
101 The City Drive
Building 44, Route 81
Orange, CA 92668-3297

RICHARD C. MOON
IIT Research Institute
Life Sciences Research
10 West 35th Street
Chicago, IL 60616

MICHAEL W. PARIZA
Department of Food, Microbiology,
    and Toxicology
University of Wisconsin
Madison, WI 53706

KEDAR N. PRASAD
University of Colorado
Health Sciences Center
4200 East Ninth Avenue
Denver, CO 80262

LEONIDA SANTAMARIA
C. Golgi Inst. for Gen. Path
Piazza Botta
10 Univ. of Pavia
Pavia, Italy 0382-25356

RAYMOND J. SHAMBERGER
CIBA Corning Company
132 Artino Street
Oberlin, OH 44074

RAMESHWAR K. SHARMA
Department of Brain and Vascular
    Research
The Cleveland Clinical Foundation
9500 Euclid Avenue
Cleveland, OH 44195

H. F. STICH
British Columbia Cancer Research
    Center
601 West 10th Avenue
Vancouver, BC V521L3
Canada

CHUNG S. YANG
Department of Chemical Biology
    and Pharmacology
College of Pharmacy
Rutgers University
Piscataway, NJ 08855-0789

Author Index

Subject Index